NOVA SCOTIA
and the
Great Influenza
PANDEMIC
1918–1920

NOVA SCOTIA
and the
Great Influenza
PANDEMIC
1918–1920

※◦(✿)◦※

A REMEMBRANCE OF THE DEAD
AND AN ARCHIVE FOR THE LIVING

Compiled and Edited by Ruth Holmes Whitehead
With contributions from Allan Everett Marble, Gordon Hammond,
Martin Hubley, Harriet McCready, Gabriel LeBlanc, Lori Poirier Forgeron,
Lena Samson, Viola Samson, Caitlin McCready-Carswell, Nicholas Boudreau,
Ruth Legge and the Borden Descendents, Lewis MacIntosh, Lloyd Sinclair,
Don Gordon, Jim St. Clair, Rannie Gillis, Janet Baker, Elizabeth Peirce,
Dale Swann, Ashley Sutherland, Jocelyn Gillis, Liam Cogger,
Rosemary Barbour, Garry Shutlak, Phillip Hartling, Barry Smith,
Darlene Brine, Bernie Francis, Karen Smith, Jim Burant, Bennett McCardle,
Heather Ludlow, Roger Lewis, Scott Robson, Sharon MacDonald,
Deborah Trask, Gwen Trask, David States, Joleen Gordon,
Catherine Cottreau-Robins, Kevin Robins, Eli Diamond, Roger Marsters,
Pauline MacLean, Lois Ann Dort, Leslie Pezzack, Doug Pezzack,
Edward Crane Gilbert, Linda Littlejohn, Linda Rafuse, Frank Allen,
Charles Thompson, Chris Henkelmann, Brigitte Neumann, Angela Buckles,
Susan McClure, Chara Kingston, Mark Lewis, Lisette Gaudet, Dale Mills,
Eric Mills, Sarah Whitehead, and Sam Everett Howard.

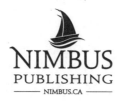

NIMBUS
PUBLISHING
— NIMBUS.CA —

Nimbus Publishing Limited
3660 Strawberry Hill St, Halifax, NS, B3K 5A9
(902) 455-4286 nimbus.ca

Printed and bound in Canada
NB1543

All royalties from this book are donated to
MSF/Doctors Without Borders.

Excerpts from THE GREAT INFLUENZA: THE EPIC STORY OF THE DEADLIEST PLAGUE IN HISTORY by John M. Barry, copyright © 2004 by John M. Barry. Used by permission of Viking Books, an imprint of Penguin Publishing Group, a division of Penguin Random House LLC. All rights reserved.
Excerpt from "Outbreak: The little-known story of the 1918 Spanish Flu and how we're preparing for the next great pandemic," by Alanna Mitchel. *Canadian Geographic;* September/October 2018, p. 53.

Cover: Holy Cross Cemetery, Halifax. (*Ruth Holmes Whitehead*)
Editor: Elizabeth Eve
Editor for the Press: Angela Mombourquette
Cover & interior design: Heather Bryan

Library and Archives Canada Cataloguing in Publication

Title: Nova Scotia and the great influenza, 1918-1920 : a remembrance of the dead and a sourcebook for the living / compiled and edited by Ruth Holmes Whitehead ; with contributions from Allan Everett Marble [and 62 others].
Names: Whitehead, Ruth Holmes, editor.
Description: Includes bibliographical references.
Identifiers: Canadiana (print) 20200280759 | Canadiana (ebook) 20200280945
ISBN 9781771089159 (softcover)
ISBN 9781771089166 (EPUB)
Subjects: LCSH: Influenza Epidemic, 1918-1919—Nova Scotia—Sources. | LCSH: Influenza—Patients—Nova Scotia—Biography—Sources. | CSH: Nova Scotia—History—1918-1945—Sources. | LCSH: Nova Scotia—Biography—Sources.
Classification: LCC RC150.55.C32 N86 2020 | DDC 614.5/180971609041—dc23

 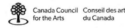 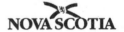

Nimbus Publishing acknowledges the financial support for its publishing activities from the Government of Canada, the Canada Council for the Arts, and from the Province of Nova Scotia. We are pleased to work in partnership with the Province of Nova Scotia to develop and promote our creative industries for the benefit of all Nova Scotians.

In memory of those who died,
and
those who were left to mourn.

TABLE OF CONTENTS

Prologue: Dr. Martin Hubley ix
Legend of Symbols...x
Preface: Dr. Allan Marble..xi
Introduction: Dr. Ruth Holmes Whitehead..........xiii

Chapter I   THE GREAT INFLUENZA 1
Chapter II   ANNAPOLIS COUNTY 21
Chapter III   ANTIGONISH COUNTY 3o
Chapter IV   CAPE BRETON COUNTY 42
Chapter V   COLCHESTER COUNTY 71
Chapter VI   CUMBERLAND COUNTY 106
Chapter VII   DIGBY COUNTY.. 138
Chapter VIII   GUYSBOROUGH COUNTY 158
Chapter IX   HALIFAX COUNTY...178
Chapter X   HANTS COUNTY 224
Chapter XI   INVERNESS COUNTY.......................................237
Chapter XII   KINGS COUNTY.. 251
Chapter XIII   LUNENBURG COUNTY 261
Chapter XIV   PICTOU COUNTY..273
Chapter XV   QUEENS COUNTY 283
Chapter XVI   RICHMOND COUNTY 288
Chapter XVII   SHELBURNE COUNTY 310
Chapter XVIII   VICTORIA COUNTY...327
Chapter XIX   YARMOUTH COUNTY.................................... 332
Chapter XX   SUMMATION...348

Coda..353
Acknowledgements 356
Appendix 358

PROLOGUE

※〜❦〜※

MORE THAN TWO thousand Nova Scotians died during the Great Influenza pandemic of 1918–20. Over the intervening decades, their fates and the struggles faced by families and communities during the pandemic have largely been forgotten. One hundred years later, the Nova Scotia Museum decided to undertake a small virtual exhibit on the subject which relied on research drawn from historians such as Dr. Allan Marble, and also from community contributors across the province. Individual experiences were used to cast light on the course of the pandemic, the courage of Nova Scotians facing it, and the legacies left in a changed public health system— among others the importance of vaccination to prevent future such catastrophes. "Remembering the Forgotten Dead: Nova Scotia and the Great Influenza Pandemic of 1918-1920" can be found online at museum.novascotia.ca/collections-research/ virtual-exhibits/remembering-forgotten-dead.

The constraints of time, space, and resources allowed only a handful of the stories which were brought to light to be profiled in that exhibit. Dr. Ruth Holmes Whitehead, Curator Emeritus and Research Associate, has compiled here many more narratives of the experiences of individual Nova Scotians and their families during the pandemic. These, and the comprehensive county lists of those who died, will be useful not only to genealogists and historians, but to anyone tracing their family history during this difficult and little-known period of Nova Scotia's past, and hoping to learn more about it. There is still much more to be learned about the Great Influenza pandemic in Nova Scotia, but readers will find here a comprehensive starting point. This work forms a fitting tribute to both the memory of those who lost their lives to the flu in those bleak years and to the doctors, nurses, and everyday Nova Scotians who struggled to care for the many thousands more who fell ill with influenza.

Martin Hubley, PhD
Curator of History
Nova Scotia Museum

LEGEND OF SYMBOLS

 Author text

 Newspaper excerpts

 Death records and other government documents

 Book excerpts

 Magazine excerpts

 Historical records

 Personal communications

PREFACE

THE WORD INFLUENZA is derived from the medieval Latin word *influentia*. In the Middle Ages, it was believed that disease developed because of the influence of the stars. In more modern times, the word influenza has been used to describe any inflammation of the upper respiratory tract and is frequently referred to as the flu. Patients with influenza present with severe fever, protracted aching, and also catarrh. In 1918, the influenza pandemic was initially attributed to *Bacillus Influenzae* or *Pfeiffer's Bacillus*, that is, due to bacteria. It was not until Richard Shope isolated the influenza virus in swine in 1931, and Christopher Andrewes isolated the influenza virus in humans in 1933, that epidemiologists concluded that the causative agent in the 1918 influenza was viral rather than bacterial.

There are at least three theories about the origin of the 1918 flu. Some historians believe that it originated in China, while others have suggested that it first appeared among the soldiers in Europe during the First World War. The best-documented and most likely origin of the 1918 flu, however, shows it first occurred in the state of Kansas in the United States. In February 1918, Dr. Loring Miner, a physician practising in Haskell County, Kansas, noticed that "dozens of his patients—the strongest, the healthiest, the most robust people in the county—were being struck down [by influenza] as if they had been shot."* He administered diphtheria and tetanus antitoxins to these patients but neither had any positive effect in relieving the symptoms of their illness. Dr. Miner sent a report to US public health officials in Washington indicating that he had a severe influenza epidemic on his hands.

Camp Funston, the second largest army camp in the US, was located in Haskell County, and housed fifty-six thousand soldiers in overcrowded and unheated barracks and tents. On March 4 the influenza appeared among soldiers in Camp Funston and within three weeks eleven hundred soldiers had contracted the influenza.

In April, soldiers from Camp Funston were transported to the east coast of the US and sailed for Brest, France. By the middle of April, a major influenza epidemic had broken out among the French and British Armies. In June, British soldiers returning to England introduced the influenza to their country. On the European continent, German Commander Erich von Ludendorff postponed and later cancelled a major

---

* John M. Barry, *The Great Influenza: The Story of the Deadliest Pandemic in History* (New York: Viking) 2nd ed. 2009, 92.

offensive because so many German soldiers were ill with influenza. By July, the influenza had spread to Italy, Holland, Norway, Sweden, Portugal, and Spain.

Every country involved in the First World War censored their newspapers in an attempt to keep information about the influenza's severity away from the general public. It was believed that if families were aware that influenza was rampant in army camps, parents would prevent their sons from joining the army. Spain was not involved in the War and therefore did not censor its newspapers from carrying news of the influenza. During the pandemic there were over five million deaths in Spain, and, because the influenza was constantly mentioned in their newspapers, it became known as the Spanish Influenza. Approximately thirty-five thousand died from the Spanish flu in Canada and about thirty-five million throughout the world.

Information about the impact of this influenza on Nova Scotians was initially gathered from death certificates for summer 1918 through late spring 1919, recorded in the Nova Scotia Vital Statistics Office in Halifax. The death certificates indicated that a total of at least eighteen hundred Nova Scotians died from a combination of the influenza virus and pneumonia. An additional three hundred–plus succumbed to the flu without their death certificates being recorded—their deaths, however, were announced in provincial newspapers.

This book includes a third and most important source for information on those who died from this influenza. Individuals and families from many of the eighteen counties of Nova Scotia were interviewed about the impact of the flu on relatives who were alive in 1918 and 1919. Those interviewed related heart-wrenching stories about the suffering and tragic loss of family from this influenza during September to December 1918 and from January to April of 1919 [and parts of 1920]. Every city, town, village, and isolated settlement was affected. It is very likely that the reason it has taken over one hundred years to produce this important volume is because the Great Influenza was such a tragic incident in Nova Scotia's history that people wanted to forget that it occurred.

Dr. Allan E. Marble
Chair, Medical History Society of Nova Scotia

INTRODUCTION

A NUMBER OF books have examined the Great Influenza in relation to its nature, the damage it did, and the aftermath of the epidemic. They explain how the virus was later isolated and the genome decoded. Its worldwide effect on society, the military, world politics, and on the course of the First World War have been scrutinized. Books and articles have looked at the economic context, housing conditions—especially in industrial urban centres—the efficacy of quarantines, the heroic undertakings of doctors and nurses, the dangers to pregnant women, the frighteningly high number of orphans, and the types of neurological damage this pandemic influenza could do to ruin the lives of survivors. With the arrival of the centenary, there was a blossoming of articles and books about this three-year pandemic, which shed light on the inability of governments to control this outbreak, and thus, what measures should be taken to cope with the next global pandemic. As one unnamed reporter wrote in 1918, "We must not again be caught unprepared." The reporter was thinking of 1919, but modern science must plan for the next hundred years.

This book is a local history, organized by Nova Scotia counties. It is a compilation of what we know about those who died in this province during the outbreak. We list the names of those who perished in Nova Scotia during the catastrophic three years from 1918 to 1920, when influenza destroyed whole families, brought towns to a standstill, and terrified almost everyone. Sometimes looking at individuals gives us a more vivid sense of history than do broad overviews and statistics. This book has its share of both things, but its heart belongs to the stories and the people. It is a commemoration of the dead that shows something of their lives, their relationships, and their last moments. It is a sourcebook and a springboard for further research.

Although the term "Spanish Influenza" is frequently used to describe this illness, it is based on a misconception. Except when quoting directly from a source, this book utilizes the Great Influenza, a more recent designation.

It is also worth noting that the less severe First Wave of this epidemic spread rapidly, particularly within and from overcrowded army training camps. The severe Second Wave expanded the epidemic in Nova Scotia, and this was followed by the marginally milder Third Wave in 1920. Estimates of worldwide death-rates range from 50 million to 100 million.

The basic information about deaths during the epidemic in Nova Scotia comes from the provincial death registers, which were kept county by county. And since every death requires what was called a "return of information" to the local registrar, with the name of the deceased, the date, location, and cause of death, along with other identifiers like birthplace, residence, attending physician, undertaker, place of burial, and religion, these registers are the primary source of data.

Names of pandemic influenza victims in Nova Scotia during those three years were extracted from each county's register by Dr. Allan Marble, chair of the Medical History Society of Nova Scotia, using the original ledgers, now housed in the Nova Scotia Archives, Halifax. He copied these registers county by county, record by record, mistakes included, exactly as they appeared on the ledger pages. As Dr. Marble was writing a chapter on this epidemic for his forthcoming book, *History of Medicine in Nova Scotia, Volume Three,* he left out some details that were unnecessary for his research, such as father's name (after 1919, mother's names were added), birthplace, religion, place of burial, undertaker's name, and so on.

Some of this biographical information has since been extracted using the Historical Vital Statistics/Death Register (HVS) website of the Nova Scotia Archives, as access to the originals is now limited due to their age and frailty. In the future, more data will add such details for every one of the dead here listed. I could not do this for all two thousand-plus people, but I looked at the online records of the eighteen counties every time I encountered an odd-sounding name, or puzzling entry, correcting where possible, or merely making suggestions. The occurrence of a person having a death record in two different counties has now been remedied. Each of the edited lists appears in this book at the end of the appropriate chapter.

The second major sources of names are newspapers of the period. Dr. Marble made a list of all the Nova Scotia papers published between 1918 and 1920 (his second list, which was handwritten), adding their microfilm numbers at the archives. Using this as his guide, he went back and began reading through the papers—through almost all of them, he says—and thus created his third list: notes (but not full text, in many cases) of any useful articles or reportage in Nova Scotia newspapers were presented in sections, arranged by each paper's county of publication.

The full texts of most of these articles were photocopied at the archives by Sam Howard, who also did supplemental research on any further avenues of exploration suggested by such articles. I then digitally entered the verbatim text into this manuscript.

The research for the edited county lists was supplemented by a collection of obituaries made by the Colchester Historeum, Truro, and the Antigonish Heritage Museum. Both included a number of deaths of Nova Scotians who died out of the province, which were new to us. While outside deaths were not included in the county lists, these obituaries or death notices appear chronologically in the county chapters.

From archival sources, Dr. Marble began compiling his final list of Nova Scotia's influenza victims, sorting them alphabetically by surname. This data shows mentions of most local deaths, from whatever source, and some of the names of those who died elsewhere of influenza, but who received mention in the papers back home in Nova Scotia. His final unedited list, combining these newspaper accounts, as a different type of death notice source, with the names from the county registers shows a higher number of deaths in the province than do totals from the county lists. This master list is a singularly important piece of research, but is not the final word on the total number of influenza deaths.

Dr. Marble cautions that there were certainly uncounted *other* deaths, apart from those on his lists—some perhaps overlooked in the registries or the newspapers, as well as persons who never had *any* "return of information" submitted to the registrar in their county. Research for this sourcebook has already produced some of those names, by rechecking registries where possible, or via oral histories and unpublished family memoirs. These names are not included in the edited county lists, but appear in the relevant county chapters. See the chapter on Kings County, in particular.

In this book, therefore, I have included the following from Dr Marble's research: my edited version of the county-deaths lists, and information from three years of newspaper articles.

Please note that newspaper articles have been transcribed exactly as printed, including the misspelled words. For example, starting in October 1918, the *Truro Daily News* began exhibiting some very strange orthography, such as "deth," "ded," "helth," "offiser" et al. As verbatim quotations, they were not corrected, however some names are given in a corrected form in brackets.

Keep in mind, however, that just as we are unsure about the total number of Nova Scotia's losses due to influenza, I have even less data on the numbers of those who were infected and survived. Enormous numbers of people collapsed with influenza all over the province, with the possible exception of Victoria County. I know that further cross-referencing, checking of original sources, and additional research is needed.

Memoirs, Letters, Newspapers, Reports, Oral Histories, Biographies, Photographs, and Fieldwork

Glimpses and stories, unpublished memoirs—the heart of this work came from the people of Nova Scotia. The county chapters and other features of the sourcebook were greatly enhanced by the labour and the generous contributions of data sent in by many people, including museum people, archivists, genealogists, grassroots researchers, and Nova Scotians from all walks of life, often working with community knowledge and family histories. Some of the knowledge they shared could never have been found by archival research as it existed only in memory. Local historians cheerfully contributed research they had been amassing for years. They sent in illustrations to go with their data, modern or historical. They found small self-published books and unpublished memoirs. They took me to visit tiny hidden cemeteries, photographing gravestones. Chance-met people began telling me stories at parties or in dental office waiting rooms as soon as I mentioned what I was working on. If Dr. Marble's lists were the backbone of this book, these contributions are the real heart of the work. With this additional data in hand, patterns began to emerge, connections were made, and the book began to take shape.

I have felt compelled more and more to do this sort of oral history collecting, before such accounts pass out of living memory. I started by contacting people I had met in my forty-eight years at the Nova Scotia Museum, and expanded this to contacts I was newly given. During this time, I was continually amazed at the energy this investigation generated. I have *never* participated in a project that caught the imagination of so many people, all over the province. I used to wonder about it, and to ask people why they were so enthused about it.

"It's because it's about *us.*" That's what they said, every last one of them. "It's about us."

Nothing today better demonstrates how the Great Influenza pervaded the whole province during the years 1918–20 than this outpouring of responses from all over Nova Scotia, sometimes from even the smallest of communities. Influenza had infected and affected throughout Nova Scotia during those terrible three years of pandemic.

So this book is for everyone, but particularly for Nova Scotians, in hopes that it will prove to be an informative history and a spur to future research, with a host of riveting stories about ordinary people doing their best to help one another in a most frightening time.

Dr. Ruth Holmes Whitehead, ONS
Halifax, Nova Scotia, 2018–20

For Wade Cullen Humphreys, 1901–18,
dead of influenza at seventeen.

Chapter I

THE GREAT INFLUENZA

I BEGAN THIS research literally trying to understand how my uncle Wade died of influenza. What had been his experience? I began by thinking that influenza and the pneumonia which it created must have been rather like the double pneumonia I had at age fifteen, though perhaps a little more intense. I couldn't have been more wrong. I had antibiotics; he had nothing. He just intensely suffered. And then he died. I really wanted to know what it was like to die of influenza.

The course of this pandemic throughout the world seems to have been more like an endless loop from a horror movie, as the illness raced through homes and hospitals, towns and countryside. It was a disease so savage, so shocking, it demanded hyperbole, as the article at the top of the next page attempts to convey.

An example of a typical death record held at the Nova Scotia Archives—in this case, for Robert Auntivine, influenza victim, and other seamen, Sydney, NS. *(Nova Scotia Archives)*

It started innocently enough, with sniffles and a cough. Then the fever pounced. Every muscle, every joint, ached. Blood poured from the nose. Teeth fell out. So did hair. The stench was indescribable. Vomiting and diarrhea were common, as was delirium. Extreme anxiety led some sufferers to take their own lives. Others shrieked in terror, prey to technicolour nightmares. Breathing became laboured. Then the dreaded mahogany-coloured patches appeared over each cheekbone. The skin took on a deep plummy red colour—doctors dubbed it "dusky heliotrope"—then began to darken to blackish purple as the lungs filled with fluid. When the fingertips and toes turned inky, the game was up. The end came swiftly. People fought to catch a breath only to drown in their own bodily fluids. This was death by Spanish Flu.

> Alanna Mitchell, "Outbreak: The little-known story of the 1918 Spanish Flu and how we're preparing for the next great pandemic." *Canadian Geographic*, September/October 2018, 53.

John Barry opens his meticulously researched book, *The Great Influenza*, by describing a moment when scientist and medical doctor Paul Lewis, a lieutenant commander in the U.S. Navy, first encountered this disease:

The clinicians now looked to him to explain the violent symptoms these sailors presented. The blood that covered so many of them did not come from wounds....Most of the blood had come from nosebleeds. A few sailors had coughed the blood up. Others had bled from their ears. Some coughed so hard that autopsies would later show they had torn apart abdominal muscles and rib cartilage. And many of the men writhed in agony or delirium; nearly all those able to communicate complained of headache, as if someone were hammering a wedge into their skulls just behind the eyes, and body aches so intense they felt like bones breaking. A few were vomiting. Finally the skin of some of the sailors had turned unusual colors; some showed just a tinge of blue around their lips or fingertips, but a few looked so dark...[t]hey looked almost black.

> John M. Barry, *The Great Influenza: The Story of the Deadliest Pandemic in History* (New York: Viking) 2nd ed. 2009, 2.

Initial Disease Vectors in Nova Scotia, 1918–20

News of the spread of the epidemic in the United States was waking Nova Scotians to the fact that something unusual, massively contagious, lightning-fast, and lethal was happening in the outside world. In September, things in Massachusetts got so bad that they begged other states for help. They even sent word to Halifax, asking for assistance in the form of doctors and nurses. Lieutenant-Governor McCallum

5,500 New Cases of Influenza are Reported in the State of Massachusetts

BOSTON, September 30.—Governor McCall to-night received from Lieutenant-Governor McCallum Grant, of Nova Scotia, the following telegram:—

"This province cannot fail to recall with gratitude the magnificent and immediate resource Massachusetts made in the time of our urgent need at Halifax. Some nurses have already gone to help you and more both of doctors and nurses will follow as you may require them."

The aid extended by federal and other outside workers in Massusetts to the state authorities in organizing the campaign against influenza, led the state department of health to-night to express its expectation that the epidemic would be checked before gaining further headway. The department reported conditions in Boston to-day as improved, but the disease was more prevalent in cities and towns in the metropolitan district and thruout the state.

State Health Commissioner E. R. Kelley, in a telegram to Surgeon-General Blue, of the United States public health service, covering the situation up to one o'clock to-day, says: "Reports from 55 cities and towns outside Boston total 5,500 new cases of influenza. There are at least 75,000 cases of influenza in Massachusetts to-day, excluding the number in Cantonments. Nurses and doctors most urgently needed."

The state department of health to-night announced an offer of $10 a day and expenses to registered physicians not in government service who will come to Massachusetts. Transportation will be refunded to physicians within a 24-hour travelling radium of Boston. Before starting, physicians should wire the department for instructions.

"5,500 New Cases of Influenza Reported in Massachusetts." *(Nova Scotia Archives)*

Grant wrote Governor McCall a letter saying that Nova Scotia remembered the help Boston sent them in the aftermath of the Halifax Explosion in 1917, that aid in the form of nurses had already been sent to Boston, and that other nurses and doctors would follow, "as you may require them." A copy of this letter appeared in Halifax newspapers on September 30 and October 1. It included portions of a telegram by Massachusetts State Health Commissioner E. R. Kelley to Surgeon-General Blue of the US Public Health Service, underlining the state of emergency:

Reports from 55 cities and towns outside Boston total 5,500 new cases of influenza [in 24 hours]. There are at least 75,000 cases of influenza in Massachusetts to-day, excluding the number in Cantonment.

Halifax Evening News, 1 October 1918, 7.

☞ Cantonment refers to the army camps which were woefully jammed way beyond their capacities, and flooded with sick recruits. Nova Scotia officials evidently queried this, privately, and received the following report from three of their doctors who had gone down to Massachusetts to assist. They had it printed for dissemination to medical personnel only:

✒ EPIDEMIC INFLUENZA (Issued by the Department of the Public Health, Nova Scotia.)
The following report of the Halifax physicians who went to Boston to assist in fighting epidemic influenza in that city, is, by the courtesy of the Mayor of Halifax, issued for the information of the medical profession of Nova Scotia:

Boston, Oct. 4, 1918

His Worship Mayor Hawkins:

Dear Sir:

As we received no special appointment from the Massachusetts Board of Health, we decided to investigate the epidemic from a general standpoint in order that measures to combat the disease, should it visit Halifax, might be inaugurated. During this investigation we have visited various emergency hospital[s] and consulted with representatives of various health organizations, and with those in charge of district work.

1. All authorities emphasize the suddenness of the onset of the epidemic; the immediate infection of over 5,000 in the first 24 hours and higher figures in the following successive days. The rapidity of the spread where people were massed (ship-building plants, factories) is practically without parallel.

2. The severity of the infection—the high grade of virulence of the infection, many cases dying within the first twenty-four hours or forty-eight hours—death being due in this type to toxaemia. The appalling death rate in the later stages we learn to be due to a broncho-pneumonia, occasionally one of the lobar type. The organism found in 90 cases out of 110 autopsies was that of influenza. Pure streptococci and pneumococci were also incidentally found in the remaining 20. From these figures it is obvious that the real factor in the epidemic is the influenza bacillus [virus] and not, as was the previous impression, that streptococci are the cause of the high death rate.

3. The symptoms are sudden—practically immediate onset with headache, muscular pain in the back and limbs, tendency to nausea, chills, rapid rise of fever (103–105 deg.) with or without the involvement of mucous membranes shown by coryza and bronchitis.

4. Physical examination of the chest should always be made. Evidence of pneumonia has been frequently found where it was unsuspected until this examination had been made.

5. Mortality as above noted is largely due to (a) an overwhelming toxaemia, (b) a broncho-pneumonia. This broncho-pneumonia may be an initial feature, or may not manifest itself for some days. Relapses during convalescence usually show pneumonia. Exact figures of mortality are not available, but it should be particularly noted that those cases who continued at their work, so-called 'fighting the disease,' showed an appalling mortality.... Death rate of pneumonia is considered not less than 50%.

☞ Doctors McDougall, Thomas, and Lessel told the mayor of Halifax, "We advise that with the first appearance of the disease, the utmost limit of preventive measures should be used—such measures as would be used in dealing with any of the dangerous epidemic diseases—and used at once."

They went further, giving measures in effect in Boston. "We endorse the compulsory reporting of all cases promptly...Only patients on the danger list are permitted visitors. No public funerals are permitted," they wrote, adding something which now seems almost unbelievable: "All emergency hospitals [in Boston] are under armed guard, with fixed bayonets."

Finally, they closed with, "We recommend that the above or any portion thereof be used for the public good and brought to their attention in whatever form you see fit. We also wish to state that the press reports were in no way exaggerated and from what we personally know of the epidemic we cannot too strongly urge the co-operation of all to protect the city and province from this terrible scourge."

J. G. McDougall, Lewis Thomas, J. Fred Lessel. For a copy of the pamphlet, see
Nova Scotia Archives, V/F Vol. 86 No. 20 (original); No. 20a (the photocopy).

☞ According to Garry Shutlak, of the Nova Scotia Archives, this is a printed pamphlet, probably commissioned by the municipality of Halifax (even though it says Department of Public Health), as it doesn't appear in any relevant Legislative Assembly of Nova Scotia Journals for 1919, 1920, and 1921.

Setting up these preventive measures here in Nova Scotia was more successful in some areas than in others. People might have taken such measures much more seriously, however, if the above communication had been printed in the newspapers. I cannot find that it ever was. Rosemary Barbour, Senior Archivist at the Nova Scotia Archives, told me this: "There is an interesting note about the first cases of the flu in Inverness County in the 26th Annual Report of the Department of Public Health for the year ending 30 September 1918 (Journals of the House of Assembly 1919). It is worth noting the number of people who fell ill compared to the number who died." This note is as follows:

A few weeks ago epidemic influenza made its appearance in Inverness and its neighbourhood. Some 1200 cases developed in the town of which ten resulted fatally. Neighbouring communities suffered to a lesser extent. The plague has apparently been stayed in that part of the province, but as this report is being written word comes that other districts are being invaded. The extremely serious condition being reported from Massachusetts and neighbouring states arouses the fear that we may have great difficulty in coping with this disease should it become widespread in our province. Warning letters have been sent out to medical health officers and physicians, urging immediate organization and development of plans for dealing with the scourge should it make its appearance. It must be confessed that the incompleteness of the organization which has been effected in our province makes me most apprehensive at this juncture.

26th Annual Report, Department of Public Health, 30 September 1918 (Journals of the House of Assembly 1919); Rosemary V. Barbour, Senior Archivist, Preservation Services, Nova Scotia Archives, to Ruth Whitehead, email, 10 July 2018.

Death Comes in Crowded Situations

That was the hardest lesson the authorities had to learn. Anywhere there were crowded conditions—barracks, hospitals, jails, asylums, poorhouses, ships, the fishing vessels, factories, mines, lumber camps, internments camps of the First World War—these were breeding grounds for the quick transferral of the influenza virus from one victim to many victims, spreading exponentially. Even in smaller venues such as banks, grocery stores and pharmacies, pool halls and barber shops, bowling alleys, dance halls, live theatre and the movies, or gatherings at churches, schools, or where whole communities joined celebrations of the end of the war, there were fertile grounds for infection to spread. And spread it did.

Shipping, General

In early August 1918, according to author John Barry, "the crew of a steamship proceeding from France to New York was hit so hard with influenza 'that all of the seamen were prostrate on it and it had to put into Halifax.'".

John M. Barry, *The Great Influenza: The Story of the Deadliest Pandemic in History* (New York: Viking) 2nd ed. 2009, 181. (Name of the vessel unidentified.)

Shipping, where people were confined together for weeks or months on end, was responsible for major contagions in Nova Scotia, notably in the largest ports—Halifax and Sydney. Major disease vectors (the lines down which infection travels) in this category are reported in Halifax and Cape Breton Counties. Halifax, being the largest port with the greatest amount of shipping, had the highest numbers of provincial deaths from the Great Influenza. Accounts in Halifax newspapers of the period quote health officials as blaming the arrival of influenza in the city on shipping.

DR. N. E. MACKAY WILL PROTEST TO OTTAWA AGAINST ALLOWING STEAMERS TO BE SENT HERE WITH CASES OF SPANISH INFLUENZA ON BOARD—A SERIOUS MATTER

HALIFAX, October 8. The apparent disregard of health regulations by the shipping authorities at Montreal and New York, will be reported to the Canadian director of health at Ottawa, by Dr. N. E. MacKay, Dominion government quarantine officer at Halifax. Steamers given their practique (clear bill of health) at these ports are continually reaching Halifax with large numbers of cases of Spanish influenza on board. The belief is that the disease was introduced into Halifax through this source, and a protest will be made to the Dominion director of health. Yesterday a steamer reached Halifax with a large number of influenza cases on board. The ship was from Montreal, where she had been given her practique. On a very recent occasion a steamer arrived from New York with a number of cases of the disease, even the captain being very ill with it. His temperature was 105 [degrees Fahrenheit]. Dr. MacKay regards the practice of allowing steamers to come to Halifax, under the conditions referred to, as dangerous to the health of the citizens. Other instances equally as serious, indicating an utter disregard for the health of our citizens, have been reported.

Halifax Evening Mail, 9 October 1918, 2.

Troopships

At first the deaths of men were separated by a few hours....But a week after leaving New York, the officer of the day [aboard troopship *Leviathan*] was no longer bothering to note in the log "died on board," no longer bothering to identify the military organization to which the dead belonged, no longer bothering to note a cause of death; he was writing only a name and a time, two names at 2:00 A.M., another at 2:02 A.M., two more at 2:15 A.M, like that all through the night, every notation in the log now a simple recitation of mortality, into the morning a death at 7:56 A.M, another at 8:10 A.M , at 8:25 A.M.

John M. Barry, *The Great Influenza: The Story of the Deadliest Pandemic in History*
(New York: Viking) 2nd ed. 2009, 306.

Bodies were lined up on deck and then slid into the sea, an endless roll-call of the dead.

Sydney and Halifax, as major ports receiving sailors and soldiers shipping out to Europe before the First World War ended in November of 1918, or returning from Europe during and after the Armistice, were hard hit by influenza. Canadian troop-ships were loading in Halifax Harbour for Europe, leaving their last-minute sick behind. American ones, crammed full, would divert to Nova Scotia (last stop before the deep Atlantic), and unload their influenza cases.

Ships are still arriving in the port of Halifax with infected crews. Yesterday several more sailors were admitted as patients in hospital at Lawlor's Island. An American ship also put in with a number of cases. The introduction of Spanish influenza to Halifax is supposed to be owing to the arrival of ships whose men were suffering from the disease....DEPARTMENT OF THE PUBLIC HEALTH OF NOVA SCOTIA. Halifax, October 8.

Halifax Morning Chronicle, 10 October 1918, 5.

Sydney, on the other hand, took in five hundred cases on a single day—September 22, 1918—who were U.S. Army recruits being shipped to Europe, and the ship's crew. The need for stringent quarantine was not yet fully understood. Inevitable disaster followed.

"The transports became floating caskets," writes John Barry. "Shipping more men who required medical care into this maelstrom [the theatre of war] made little sense." In Europe, said Barry, they were swamped taking care of their own and their allies' influenza cases already.

It is impossible to state how many soldiers the ocean voyages killed, especially when one tries to count those infected aboard ship who died later on shore. But for every death at least four or five men were ill enough to be incapacitated for weeks. These men were a burden rather than a help in Europe.

John M. Barry, *The Great Influenza: The Story of the Deadliest Pandemic in History* (New York: Viking) 2nd ed. 2009, 306-307; referencing Alfred W. Crosby, *America's Forgotten Pandemic*, (Cambridge: Cambridge University Press) 1989,166.

The U.S. Army, however, kept shipping troops anyway. Why was this insanity continued? President Woodrow Wilson and his personal physician, naval admiral Dr. Cary Grayson, tried to argue down army chief of staff General Peyton March on the subject. They wanted him to stop troop movement until the influenza was controlled. Grayson and Wilson met with Gen. March on October 7, 1918, but March declined to halt troop shipments. Barry sums this up: "He insisted that every possible precaution was being taken. The troops were screened before embarking and the sick winnowed out." And then—*get this!*—General March reassured the other two that, as a final precaution, "Some ships even put ashore in Halifax, Nova Scotia, those who fell seriously ill before the actual Atlantic crossing began."

There was no need to halt shipments, because, Barry reports, as General March told the US president, "Every such soldier who has died just as surely played his part as [did] his comrade who died in France." But what about the collateral damage?

I can't find that Nova Scotia's provincial government was ever apprised of this plan to make Halifax (or Sydney) last-chance dumping grounds for American troops or ships' crews ill with influenza. No word of warning about needing to prepare was whispered in an ally's ear. Mariners have always assisted other mariners, and to Nova Scotians, assisting such, no matter the circumstances, was just business as usual—and, besides, there was a war on.

This American policy left Nova Scotia with the financial and physical burden of care for all these many infected troops and ships' crews being foisted upon them. But there would be a darker legacy. According to John Barry, it was October 7 when General March refused to stop shipping troops to Europe, sick or not. The Armistice and war's end came on November 11, a little over a month later. By then the disease, which has been called the "deadliest pandemic in history," was already firmly established in the province, and would continue here into the late spring of 1920. Peyton March had signed a death warrant for thousands of troops, and for quite a lot of Nova Scotians as well, but the general was prepared to sacrifice all of them. To do otherwise, he said, would be bad for morale.

My own grandfather was on one of those American troopships. He could never speak about it afterwards.

FIVE HUNDRED U.S. SOLDIERS IN PORT

Landed on Sunday, Most of them Suffering from Spanish Influenza

About five hundred American soldiers arrived at an Atlantic port [Sydney] yesterday [September 22] suffering from Spanish Influenza, and were removed to hospitals ashore for treatment. The curling rinks, and some of the church halls were commandeered by the military authorities and turned into emergency hospitals, with nurses taken from anywhere about the place. The worst cases have been taken to one of the military hospitals. It is understood that the first aid and the home nursing class graduates will offer for service at the hospitals, and will assist with the care of the men. The chief difficulty was to get beds for the cases and all day the authorities were busy with the work of procuring and preparing beds for the sick to sleep in tonight. The men will remain for several weeks.

Sydney Daily Post, 23 September 1918, 1.

☞ The port's name was withheld as it was still wartime, but further newspaper accounts made it obvious that it was Sydney and the chapter in this book on Cape Breton County tells the whole story.

Fishing Vessels

☞ The influenza epidemic seems initially to have arrived in the counties of Yarmouth, Digby, Shelburne, Guysborough, and Richmond via fishing vessels, a considerable number of them operating out of Gloucester, Massachusetts, which at one time had the second largest fishing fleet in the world. Gloucester companies were buying Nova Scotian catches, and in return selling supplies of salt and equipment to fishing boats or fish plants there. Massachusetts vessels began offloading sick crew members to Nova Scotia hospitals and the deceased into graves.

The chapters on Yarmouth and Richmond counties give more detailed information and for more about the Gloucester fleets, see Joseph E. Garland's *Down to the Sea: The Fishing Schooners of Gloucester*, published by David R. Godine, Publisher Inc., in association with Cape Ann Historical Association, in 1983.

DEATH IN YARMOUTH FROM INFLUENZA

Gloucester Man Succumbs to the Disease after a Couple of Weeks Illness

YARMOUTH, October 1. The death took place at Yarmouth hospital today of Augustus Thompson, of Gloucester, Mass. The deceased was one of the two members of the crew of the Gloucester fishing schooner Nathalie Hammond which that vessel left in Yarmouth two weeks ago today seriously ill with Spanish Influenza.

Halifax Morning Chronicle, 2 October 1918, 13.

ALBERT SAULNIER. Albert, son of Mr. and Mrs. Monde Saulnier, died at their home at Saulnierville, Digby Co., on Saturday after only four days' illness of pneumonia, which developed from a severe attack of influenza. He was a ship carpenter of considerable ability and as such was well known all along the St. Mary's Bay shore. Mr. Saulnier was 30 years of age.

Digby Courier, 26 March 1919, 5.

WHOLE CREW HAD DISEASE
Gloucester Schooner Made Cape Breton Port with Difficulty—One Man Died. Special to the Morning Chronicle

A CAPE BRETON PORT, September 28. The Gloucester schooner *Athlete*, Capt. Berhan [Bonham], arrived here last Tuesday [September 24] to load fish for the Gordon Pew [Gorton-Pew] Fish Co., of Gloucester, the cargo having been bought by them from our Bay fishermen. Shortly after leaving Gloucester sickness developed among the crew, and when the vessel arrived it was with difficulty she was sailed into port, as all the members of the crew were afflicted with the disease, which the doctors have pronounced Spanish influenza.

Halifax Morning Chronicle, 2 October 1918, 1.

☞ This fishing schooner from Massachusetts infected huge numbers of people in Richmond County, via those in Petit-de-Grat, who innocently unloaded her cargo of salt at Comeau Brothers fish plant, then loaded the return cargo of salted fish aboard a vessel full of sick crew.

It should be noted that the small Mi'kmaw population living in Barra Head, Richmond County, was also affected by this influenza, its onset beginning in late September 1918, peaking in October of that year. Because of the identical timing of the outbreak in Petit-de-Grat, it is quite possible that these victims were exposed directly or indirectly to the sick crew of the fishing schooner *Athlete*, moored in the harbour of Petit-de-Grat. There were five deaths. All we know for sure is that the Mi'kmaw community had become infected at around the same time as did Frank Poole, crew on the *Athlete*, who fell ill September 20th at sea, and died eight days later on board his infected schooner in the Petit-de-Grat harbour. Parts of Richmond County would shortly thereafter reach epidemic status.

One case of the disease at Cape North is understood to have been traced directly to Spain in its origin, having been contracted from a Newfoundland man who had returned from a voyage to Spanish ports.

Sydney Record, 24 September 1918, 2.

☞ This is the first reference to influenza in Victoria County. That county's first death also occurred in Cape North: Henry Christie, aged 15, contracted a fatal dose of flu after he became ill on October 31.

SITUATION IN NOVA SCOTIA
The situation is bad in certain localities of the province. Lockeport is in a very bad influenza condition. Dr. W. H. Hattie, provincial health officer, reports a total of 300 cases to date in that small town, four deaths from the disease, and 28 attacks which have resulted in pneumonia. Dr. Hattie has sent out an urgent call for nurses for Lockeport.

Sydney Daily Post, 17 October 1918, 6.

☞ George McIntosh, the first person to die in Lockeport, was a fisherman. He brought his infection home from wherever he picked it up, and he died on October 2. He passed it to his daughter Minnie, who died on October 18. This was a particularly virulent phase of this influenza, perhaps fresh out of Massachusetts. It attacked Lockeport either in late September or early October, however introduced, and began spreading outward to the rest of the county and beyond—and in a number of cases, via infected fishermen.

Quite a few Shelburne County fishermen fell victim to this flu, including a large cluster on Cape Sable Island, in the villages or hamlets of Cape Island and of South Side Cape Island; Clarks Harbour, Newellton, The Hawk, North East Point, West Head, and Stoney Island. The first death occurred on Cape Island: Edward Quinton, 18, died 15 October 1918; he showed symptoms first on 4 October. Percy Nickerson, 35, fell ill 24 October, and died on the twenty-eighth. Judah Nickerson, a fisherman at South Side Cape Island, died November 2, aged 31. At Clarks Harbor, the dead included Russell Nickerson, aged 30, who became ill October 11 and died on the seventeenth.

Nova Scotia Death Register, Shelburne County, 1918, Book 49.

Some weeks ago the trawler 'Ran' arrived in Canso, reporting some of her crew ill, and while the disease could not at that time be recognized as Spanish Influenza, precautions were taken to isolate the steamer and other means were taken to guard against contagion. Two or three other cases in the town apparently developed but with the exception of one case, these were very mild, and we are glad to report that all have recovered.

Canso News, 26 October 1918, 1.

☞ This freedom from flu did not continue for long. Canso lost a number of people from the community, many of whom were fishermen.

FRANK SUTHERLAND. Not only on the battlefields of Europe are Canso's young men giving up their lives, but on this side of the water, far removed from the danger of cannon balls and bullets, many of Canso's young men are being taken off. The death of Frank Sutherland, son of Mr. and Mrs. Roderick Sutherland of Canso, took place in Gloucester [Massachusetts] recently, caused by Spanish Influenza. Frank Sutherland was a capable, straightforward, manly young fisherman, whose prospects of success in life were very bright, but like so many men in like circumstances he contracted the dread disease and his young life was quickly snuffed out.

Canso News, 26 October 1918, 4.

☞ Canso fishermen were still in regular contact with the fisheries at Gloucester, Massachusetts, sometimes with fatal consequences. Did they bring the contagion home with them?

AUGUSTUS HANLON. Among the sad events in connection with the visit of influenza in Canso was the carrying off of several young men, among whom was Augustus Hanlon, who died on November 28th. Mr. Hanlon was a successful young fisherman and leaves a wife and one child.

Canso News, 28 December 1918, 2.

Chignecto Mines, Cumberland County

INFLUENZA IN CUMBERLAND. The Mines at Chignecto have been temporarily shut down owing to the epidemic at that place. There is hardly an occupied house in that village, but has one or more persons suffering from influenza. There is also a serious outbreak in River Hebert, but so far the Joggins Mines is free from the disease.

Amherst Daily News, 22 October 1918, 3.

☞ With 150 men ill at once, mining ceased. The workings mentioned above, as well as those at Maccan upriver from Chignecto and various others, were established to mine the same extensive coal seam running from Spring Hill down to Joggins. One by one, all over the county, miners and their families began to come down with influenza. The mines' crowded working conditions made it easy for the contagion to pass on, and poor air quality (low in oxygen and high in coal dust) affected the lungs, even before the horrific pneumonia which accompanied the influenza struck the men. Ill, with nowhere to go but home, they took the disease with them. Contagion spread outwards from the mines.

Fort Edward, Hants County

⟜⟞ In the crowded conditions of this training camp for new recruits to the British Expeditionary Force, influenza found conditions ideal for infecting great numbers of soldiers at once. Some of the camp's early fatalities don't appear on Dr. Allan Marble's lists because the immediate cause of death wasn't given as influenza. The West Hants Historical Society website, on the other hand, states the cause of death *was* epidemic influenza.

It is well known that individuals trained at Fort Edward during the First World War but did you know that not all these soldiers survived to fight in Europe? In October of 1918 Windsor was visited by the Spanish Influenza. It took many lives amongst the civilian population along with several soldiers, killing 9 recruits of the B.E.F. in six weeks.

West Hants Historical Society / Posted on 14 December, 2015.

⟜⟞ For names of the dead, and more detail, see the Hants County chapter.

Amherst POW Internment Camp, Cumberland County

⟜⟞ The conditions at the camp were best described by its most famous internee, Leon Trotsky, who stayed there until his release was requested by the new Russian government.

The Amherst Concentration camp was housed in an old and very dilapidated iron foundry that had been confiscated from its German owner. The bunks were arranged in three tiers, two deep on each side of the hall. About 800 of us lived in these conditions. The air in this dormitory at night can be imagined. Men hopelessly clogged the passages, elbowed their way through....In spite of the heroic efforts of the prisoners to keep themselves physically and morally fit, five of them had gone insane. We had to eat and sleep in the same room with these madmen.

My Life, by Leon Trotsky. New York: Charles Scribner's Sons, 1930.

⟜⟞ Pandemic influenza flourished in crowded situations such as this camp. At its peak, the facility held 834 prisoners. They were crammed into a building a quarter of a mile long, but only one hundred feet wide. In addition, there were up to 256 guards, most of them Amherst men. For more detail, see the Cumberland County chapter.

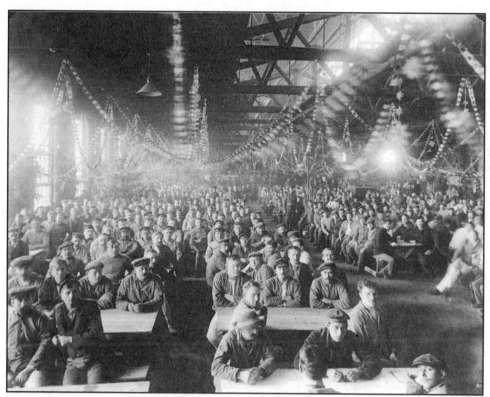

Amherst Internment Camp for First World War prisoners of war, showing the crowded conditions which readily enabled the spread of influenza. *(Library and Archives Canada)*

INFLUENZA OUTBREAK. There has been a serious outbreak among the interned prisoners. There are over one hundred and twenty cases in the Military hospital in the Drill Hall, and there are a number of prisoners in the hospital in connection with the camp which will be transferred to the Drill Hall as soon as possible.

Amherst Daily News, 12 February 1919, 3.

Factories and Large Businesses

Mr. Smith of the Kingston canning factory informed us that despite the 'Flu', which at one time bowled out the entire staff, a satisfactory season's output was secured. About 30,000 barrels of apples were purchased, 20,000 of which were sold whole, 10,000 barrels going into the cannery.

Bridgetown Monitor, 25 December 1918, 4.

Lumber Camps

INFLUENZA DISORGANIZES LUMBER CAMP

Because of the outbreak of influenza in a large Nova Scotia lumbering camp, all operations have ceased. This means not only a very serious loss to operators, but will materially lessen the lumber output – a matter of no small concern to the people at large. As the men are said to have returned to their homes, there is reason to fear that a number of new communities may be infected by the disease. It is understood that instructions are being sent to all mill operators by the Provincial Health Officer with leaflets for distribution amongst the men.

Halifax Morning Chronicle, 23 November 1918, 2.

The deaths occurred at the Lumber Camp at Folleigh Lake, of two of our young men, of Spanish Influenza Saturday morning Dec. 14th, Fred Chisholm, aged twenty four years passed away at eleven o'clock. His remains were brought to our Village and interred in the family plot of the Mahon Cemetery. This young man is survived by his father Mr. Avon B. Chisholme, two sisters, Mrs. Ferguson Hill, and Mrs. Wm. Urquhart, of our Village, a younger brother, Lou, at home, and two brothers, Burnham and Judson, overseas.

Norman Tipping also succumbed to this terrible disease on Sunday the 15th his remains was laid away in the Mahon Cemetery today, he is survived by his father Mr. Robert Tipping, a brother Stuart, who is ill at present at Londonderry Stn. of influenza.

Truro Daily News, 18 December 1918, 1. Courtesy the Colchester Historeum.

Influenza has paid a second visit to Tracadie, Antigonish. Two weeks ago all the workmen at a lumber camp were taken sick. Thirty men comprised the camp, which was operated by Mr. Haggerty of Mulgrave, and was in charge of Mr. George Cameron of Melrose, Guysborough Co.

Antigonish Casket, 27 March 1919. Courtesy the Antigonish Heritage Museum.

Churches

Sometimes all it takes is one person to infect a whole community, but often there is no record of who that person was, or how it all happened. The story of the Eight Island Lakes victims is therefore of interest. Three people died at this Guysborough County hamlet in late 1918. This was a very isolated community, and the three all became ill at around the same time. A search for anything on Eight Island Lake's victims in the HVS death registration database revealed that all three victims were buried as Baptists, at a cemetery a few miles up the road, used by the Goshen Baptist Church.

This was confirmed by Western Guysborough historian and author Ruth Legge, and informant Lewis MacIntosh.

Using Allan Marble's newspaper references list, the following article from a neighbouring county newspaper on Goshen was found, showing the smoking gun.

 [F]rom Goshen, Guysboro County, comes a story that indicates how alarmingly contagious an infection influenza really is. A Baptist clergyman visited the Mission to hold Divine Service on a recent Sunday. He had the disease in its incipient state. Apparently all who attended the service became sick, also all the members of the household at which he was a guest. Altogether there were some fifty cases of influenza at Goshen. At least one death has occurred there [probably that of Mrs. Henry Mason of Eight Island Lake on November 30] from influenza.

Pictou Advocate, 6 December 1918, 4.

☞ Evidence points to Sunday, October 24, 1918, as the date the minister infected the congregation of the Baptist church. Once again, a large crowd of people: add one infected person, and get fifty ill and three deaths. A contributing factor must have been that the Goshen Baptist church had burned down in August 1918, and the people were holding services crammed into a small schoolhouse at Eight Island Lake. And because pastoral visits were infrequent, perhaps every church member strove to attend this service, bringing their infants and children.

Thanks to Lewis MacIntosh and Lloyd Sinclair for information re: church.
Cemetery locations: Ruth Legge to Ruth Whitehead, email, 16 May 2018.

Schools

There passed peacefully to rest at Edgehill College, Windsor, N.S., on Oct. 28th, Miss Maizie Viola Corkum, youngest daughter of the late Almon Corkum of East Middle LaHave. The deceased had gone to Edgehill College when the school opened in September. When influenza made its appearance among the inmates of the College, she too became a victim of the disease, which finally developed into pneumonia.

Lunenburg Progress Enterprise, 6 November 1918, 5.

Crowded Celebrations and Events

YARMOUTH HOLDS RED CROSS FETE. MONSTER PARADE IN THE AFTERNOON AND MINSTREL SHOW IN THE EVENING

Special to the Morning Chronicle

Yarmouth, Sept. 26. One of the greatest demonstrations in aid of the local Red Cross work took place this afternoon and evening. The firemen of the town who for the past week or two having been working most arduously for the cause turned out a monster parade with beautifully decorated floats....The town throughout the day has been in holiday attire....The parade was witnessed by thousands of people from all parts of the country and the "rag girls" did a big business. The affair concluded this evening with a grand minstrel show in the people's theatre, the entire seating capacity of which was sold out early this afternoon.

Halifax Morning Chronicle, 27 September 1918, 2.

 INFLUENZA IS AGAIN MENACING
Department of Public Health States There Have Been 700 Deaths Since October 1st

Several communities in which the influenza situation had improved to an extent which seemed to warrant the removal of restriction are again reporting a rather alarming prevalence of the disease. It was impossible for us to restrain our feelings when the news of peace came, and the free mingling of the people in our celebration of the great event is doubtless responsible for the recent increase in the number of cases....Incomplete returns show that we have had more than 550 deaths from this disease in Nova Scotia since October 1st.

Halifax Morning Chronicle, 23 November 1918, 2.

Death Comes Riding on the Rails

COMING HOME FOR BURIAL
A gentleman, who returned from the United States Saturday morning, states that the train on which he travelled brought ten caskets containing Nova Scotia victims of the scourge. He also states that twenty-five Nova Scotian young ladies, who were professional nurses in the States, succumbed to the disease.

Bridgetown Monitor, 23 October 1918, 7.

All over Nova Scotia, as the epidemic took hold, bodies were being shipped home for burial, both within and from outside the province.

The body arrived here by train yesterday of Miss Lillian Wagstaff who had died in Chicago at the age of 41. The body was consigned to her sister, Miss Edith Wagstaff, and funeral services were held in the Baptist Church here and largely attended, with interment in Woodlawn Cemetery. Deceased was a native of Granville and had been strenuously nursing others in Chicago before she herself succumbed.

Annapolis Spectator, 9 January 1919, 8.

Since it is manifestly impracticable to place legal restraints upon travel, every physician should point out the serious result which may ensue if a person slightly ill with influenza should go from one community to another. October 14, 1918.

Halifax Morning Chronicle, 16 October 1918, 2.

It wasn't only the dead who rode the rails. So did the sick and the recovering, and they infected others. Once the Great Influenza began to be established at ports in the province, the train interiors took it everywhere, or brought it into the province from elsewhere. Often, the dead were accompanied on their railroad journeys by family members, who might themselves have been exposed to this disease. Others contracted the flu and then took the trains home, infecting passengers and crew on the trains, and then in their communities. People were stricken merely by traveling on the railroads.

Those who worked on the railroads in various capacities began to fall ill. The papers were full of it. Engineers, firemen (stokers), brakemen, postal clerks on the railway lines, and management were infected by daily exposures. Their families began to sicken as well. The wife of a brakeman, who was actually herself the local station agent, took ill on the train to Bridgewater and there died.

BRIDGEWATER ENTERPRISE. The death occurred here on Thursday, Oct. 13th, of Mrs. Smith, wife of Granville Smith, brakeman on the H. & S.W. Railway. Mrs. Smith, who was the station agent at Barrington, was spending a week here with her husband at the home of Mrs. Murray Richardson. The deceased took ill en route to Bridgewater [on the train] and later developed Spanish Influenza and pneumonia, which resulted fatally.

Lunenburg Progress Enterprise, 23 October 1918, 5.

The flu situation shows no improvement....The only means of guarding against the spread of the disease is for the general public to exercise precaution. In our own County people are extremely careless in regard to the disease. Patients recovering from the flu mix unconcernedly with the general public, in church and in other places of public assemblage. Though the disease has been epidemic along the I. C. Railway communities from Tracadie to Town and is spreading at Heatherton and adjoining districts, the one passenger car on the morning freight from these points is daily crowded to capacity. Among the crowd are noticed persons just recovering from the disease and persons in whose homes the disease is.

Heatherton is particularly troubled just now with the flue visitation. A few have recently died there from the disease and many others are sick. In one house at

Heatherton all the inmates, five in number, are down with pneumonia. We urge people to exercise greater care in guarding against the spread of the disease.

Antigonish Casket, 26 December 1918.

C.G.R. BRAKEMAN DANIEL McQUARRIE DIES OF INFLUENZA. There occurred early this morning the deth [*sic*] of C.G.R Brakeman, Daniel McQuarrie. The deceased had been ill with influenza and pneumonia developed which caused his deth. Mr McQuarrie is survived by his wife and three young daughters. Mrs. McQuarrie is ill with influenza at her home [on] Brunswick Street.

Truro Daily News, 24 October 1918, 4.

And so it progressed. Those who survived the Great Influenza epidemic often were burdened with lifelong health problems, depression or disorientation, tremors or other neurological damage. The disease spread outward from such initial points of introduction as mentioned above, and by the summer of 1920, it had taken the lives of at least two thousand people in the province, leaving hundreds of orphaned children, grieving families, and a disrupted economy.

Chapter II

ANNAPOLIS COUNTY

ANNAPOLIS COUNTY HAD at least fifty-six confirmed deaths from the Great Influenza. At first, physicians were saying that this was a milder version of what was raging elsewhere. Then the first fatalities started appearing in the newspapers. By far, most were farmers or housewives. Other professions included carpenters, labourers, a manufacturer, a clerk, a foreman printer, a bridge builder, and a larrigan maker! There was only one fisherman—quite a change from deaths in counties on the Atlantic side of the province.

Death record for Edward Moses and others, Annapolis County. (*Nova Scotia Archives*)

☞ The first recorded death apparently happened in Maitland Bridge. The Annapolis County Death Register does not show it, but, weirdly enough, the Queens County Register does. Her name, Margaret Cole, is on Dr. Marble's list of Queens County dead, because it appears in the Queens County death register, which he was transcribing verbatim. So, even though the register clearly says she was born in Caledonia but resided, died and was buried in Maitland, Annapolis County, her name is still in the Queens County register but her information has been added to the amended list of Annapolis County dead at the end of this chapter. Mrs. Cole, 79, died on August 31, 1918 in Maitland [Bridge], after three weeks of illness, the cause being "LaGrippe and pneumonia."

HVS, Queens County Death Register, 1918, Book 46, Page 320, Number 743.

 Death of Mrs. Harry Odell. The Annapolis Spectator says Word was received here last Saturday of the death in the United States of Mrs. Harry Odell, who succumbed to an attack of the new Spanish influofenza [*sic*] disease. Mr. Odell is a son of Mrs. Griffin Odell, this town, and Mrs. Odell is a native of Truro. They were married only about two years ago.

Bridgetown Weekly Monitor, 2 October 1918, 4.

☞ This death is the first mention, in an Annapolis County newspaper, of the "new disease" influenza, or "influofenza," as they spelled it. In cases where a death is reported in a weekly or monthly paper, it is entered here chronologically by the date of the death, *not* by the date of the publication.

BRIDGETOWN. October 8. The local Health Office reports thirty cases of influenza in Bridgetown and vicinity. No deaths have yet occurred.

Halifax Morning Chronicle, 9 October 1918, 2.

Miss Ethel Kelly, daughter of Mr. Thomas Kelly, passed away at her home in Bridgetown yesterday afternoon, this being the first fatal case of Spanish Influnza [*sic*] in this vicinity.

Bridgetown Monitor, 16 October 1918, 4.

☞ Only 23 years old when she died, Miss Kelly was buried at Gibson's Lake, Dalhousie.

Dr. M. E. Armstrong, medical health officer for the town, reports 100 cases of Spanish Influenza in Bridgetown and vicinity, with only one death. All patients appear to be improving.

Bridgetown Monitor, 16 October 1918, 4.

FREDERICK BEELER. Annapolis, October 21. The first fatal case resulting from Spanish influenza occurred at LeQuille on Sunday night, when Frederick Beeler passed away, aged fifty-three years. He was taken ill on Monday of last week, the attack developing into pneumonia....A widow and nine children survive.

Middleton Outlook, 1 November 1918, 1.

His death record gives his name as James Fred Beeler and appears in Dr. Marble's list as James Beeler. He was born in Princedale, grew up to be a manufacturer, married, and died of "Influenza/Pneumonia" after an illness of one week. A Baptist, he was buried in Annapolis Royal, at Woodlawn Cemetery.

HVS Death Register, Annapolis County, 1918, Book 27, Page 421, Number 1113.

The Influenza in Bridgetown. In an interview with the health officer, Dr. M. E. Armstrong, the MONITOR learns that the influenza in Bridgetown, which has been of a very mild type, compared with other places, is now subsiding in the town, but is quite prevalent in the rural districts. It is thought that the improvement in the town is owing to the prompt closing of the churches, schools, theatres, lodges and other societies, which will remain closed until future notice. Action along this line is now being taken in several of the surrounding villages. Few deaths have occurred.

Bridgetown Monitor, 23 October 1918, 4.

THE INFLUENZA

While there are a number of cases of influenza about town, no fatalites [*sic*] have at this writing been reported within the town limits, and professional nurses consider the disease here as of a mild type. The dwellings with cases have been placarded and the schools, churches and theatres continue closed.

Annapolis Spectator, 24 October 1918, 1.

MRS. HAROLD MASON. At Falkland Ridge, Nov. 4th, 1918, of pneumonia following an attack of influenza, Gertrude [Downey] Mason, aged twenty-four years, wife of Harold Mason. Death comes under sad circumstances, as she leaves a delicate eight months old daughter, to care for whom she left her bed when the family were stricken with the epidemic, contracting a heavy cold which ended fatally in a few days. Mrs. Mason came to this village a young bride three years ago and in her quiet, kindly way took her place in the love of her family and friends and the esteem of the village....The epidemic, and the numbers ill, made the funeral a very quiet one. A short service at the home was given by her pastor, Rev'd Harry Puddington, and the body laid to rest in the little cemetery on the hill.

Middleton Outlook, 15 November 1918, 2.

ROBIE BRUCE [James Robert Bruce]. We regret to record the death of Robie Bruce which took place at his home in [West] Brooklyn on Friday, Oct. 25. The deceased was the only surviving son of Mr. and Mrs. Elias Bruce and was 30 years of age. He had been in poor health for some months, but seemed to be improving when he contracted the influenza from which he was unable to rally.... The bereavement is doubly sad because it follows so closely upon the death of his only brother, Leslie P. Bruce only a few months ago. The funeral took place on Saturday, the 26th and interment was made at Pine Grove Cemetery. The Rev. S. J. Boyce of Lawrencetown conducted the services.

Middleton Outlook, 29 November 1918, 2.

In trying to confirm in whether this Brooklyn was in Annapolis or Queens, the death registers for Annapolis County were searched for Robie Bruce, with no results. Searching for his brother, Leslie P. Bruce, gave no results either (as the search engine had him in there as "Lester P. Bruce"). Searching only by surname, date, and county finally found him. The name on his actual death record was Leslie Parker Bruce, and his particulars matched those in the obituary for his brother. A similar search then found that "Robie" was actually James Robert Bruce, a victim of influenza and pneumonia, with details matching the obituary. This death took place in Annapolis County.

HVS, Annapolis County Death Register, Year 1918, Book 27, Page 387, Number 1040, "Lester P. Bruce"/Leslie Parker Bruce; Book 27, Page 431, Number 1153, "James Robert Bruce."

The influenza situation in Middleton remains about the same there being several cases in the town. Numerous calls for doctor's services are coming from the surrounding country where the epidemic appears to be spreading. The fact that Dr. Messinger and Dr. Kirkpatrick are ill throws a heavy task upon Dr. Miller. Dr. Phinney of Lawrencetown and Dr. DeVine of Kingston are doing extra work to improve the situation.

Middleton Outlook, 25 October 1918, 2.

Mrs. J. B. Jefferson, the first toll of the epidemic in Lawrencetown, passed away Wednesday Oct. 30th. She was only sick a few days and all hoped for her recovery....Mrs. Jefferson was a graduate of Acadia Seminary of '09 and after graduation taught for four years in the School for the Blind, Halifax.

Middleton Outlook, 8 November 1918, 2.

The Influenza Situation is about as a week ago. Dr. Kirkpatrick, the health officer, is able to get out of doors again. Dr. Sponagle rendered valuable assistance in the fight against the epidemic and returned to his duties in Halifax yesterday. The nurse, Miss Bentley, whom he brought from Halifax on Monday, is remaining and is giving valuable assistance....There have been three fatalities. The death of Miss Hannam last week was followed on Sunday by that of Ingram Marshall and on Monday by the death of Mrs. Von [Vaughn] Young.

Middleton Outlook, 8 November 1918, 2.

MRS. VAUGHN YOUNG. The death took place at Middleton last Monday, after an attack of influenza, of Flossie Kathleen, wife of Vaughn Young of that town, and daughter of A.M. King of Annapolis Royal, leaving besides her husband a little boy only three months old.

Middleton Outlook, 15 November 1918, 2.

MRS. HALLETT ALLEN. The death of May, wife of Hallett Allen and daughter of Mr. and Mrs. George Demone, after a two weeks' illness of Spanish influenza followed by pneumonia on Monday evening, was heard with profound sorrow.

Middleton Outlook, 15 November 1918, 2.

INGRAM MARSHALL. The people of Middleton were greatly saddened on Sunday evening 3rd inst. when the word went out that Ingram, only child of Mr. and Mrs. M. P. Marshall of this town had passed away at his home on Commercial St. The deceased, who was only twenty-nine years of age, had been ill about a week with influenza followed by pneumonia. 'Ing' as he was popularly known to his friends, had been intimately identified with the 'boy life' of Middleton for a number of years, taking a great interest in athletics and sports of all kinds. He assisted his father in the boot and shoe business....[L]eaves a wife and three children.

Middleton Outlook, 15 November 1918, 2.

NORMAN WEIR. The death took place at Victoria Beach, on Tuesday, Dec. 3rd, of Norman Weir, age 18 years, son of Mr. and Mrs. Isaiah Weir. Death was caused by influenza.

Digby Courier, 13 December 1918, 2.

IMPORTANT! BOARD OF HEALTH NOTICE
As the Epidemic of Influenza is spreading rapidly in this county, many cases not reporting and some not very ill, are visiting their neighbors and spreading the disease broad cast. I hereby give notice that no public gatherings, which include church meetings, schools, lodge and society meetings are allowed in the County and no visiting from house to house that is not absolutely necessary and no social

house gathering to be held until this serious state of affairs is past, for these house gatherings are now very much to be dreaded. Every case of even a slight cold is considered this same infection and the next case may be very severe. No other form of grippe is now prevalent, that is, every case of grippe must consider themselves under quarantine until five days after all symptoms subside....W.H. Phinney, M.H.O. [Medical Health Officer] / Municipality of Anna. Co. Lawrencetown, Nov. 5, 1918.

Bridgetown Monitor, 6 November 1918, 4.

 IMPORTANT SCHOOL NOTICE
At a meeting of the Council of Public Instruction held December 18, it was ordered that Prov. Aid be paid to all teachers employed in the public schools for the time school was closed by Board of Health on account of the epidemic Influenza, altho the time should exceed the four weeks allowed by Regulations 131. Many schools having been closed for more than 20 days were intending to keep open during a part of the Xmas Holidays. They still have this priviledge. Trustees must pay the salary of the teacher for the entire period the school was closed by order of the Board. M.C. Fosster, Inspector of Schools. Bridgetown N.S., Dec. 23, 1918.

Bridgetown Monitor, 25 Dec. 1918, 4.

 At No. Williamston, Dec. 20, 1918, Ruby, wife of George Merriot [Marriott], aged 26 years.

Annapolis Outlook, 10 January 1919, 3.

☞ Ruby Banks Marriott died of the Great Influenza on December 20, 1918, in North Williamston, Annapolis County, NS. She was buried in Nictaux, probably at the Nictaux Community Cemetery, because the bulk of her family lies there. North Williamston, as a community of people, has since disappeared, leaving only a road of the same name. Ruby was the wife of George Marriott, a stone cutter. Three years after the death of his first Banks wife, George married Ruby's widowed sister, Idella Blanche Banks Martin. He moved in with her and her children at her late husband's house in Melvern Square, a community just up the road from North Williamston, perhaps one of many reasons North Williamson emptied out.

 DEATH OF WILLIAM E. BENT
A Prominent Resident of Belle Isle Has Passed Away
The community of Belle Isle and surrounding districts was profoundly shocked and grieved, on the morning of Feby. 28th, when word was passed around that at an early hour of that day, William E. Bent had passed away. Stricken with that dread disease Influenza, some ten days before, Mr. Bent put up a brave struggle for life against this malignant foe. But in spite of all the physcans [*sic*] skill, tender

nursing and kind friends could do, pneumonia developed, and on the morning of the forty-first anniversary of his birth, his soul passed out into the spirit world.... Deprived of a Father's care and protection at the early age of fourteen, he assumed the entire inanagement [management] of the homestead farm on which he spent his whole life, with marked success. He is survived by a sorrowing widow who lies critically ill at the present time, of the same disease, and five small children.

Bridgetown Monitor, 5 March 1919, 1.

Death of Dorothy Bent. The community of Belleisle was saddened early Ash-Wednesday morning, March 5th, when they learned of the 'passing on' of little Dorothy LaVaughan, second child of Mr. and Mrs. Henri H. Bent, at the early age of eleven years, and three months. The little one was stricken with influenza on Feb. 18th, which developed into pneumonia.

Bridgetown Monitor, 19 March 1919, 4.

Annapolis County had twenty-five deaths from flu in 1918, twenty-five in 1919, but only five in 1920. Charles Messenger, aged 72, had been a farmer all his life. He was born, lived, and died at Tupperville. His daughter Ann M. Messenger gave her father's parents as Sarah A. and Major [first name, not title] Messenger, and said that he had died at 3:00 A.M. the morning of May 3. Dr. A. A. Dechman of Bridgetown signed the death certificate, having treated this patient from May 1st to 3rd. The cause of death had been "La Grippe," complicated by five years of vascular heart disease. Dechman did the paperwork and sent the certificate on May 4 to the District Registrar, Ethel B. Davies, who entered it in the registration book the same day. The body of Charles Messenger was buried that day also, as required with influenza victims. His was the last recorded death from the Great Influenza in Annapolis County.

HVS, Death Register, Annapolis County, 1920, Book 52, Page 188.

ANNAPOLIS COUNTY, VITAL STATISTICS, DEATH REGISTRY, BOOKS 27, 52:

1918

1. Margaret Cole, d. 31 August 1918, in Maitland [*Bridge*], Annapolis County. [*This woman does not appear in Dr. Marble's list of Annapolis County dead; she is not in the Death Register for Annapolis County, 1918. Marble records her in his Queens County list, as that register is where he found her. I am assuming that by "Maitland, Annapolis County," the registrar meant Maitland Bridge, as "Maitland" proper is in Hants County. Since the entry in the Queens County register clearly states that she lived and died and was buried in "Maitland" [Maitland Bridge], Annapolis County, it may be a clerical error that put her in the wrong register. She has been added here to reflect an accurate death count for the county.*]

2. Edward Moses, 17, d. 17 October 1918, Lequille, labourer.

3. Charles Hamm, 17, d. 18 October 1918, Lequille, farmer.

4. James Beeler, 53, d. 20 October 1918, Lequille, manufacturer.

5. Donald Lohnes, 8, d. 2 November 1918, South Milford.

6. Winnie Oickle, 25, d. 14 November 1918, Victory, housewife.

7. Fred Hewey, 27, d. 19 November 1918, Victory, farmer.

8. Eva L. McCaul, 32, d. 28 November 1918, Delap's Cove.

9. Norman Wear, 17, d. 3 December 1918, Victoria Beach, fisherman.

10. Helen Lowe, 23, d. 19 October 1918, Bridgetown.

11. Charlotte Emery, 92, d. 14 November 1918, Bridgetown.

12. Augusta Tyler, 38, d. 31 December 1918, Inglewood.

13. Ethel Keddy, 23, d. 15 October 1918, Bridgetown.

14. James F. Bruce, 31, d. 25 October 1918, West Brooklyn, farmer.

15. Mary M. Jefferson, 28, d. 30 October 1918, Lawrencetown, housewife.

16. Aubrey Scott Sawler, 29, d. 12 November 1918, New Albany, carpenter.

17. Etta Hannam, 24, d. 19 October 1918, Middleton.

18. Ingram Marshall, 29, d. 3 November 1918, Middleton, clerk.

19. Kathleen Young, 28, d. 4 November 1918, Middleton.

[*Below this entry, Dr. Marble's numbering skips to 20, but this has been corrected here; Dr. Marble eventually corrected his number of deaths at the end of the 1919 entries here.*]

20. Dolly Mosher, 35, d. 11 November 1918, Middleton.

21. Annie DeAdder, 18, d. 22 December 1918, Middleton.

22. Helen Lightfoot, 5, d. 28 October 1918, Prince Albert.

23. Adelia Cropley, 62, d. 9 November 1918, Nictaux.

24. James Parks, 82, d. 22 December 1918, Port George, bridge builder.

25. Ruby Marriott, 27, d. 20 December 1918, North Williamston.

1919

26. George Bailey, 4, d. 30 January 1919, Round Hill.

27. Fred Cress, 40, d. 2 February 1919, Round Hill, farmer.

28. Rita Dunn, 3 weeks, d. 18 February 1919, Upper Clements.

29. Alma Rice, 12, d. 31 March 1919, Lake La Rose.

30. Harvey Oickle, 25, d. 11 February 1919, Greenland, farmer.

31. Dora Hill, 14, d. 20 February 1919, Bear River.

32. Ruth Oickle, 4 months, d. 26 February 1919, Greenland.

33. Charles Robinson, 27, d. 23 January 1919, Bridgetown, labourer.

34. George Robinson, 64, d. 28 January 1919, Bridgetown, labourer.

35. Harry Hicks, 56, d. 23 March 1919, Bridgetown, farmer.

36. David Taylor, 32, d. 11 January 1919, Bridgetown, farmer.

37. William Bent, 41, d. 27 February 1919, Belleisle, farmer.

38. Joseph De Vany, 35, d. 28 February 1919, Centerlea [sic], farmer.

39. Walter Waterman, 7, d. 13 January 1919, Middleton.

40. William Taylor, 47, d. 26 January 1919, Middleton, foreman printer.

41. Leveret Keddie, 37, d. 28 January 1919, Middleton, cooper.

42. Alonzo Durling, 19, d. 10 January 1919, Nictaux South, farmer.

43. John Hartley, 89, d. 13 January 1919, Middleton, farmer.

44. Percy Morse, 37, d. 25 March 1919, Bloomington, farmer.

45. Ralph Troop, 32, d. 13 May 1919, Granville Ferry, farmer.

46. James McLaughlin, 27, d. 15 January 1919, Bridgetown, larrigan maker.

47. Joseph Marshall, 16, d. 11 December 1918, Hampton. [This young man has a death record dated 11 December 1918, even though it is recorded in the death register for Annapolis County, Year 1919, Book 27, Page 475, Number 1293. This is most likely because the local registrar for Hampton sent this return, dated December 1918, in late.]

48. Howard Vidito, 4, d. 1 April 1919, Torbrook.

49. Alfred Cunningham, 2, d. 6 May 1919, Torbrook.

50. Elizabeth Spurr, 71, d. 9 April 1919, Melvern Square, housewife.

51. Jessie Hamilton, 31, d. 30 April 1919, Wilmot, housewife. [In the margin, Dr. Marble, correcting himself, has written that this record is Number "50 / no # 19."]

[Emily M. Johnson, 12, d. 5 March 1920, Halifax, Victoria General Hospital, student. Neither Annapolis nor Halifax have a death record shown for her in the HVS database. Dr. Marble found her in the Annapolis death records, original ledger. Likely her home was in Annapolis County, but she died in the VG Hospital, Halifax. She may even have two death records, the second being in the Halifax original ledger. Since she died in Halifax, her entry has been transferred to that county.]

1920

52. Frances FitzRandoph, 31, d. 23 March 1920, South Williamston.

53. Mildred E. Messenger, 24, d. 6 March 1920, Middleton.

54. Russell Parker, 2, d. 6 March 1920, Bloomington.

55. Clifford Buckler, 20, d. 15 April 1920, Greenland, farmer.

56. Charles Messenger, 72, d. 3 May 1920, Tupperville, farmer.

Chapter III

ANTIGONISH COUNTY

ANTIGONISH COUNTY HAD only twenty confirmed deaths from the Great Influenza. The medical officer for the district reported in January 1919 that, relatively speaking, they had gotten off lightly compared to other parts of the province. Below are also some of the deaths that occurred *outside* the province, of Antigonish County natives—deaths that aren't on the county registration list, of course, but which appear in newspaper reports. These were gathered from the Antigonish Cenotaph Project, affiliated with the Antigonish Heritage Museum, whose goal is to research and preserve stories of First World War soldiers, and they were entered on the one hundredth anniversary of their death date. Current and previous stories are available online at antigonishcenotaphproject.wordpress.com. Extracts of those who died of influenza follow.

August 19, 1918: Private Francis 'Frank' Bouchie* / Posted August 19, 2018. Francis 'Frank' Bouchie was born at East Havre Boucher, the son of Maurice and Susan (Briand) Bouchie. Susan was Maurice's second wife....He remarried around 1887. Susan was the daughter of Joseph Briand and Osite 'Elizabeth' Coste (Decoste). Joseph, a fisherman by occupation, was born at Cape Jack, the son of Louis-François Briand, a fisherman from Isle De Miquelon, a French territory.

Frank's father, Maurice, was the son of Simon and Olivie (Pettipas) Bouchie, both of whom were East Havre Boucher natives. His grandfather, Paul Bouchie, was born at Arichat, the son of Honoré 'dit Villedieu' Bouchie, an Acadian refugee from the Grand Pré area of Nova Scotia. The Bouchie family resided on a family farm near Bennett Road, then known as Paint Road.

On May 4, 1918, Frank attested with 1st Depot Battalion, Nova Scotia Regiment, the training unit for Nova Scotian conscripts, and was assigned to Company 'D.' He spent three months completing basic training at Camp Aldershot and by late July was ready to depart for England, where he would join the 17th Reserve Battalion, the unit that provided reinforcements for the 25th and 85th Battalions, Nova Scotia's two front-line units.

On August 2, 1918, Frank departed Halifax aboard the transport *Ixion*. The crowded conditions on board provided ideal conditions for the spread of contagious disease, and a significant number of the soldiers contracted influenza and pneumonia during the vessel's two-week passage. When the ship docked at Liverpool, England, on August 15, 1918, a total of 22 soldiers were admitted to hospitals for medical treatment.

While officially taken on strength by the 17th Battalion upon arriving overseas, Frank never reported for duty. He was among the soldiers who fell sick during the voyage and was immediately transported to the Toxteth Park Auxiliary Hospital, Liverpool, for treatment of influenza and pneumonia. At the time of his admission, notes in Frank's service file indicate that he had a 'high temperature,' with 'moderately extensive pneumonic involvement of [the] lungs.' While staff administered several medications and therapies over subsequent days, Frank's condition failed to improve. He died of pneumonia at 1:20 a.m. August 19, 1918.

Private Frank Bouchie was laid to rest in Kirkdale Cemetery, Liverpool, England. He was not the only *Ixion* passenger who passed away only days after arriving overseas. Of the 22 soldiers admitted to hospital, four other young Nova Scotian conscripts died before month's end —Private Charles Abner Barss, New Harbour, Guysborough County; Private Warren L. Godfried, Little Harbour, Shelburne County; Private Pearley Parker Goucher, Albany Cross, Annapolis County.

*The 1911 Canadian census, Frank's military service file and the signature on his attestation papers spell his surname as 'Bouchie.' The 1901 census recorded the family name as 'Bouché.' Common usage today is 'Boucher.' Date of birth [December 27, 1894] obtained from 1901 census. Frank's attestation papers list his birthday as December 27, 1897.

The Antigonish Cenotaph Project Committee.

 At the Military Hospital, Newport News, Va., Oct. 20, Private Moses Everett Delorey, aged 32 years, son of Mary E. and the late Moses Delorey of Tracadie.

Antigonish Casket, 20 October 1918. Courtesy of the
Antigonish Heritage Museum.

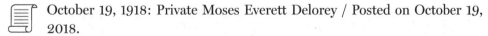 October 19, 1918: Private Moses Everett Delorey / Posted on October 19, 2018.

Moses Everett Delorey was born at Tracadie, Antigonish County, on November 2, 1885, the third of Moses and Mary Elizabeth (Delorey) Delorey's seven children and the couple's second son. The family operated a farm on or near the Merland Road, in an area sometimes called Rear Tracadie before it became known as Merland.

Around 1904, three of Moses and Ann Delorey's children—James Arthur, Annie and Ellen—departed Nova Scotia for the 'Boston States.' In January 1912, Everett— as he was known to family—joined his siblings in Brookline, MA, where he found work as a 'chauffeur.'

The United States entered the First World War in early April 1917 and immediately set about organizing the American Expeditionary Force. Everett enlisted for overseas service on August 13, 1918, and was sent to Camp Johnston, near Jacksonville, Florida, for training.

....Everett's time in uniform was brief. Military camps were breeding grounds for contagious diseases, such as measles, mumps and influenza. Everett's unit was preparing for its overseas departure when he was admitted to the Embarkation Military Hospital at Newport News, Virginia, on October 13, suffering from influenza. His illness quickly progressed to broncho-pneumonia and resulted in Everett's death at 4:19 p.m. October 19, 1918. His brother, James Arthur, accompanied Everett's remains to Brookline, where a Funeral Mass was held at St. Adrian's Catholic Church. Private Moses Everett Delorey was laid to rest in St. Joseph's Cemetery, West Roxbury, MA.

The Antigonish Cenotaph Project Committee.

October 21, 1918: Gunner Hugh John Boyd / Posted October 21, 2018.

Hugh John Boyd was born April 29, 1887, at 'Boyd Settlement,' Fraser's Mills, Antigonish County, the eighth of 13 children. His mother Ann, daughter of Alan and Janet (McIsaac) McDonald of Glen Road, Antigonish County, died at age 46 when Hugh John was only 11 years old, while his father, Angus J., passed away in 1909. The 1911 Canadian census lists Hugh John as the head of the Fraser's Mills household. Living with him at that time were his brothers James Hugh, Joseph Angus and Daniel, and sisters Margaret and Marcella. Their maternal grandmother, Janet MacDonald, age 82, also resided with the Boyd siblings.

About 1915, Hugh John left the Boyd's Settlement homestead and ventured all the way to Valdez City, Alaska, where he worked as a miner in the Midas Copper mine at nearby Solomon Gulch, along the port's south shore. The mine was the fourth largest copper producer in the Prince William Sound area.

Several years after Hugh John's arrival, however, the United States' entrance into the war in early April 1917 impacted thousands of young men. A race against time ensued, as the American Army consisted of only 25,000 regulars at the time and thousands more were required to fight in France. Following the American Congress' approval of a compulsory military draft, Hugh John completed the required registration papers at Granby, Alaska, on August 14, 1917. At the time, he was working at the Midas Copper Mine, where he was employed by the Granby Construction Company as a 'powderman.'

Based on information contained in a contemporary news item, Hugh John appears to have been called up in late September or early October 1918. Shortly afterward, he was sent to the National Army Training Camp at American Lake, near Tacoma, Washington State. The facility, later re-named Camp Lewis, was the first National Army cantonment for draftee training opened in the US during World War One. The first recruits arrived there on September 5, 1917, and 37,000 officers, cadre, garrison and trainees were on post by year's end. Camp Lewis was the largest military camp in the country at that time. Many men from the western states were processed, equipped and trained there during its operation. Hugh John Boyd was among the soldiers undergoing training in trench warfare at Camp Lewis in early autumn 1918. In mid-October, he fell ill and was admitted to the U.S. Army Base Hospital, where he died at 7:30 p.m. October 21, 1918. His death certificate identified the cause of death as broncho-pneumonia.

Hugh John's obituary in the *Antigonish Casket* stated:

"At Camp Lewis, Washington, on October 21 after a short illness of pneumonia, Gunner Hugh J. Boyd died. The deceased, who was the son of A. J. Boyd, Fraser's Mills, Ant., enlisted in Alaska a few weeks previous. His remains, accompanied by his cousin, Pte. J. A. Boyd, were brought to his native home and buried in the family lot at South River Cemetery. Four sisters and three brothers, two overseas, survive to mourn their loss."

The Antigonish Cenotaph Project Committee.

At Halifax, in the 26th year of her age, Mary McDonald, youngest daughter of Mr. and Mrs. Duncan J. McDonald of Cape George Point.

Antigonish Casket, 29 October 1918. Courtesy of the Antigonish Heritage Museum.

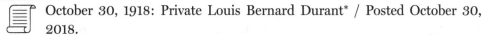

October 30, 1918: Private Louis Bernard Durant* / Posted October 30, 2018.

Louis Bernard's mother, Saraphine 'Sarah,' was a daughter of Costain and Irene (Landry) Duon; his father was John B. Durant. In 1901, John and Sarah were living at Pomquet, NS. Five children—three sons and two daughters—also resided in the household, Louis Bernard being their youngest child. Sometime after 1911, Louis' older brother, Levi, emigrated to Boston, MA. In May 1918, 19-year-old Louis joined him and found work as a carpenter.

While he was a British subject by birth, Louis filed for American citizenship on August 8, 1918. As required of all men his age at the time, he also registered for the US military draft on September 12, 1918. Rather than serve with the American Expeditionary Force, however, Louis chose to enlist with the Canadian Expeditionary Force at Boston, MA, on the same day. He immediately travelled by train to Nova Scotia and by September 18 had arrived at Camp Aldershot, near Kentville, for training,

Within days of his arrival, health concerns interrupted Louis's training. Initially hospitalized at Camp Aldershot...he was transferred to Military Hospital, Halifax, on October 4 for treatment of psoriasis and admitted to a medical facility at Pine Hill three days later. While under medical care, Louis contracted influenza—specifically, the highly contagious 'Spanish flu' that was spreading across the province at the time—and was admitted to Rockhead Military Hospital on October 23. Private Louis Bernard Durant failed to recover, passing away at 10:35 a.m. October 30, 1918. His remains were returned to Pomquet and laid to rest in St. Croix Parish Cemetery.

Louis was one month shy of his twentieth birthday at the time of his death.

*The surname Durant' is a phonetic rendition of the name Doiron'. Louis' family name was recorded as "Dorant' on his attestation papers and all other documents in his service file.

The Antigonish Cenotaph Project Committee.

 Durant was one of many who became infected by this influenza while in hospital for something else. Meanwhile, back in Antigonish County, the Medical Health Officer, Dr. Cameron, was being deluged by complaints from people who did not want their businesses closed down, or their churches, or their social lives abridged. He smote them with the rod of righteous indignation, as one sees in the following newspaper article:

INFLUENZA SITUATION
(By Dr. Cameron, Health Officer)

In this as in every other community there are persons of high and low rank who make it their business to suppress the fact that there is any infectious or contagious disease in their family, supposedly to save the inconvenience of quarantine—a perfectly selfish and inhuman attitude. Or, again, the ignorant may think it a disgrace—a reflection on their lack of cleanliness, or even on their ascendents [ancestors]. Such notions are not well-founded. Infectious or contagious disease is no respector [sic] of persons, and that being the case, any person who has the faintest suspicion that he has a case in his household should at once consult his family physician and report his findings to the Health Officer.... In addition to the duty of notification it is also the duty of each person whose case is diagnosed 'Influenza' to remain in quarantine until such times as the doctor in attendance, or the Health Officer, gives him permission to mix up [sic]....

Now, this influenza is a most complex and difficult disease to investigate....I am, however, offering this on the side, as a measure of self-defense, as many people blame the Health Officer for the spread of this disease...we have many cases of Influenza and the Health Officer is to blame. Why, I had an anonymous letter the other day from one of the Antigonish Cardinals outlining my duties, and accusing me of being in league with his satanic majesty because, forsooth, I had closed the churches. Needless to say that this pin-head bigot in her (his) six pages of instruction and diatribe is unworthy of notice.

Antigonish Casket, 31 October 1918. Courtesy of the Antigonish Heritage Museum.

 Antigonish and Pictou health officers did not seem at all reluctant to say in print exactly what they were thinking.

At Linwood, on Nov. 12, 1918, Annie, beloved wife of Benjamin Mattie, at the age of 31 years, passed peacefully to her eternal reward. Death was due to pneumonia, following an attack of Spanish influenza. The sympathy of the community goes out to the bereaved husband and seven little children.

Antigonish Casket, 12 November 1918. Courtesy of the Antigonish Heritage Museum.

At Havre Bouche [*sic*], on Nov. 23rd, Clarence Anderson, at the early age of 20 years. Death was due to pneumonia, following influenza. Deceased always led a good, kind, and industrious life, which merited for him a most edifying death.

Antigonish Casket, 23 November 1918. Courtesy of the Antigonish Heritage Museum.

At West Arm, Tracadie, on the 29th NOV after a brief illness from Spanish influenza, followed by pneumonia, William, son of Hubert Myette.

Antigonish Casket, 29 November 1918. Courtesy of the Antigonish Heritage Museum.

FATHER AND MOTHER DIE

Mr. Joseph Pettipas of Tracadie passed away two weeks ago. He had an attack of influenza which developed into pneumonia. On Monday of this week Mrs. Pettipas succumbed to the same disease. They leave three small children.

Antigonish Casket, 12 December 1918. Courtesy of the Antigonish Heritage Museum.

Influenza continues more or less epidemic. It is the occasion still of numerous deaths and of widespread sickness. Relaxing efforts to stamp out the disease seemingly is causing renewed outbreaks. Communities in which the trouble was supposed to be overcome, have had second and severe visitations of the scourge....In the outside districts of the County a more severe type of the disease is prevalent, at least in a number of districts. Five deaths occurred in Tracadie from the flu and many were sick. Happily, the epidemic has now passed from there, only a few people being still affected. Heatherton, Frasers Grant and adjoining communities are at present affected, the disease having developed in that portion of our County recently, and has assumed epidemic proportions.

Antigonish Casket, 19 December 1918. Courtesy of the Antigonish Heritage Museum.

THE FLU IN ANTIGONISH

Influenza continues more or less epidemic. It is the occasion still of numerous deaths and of widespread sickness. Relaxing effort to stamp out the disease seemingly is causing renewed outbreaks. Communities in which the trouble was supposed to be overcome, have had second and severe visitations of the source…. Promiscuous visiting during the holidays, they say, will be a means of continuing and of creating a recurrence of the epidemic, and they urge upon people generally the advisability of discouraging this custom just now….Five deaths occurred in Tracadie from the flu and many were sick. Happily the epidemic has now passed from there, only a few people being still affected. Heatherton, Frasers Grant and adjoining community are at present affected, the disease having developed.

Pictou Advocate, 20 December 1918, 5. Reprinted from the *Antigonish Casket.*

At Fraser's Grant, Ant. Co., on Dec. 24th, 1918, after a brief illness of pneumonia, Florence MacPhail, aged 33 years. Strengthened by the last Sacraments she passed peacefully to her reward, leaving three sisters and two brothers to mourn the loss of a faithful and affectionate sister.

Antigonish Casket, 24 December 1918. Courtesy of the Antigonish Heritage Museum.

The flu situation shows no improvement….The only means of guarding against the spread of the disease is for the general public to exercise precaution. In our own County people are extremely careless in regard to the disease. Patients recovering from the flu mix unconcernedly with the general public, in church and in other places of public assemblage. Though the disease has been epidemic along the I. C. Railway communities from Tracadie to Town and is spreading at Heatherton and adjoining districts, the one passenger car on the morning freight from these points is daily crowded to capacity. Among the crowd are noticed persons just recovering from the disease and persons in whose homes the disease is.

A gentleman from one of those districts, who is in a position to know conditions, says it was possible to anticipate in what house the disease was next to break out, just because of the carelessness of people in visiting and loitering around houses having the disease. Heatherton is particularly troubled just now with the flue visitation. A few have recently died there from the disease and many others are sick. In one house at Heatherton all the inmates, five in number, are down with pneumonia. We urge people to exercise greater care in guarding against the spread of the disease.

Antigonish Casket, 26 December 1918. Courtesy of the
Antigonish Heritage Museum.

THE 'FLU' IN ANTIGONISH

The influenza epidemic is not a thing of the past by any means. In fact, leading physicians of America say it will recur in 1919, and possibly in 1920. In support of this view, they claim that on the occasions of past visitations, influenza recurred in the year following the first outbreak. A few weeks back there was decided improvement in the "flu" situation in Nova Scotia. Encouraged by this improvement Health authorities relaxed regulations to control disease, and permitted public assemblage. As a consequence, many communities have had renewed epidemics. In New Glasgow there was serious spread of the disease following the lifting of the ban on public meetings, Sydney Mines has had to reclose public places and forbid meetings of upwards of ten people. Halifax also had many new cases after the regulations were withdrawn. In our own County the situation has grown worse. Three deaths from flu occurred at Tracadie last week and many are ill there with the disease. One family of nine members were all sick. One of the number died and another has pneumonia. At Harbor Bouche, the schools have been closed.

Pictou Advocate, 6 December 1918, p. 4; reprinted from the *Antigonish Casket.*

On January 1, 1919, of Spanish influenza, followed by pneumonia. Christie Ann, daughter of the late William MacPhail of Fraser's Grant, Ant., at the age of thirty-six....The deceased had been in the United States for the past number of years. Five weeks ago, she was summoned home to take care of her near relatives, who were suffering from the epidemic of influenza. Shortly after her arrival home, she herself contracted the disease, and after a few days illness she passed away. ....[T]he remains were interred at Heatherton beside those of her sister [Florence] who preceded her the week before.

Antigonish Casket, 1 January 1919. Courtesy of the Antigonish Heritage Museum.

To the Wardens and Councillors of the Municipality of the County of
Antigonish

Gentlemen—I have the honour to submit to you my second annual report
as Medical Health Officer of the County, and so far as I could ascertain,
conditions were as follows:

During the year Diphtheria broke out in one section of the County, namely,
Pleasant Valley. Five cases were treated and quarantine measures confined
the disease to that locality alone.

Three cases of Small Pox broke out at Arisaig and one at William's Point.
The houses in both places were promptly quarantined and later on fumigated. No outbreak followed.

The County was peculiarly free from Typhoid Fever, no cases having been
reported for the year.

A few cases of Measles were reported from different sections of the County,
but in no instance were there any of serious nature.

Complaint was lodged against the pollution of a stream at Glen Roy. I
investigated the matter and so far as I could ascertain some person or persons deposited a dead horse and a dead cow on the banks of that river,
thereby endangering the health of those using the water farther down
stream. There is a more sanitary way of disposing of dead animals than
that adopted in the above case. It would be to the public interest that car-
cases should be either burned or buried in a suitable place, and that any
one who disposes of dead bodies of animal as was done in the case complained of should be dealt with according to law.

So far as Tuberculosis is concerned, I have only to repeat what I said in my
last report; in every house where the inhabitants know Tuberculosis exists,
they are anxious to take all precautions to prevent the spread of the disease.

The influenza situation in the County was quite serious for a while. Schools
and churches had to be closed. Pomquet, Tracadie, Harbor-au-Bouche,
Fraser's Grant and Heatherton suffered the most, resulting complications
were the cause of a number of deaths. It may be said, however, that relatively to other places in which the disease has raged, the County has fared
off [*sic*] fairly well.

I have to thank the Warden, Chairmen and Members of Local Boards of Health as well as the Clergymen of the County for their prompt assistance in checking the spread of the influenza epidemic.

L. MCPHERSON, Medical Health Officer.

Report of Medical Health Officer, Proceedings of the Municipal Council, Casket Print, Antigonish, N. S., January Sessions, 1919: 22. Thanks to Jocelyn Gillis, Antigonish Heritage Museum, for finding the reference.

The Influenza has not given serious trouble in this County since a month. But few cases were lately reported, and hopes were expressed that the disease had been overcome here. These hopes are too sanguine, and should not be entertained. Cases of "flu" are still fairly common, and this week five cases of flu and pneumonia developed in Town.

Antigonish Casket, 13 February 1919. Courtesy of the Antigonish Heritage Museum.

A recurrence of the influenza epidemic is taking place in this Town and County. In the Town at least, the recent visitation is more serious than was the first....Harbour au Bouche [*sic*], Linwood, Maryvale and the Ohio are the districts most severely afflicted. Twenty-four new cases were reported last Saturday at Havre Boucher [note different spellings] and Linwood. At Marydale [Maryvale] and the Ohio district, the patients have a bad type of the disease.

Antigonish Casket, 27 February 1919. Courtesy of the Antigonish Heritage Museum.

Influenza has paid a second visit to Tracadie, Antigonish. Two weeks ago all the workmen at a lumber camp were taken sick. Thirty men comprised the camp, which was operated by Mr. Haggerty of Mulgrave, and was in charge of Mr. George Cameron of Melrose, Guysborough Co. The workmen were also from Guysborough County districts—East River, St. Mary's, Melrose and vicinity. Herbert Maclachlan [*sic*], one of the workmen, developed pneumonia. He was conveyed to Antigonish for treatment. Owing to the Hospital being overcrowded, other accommodation was found, a vacant office. Two nurses attended him, and every attention was given him, still he passed away on Wednesday evening, a few minutes before his wife reached his bedside. Besides his wife, he leaves five children. As the men recovered strength, they returned to their several homes, so the camp is now practically deserted.

Antigonish Casket, 27 March 1919. Courtesy of the Antigonish Heritage Museum.

With only twenty deaths from pandemic influenza in three years, Antigonish was certainly one of the more fortunate counties in the province. Nevertheless, it had its share of tragedies. Many of its families suffered losses of kin, dying from influenza elsewhere. The roll-call of the Antigonish dead may also include a number of Catholic nuns who died during that time period. Jocelyn Gillis has not been able to find death records for these women, only the names and dates on their tombstones. She wrote, "Was in the cemetery and discovered a series of grave markers of CND nuns who died (cause unknown?) They fit the time period for Spanish Flu. Checked vital statistics and no deaths were recorded for these women." We think that perhaps some of them succumbed to the Great Influenza.

Jocelyn Gillis, Antigonish Heritage Museum, to Ruth Whitehead,
email, 23 June 2018.

ANTIGONISH COUNTY, VITAL STATISTICS, DEATH REGISTER, BOOKS 26, 54

1918

1. Joseph Petipas, 24, d. 30 November 1918, railway man, Tracadie. [*Book 26, Page 487, Number 1006, says he was a railroad brakeman who was born, lived and was buried in Tracadie; a Roman Catholic, his interment was at St. Ninian's. His wife (see below) sent in the return of death to the registry, ten days before she herself succumbed to the influenza.*]

2. Mrs. Joseph Petipas, 24, d. 10 December 1918, Tracadie. [*The widow of Joseph Petipas, above.*]

3. Roderick McDonald, 30, d. 19 October 1918, Point Tupper, engineer.

[*J. Herbert McDonald, d. in October 1918, Sudbury, ON. There is nothing in the HVS Antigonish Death Register for him. His name is therefore eliminated from this list, as he did not die in this province.*]

[*Mary Dolan, 27, d. 16 October 1918, Boston. See above note. No HVS death record in any NS county register.*]

[*Harriet Broadfoot, 24, d. 27 November 1918, lived in Halifax. See note to Number 3, above. No record in any NS county.*]

4. Mrs. Addie MacKinnon, 26, d. 11 September 1918, South River Road, housewife.

5. Valentine Chisholm, 36, d. 4 November 1918, St. Andrews, farmer.

6. Fred MacRae, 30, d. 22 November 1918, St. Joseph's [*sic*], farmer.

7. Edward Breen, 54, d. 31 October 1918, Cape Jack, farmer.

8. Aloysus Webb, 27, d. 17 November 1918, Harbour Bouche [*sic*], merchant. [*The original death record spells his first name "Aloysus" rather than the usual "Aloysius"; Book 26, Page 509, Number 1061.*]

9. Clarence Anderson, 20, d. 23 November 1918, Harbour Bouchee [*sic*], farmer.

10. John W. MacDonald, 2 days old, d. 23 December 1918, Heatherton.

1919

11. Herbert McLauchlin, 33, d. 19 March 1919, Lochaber, farmer.

12. Moses Somers, 28, d. 18 February, 1919, Briley Brook, farmer.

13. Veronica McPherson, 1 year 4 months, d. 23 February 1919, Williams Point.

14. Margaret McDonald, 9, d. 5 March 1919, Maryvale.

15. Alexander W. MacDonald, 16, d. 1 February 1919, St. Joseph's [*sic*].

16. Alfred Landry, 27, d. 17 February 1919, Tracadie, farmer.

17. Florence McPhail, 31, d. 24 December 1918, Heatherton, housework.

18. Annie McPhail, 36, d. 1 January 1919, Heatherton, housework.

1920

19. Kate McDonald, 35, d. 17 March 1920, Addington Forks, housewife.

20. John Rogers, 17, d. 18 May 1920, North Grant, farmer.

Chapter IV

CAPE BRETON COUNTY

CAPE BRETON COUNTY had 376 confirmed deaths from the Great Influenza of 1918–20.

LITTLE SPANISH INFLUENZA HERE
The number of cases of Spanish influenza in the city is very small. Dr. J. F. MacAuley, city medical officer, told The Record this afternoon that in some of the neighbouring districts, it was learned, elsewhere, the number of cases is large.

At New Waterford there are reported to have been some 1,200 cases in the past few weeks, and not all the doctors escaped the disease. Happily, however, no deaths resulted among the large number of cases in Inverness county, it is reported there were several deaths but among people of advanced years whose natural weakness prevented them from resisting the disease.

Sydney Record, 24 September 1918, 2.

The claim that the number of cases of is very small seems unbelievable, when one considers that another account, published *the day before* in a different Sydney newspaper, reports five hundred cases of influenza had arrived September 22, two days before this article, all from the same troopship on its way to Europe!

FIVE HUNDRED U.S. SOLDIERS IN PORT
Landed on Sunday, Most of them Suffering from Spanish Influenza. About five hundred American soldiers arrived at an Atlantic port [Sydney] yesterday [September 22] suffering from Spanish Influenza, and were removed to hospitals ashore for treatment. The curling rinks, and some of the church halls were commandeered by the military authorities and turned into emergency hospitals, with nurses taken from anywhere about the place. The worst cases have been taken to one of the military hospitals. It is understood that the first aid and the home nursing class graduates will offer for service at the hospitals, and will assist with the care of the men. The chief difficulty was to get beds for the cases and all day the authorities were busy with the work of procuring and preparing beds for the sick to sleep in tonight. The men will remain for several weeks.

Sydney Daily Post, 23 September 1918, 1.

☞ The port was not named, due to it being wartime, but following articles make it obvious that it was Sydney.

 RED CROSS ACTIVITIES FOR AMERICAN SOLDIERS
Delicacies for the Men in Hospital / Ladies Appointed at Yesterday's Emergency Meeting

Soups, ice-creams, fruits and jellies will be a few of the delicacies temptingly offered the United States soldiers who are now quartered in hospitals and billeted here, according to the ruling and request of the local branch of the Red Cross at an emergency meeting of the Red Cross yesterday. It is in answer to the question, "What can we do?"....All articles listed are but tid-bits to nearly every citizen in Canada, but to the soldier or sailor in quarantine they are luxuries, it was pointed out. The men are unable to leave their quarters and purchase them even though they had the money. The ladies therefore decided that they would fetch the tid-bit luxuries to the men ....[*at Moxham Hospital, Rose Hospital, St. Andrews Church, the Falmouth Street church, and the curling rink.*]

Sydney Daily Post, 26 September 1918, 1.

 GRIP EPIDEMIC AT WATERFORD
Two Deaths Reported. Notes from Mining Town

(Special Correspondence) NEW WATERFORD, Sept. 26. The prevalence of influenza here has assumed a more serious aspect, due to the sudden death of two people within a very short period. On Monday, the death occurred of Miss May Fraser of Pleasant Bay, who had arrived in town but a few days previous. On Wednesday morning, George Wareham, an employee of No. 14 colliery, also passed away after an illness of but a few days....Archie McQueen and W.C. Smith, of the official staff No. 15 colliery, are on the sick list, both suffering from influenza.

Sydney Daily Post, 27 September 1918, 5.

 DEATH OF AMERICAN SOLDIER
Private Smith Dies at Moxham Hospital from Grip

The first death among the American soldiers here occurred yesterday morning when Corporal [*sic*] James T. Smith, who had been suffering from Spanish influenza and was being treated at the Moxham hospital, died yesterday morning at ten o'clock....The flag at the curling rink was lowered to the half staff as soon as the casualty was reported.

Sydney Daily Post, 30 September 1918, 1.

FIVE DEATHS FROM EPIDEMIC

SYDNEY, N.S. Sept. 29. Five deaths have resulted here and in North Sydney during the week-end from Spanish influenza, those dying being the two children of Mr. [Mrs.] D. D. MacDonald, North Sydney; Ivan O. Hart of Sydney, and Seamean John Crilly, an American sailor attached to the Aviation Corps in North Sydney; and Corporal James T. Smith, an American soldier....During the epidemic in New Waterford, it is said that there were 1,200 cases and that one doctor attended to 500.

Halifax Morning Chronicle, 30 September 1918, 2.

PRIVATE LOWELL E. WATERS DEAD AT HOSPITAL

Fourth Death Among American Soldiers Here Occurs Last Night

The fourth fatality among the American troops here occurred last night when Pte. Lowell E. Waters died. Pte. Waters came from Colome, South Dakota, and was a member of the 309th ammunition column. A number of other cases are reported as very ill, but many of the men are well on the road to recovery.

Sydney Daily Post, 1 October 1918, 1.

DEATHS AT NORTH SYDNEY

SEPT. 30.Two more American naval seamen attached to the local aviation base died at Hamilton hospital today from pneumonia following Spanish grip. The second to succumb was W. P. Schaeffert who belonged to Austin, Minn., and was 36 years old and married.

Sydney Daily Post, 2 October 1918, 2.

The following account by a volunteer nurse on duty in a Vancouver emergency hospital during the worst months of 1918 show what the Great Influenza brought to Sydney, and why the medical infrastructure was so quickly overwhelmed. Headlined "Trying Experiences of Mary A. Chesley in Hospital," it is a vivid and horrifying account of a time when influenza overwhelmed a world totally unprepared to deal with it.

Mary Chesley wrote:

Now I will tell you some of my experiences as night nurse.... I guess I was broken in that [first] night, for the close air, smell of new drugs, etc. never made me so sick again. The next night the awful shortness of help began. One nurse who had only had two wards and three helpers the night before now had four wards with the same number of helpers. She told us at breakfast that she did not discover till morning that one woman had a temperature of 105 and then she had no time to do anything. Is it any wonder the people died off as they did?

That night I was put alone, on a ward that had twenty men patients—two of them delirious. One of them was continually sitting up in bed and I would have to make him lie down. The poor fellow died a few nights later. The other man would strip off his shirt whenever I left the room and the patient in the next bed would call 'nurse, that man's got his shirt off again' and I would have to go and put it on him....There was one poor boy of seventeen, in just the next bed, who was quite sane [not delirious], and with proper care, I think might have recovered, but there he was right beside the poor man gasping for breath for hours while another fine looking young fellow was talking nonsense all night long, and another screaming and fighting with the orderlies. Poor fellow, he [the boy] would say 'Nurse, it scares me,' and it seemed to comfort him to have me hold his hand. Well—the next night poor Milford died, and five others out of the twelve, the eight hours I was on duty. It was an awful night.

Lunenburg Progress Enterprise, 25 December 1918, 1.

☞ "I could not begin to do what was needing to be done. I felt my ignorance, and there was no one to help," she said. After only nine nights on duty, Mary Chesley herself came down with influenza. (For the full article, see the Lunenburg County chapter.)

This is what it must have been like for nurses in Sydney, Cape Breton County, with five hundred men down with influenza all at once, and the authorities being totally unprepared for what this disease was going to show them. Then it began to spread through the community like a wildfire.

No one in Sydney, at first, could have realized the extreme contagion that had been let loose on the city and the surrounding areas. All those sick men; all their doctors and nurses and orderlies, the people who cooked and cleaned, took away their garbage and delivered supplies to them, were open to infection. All those who did their laundry—staff gowns and their gauze masks which had to be boiled every two hours and dried for thirty minutes before reuse, and this sickness's bleeding, coughing, vomiting, and incontinence went through sheets, blankets and towels as well as clothing almost hourly—meant that local laundries were working in a miasma of contagion.

All of the above, as well as local ministers, or the helpful Red Cross ladies who visited, were at first not even wearing masks. Protective gloves hadn't yet been invented. The first dayshift went home, and the nightshift then picked up the virus also. Wherever those people went, outside, they put others at risk. They were trying their best to be helpful, but in the end, they were helpful to the virus most of all.

SYDNEY BOARD OF HEALTH ORDERS SCHOOL, THEATRES AND DANCE HALLS CLOSED

There were 392 children absent from school yesterday, of whom there were about 300 sick, it was stated by Supervisor Woodhill. Dr. MacAuley stated that on Victoria Road there is hardly a house that does not contain a case of influenza and Dominion street is in the same condition.

Dr. Johnston stated that there are 11 cases in the marine hospital which were brought here from Quebec in a lake boat.

Sydney Daily Post, 1 October 1918, 1.

JOHN FINDLAYSON. After a painful illness of ten days, John Findlayson of Scotchtown, New Waterford, succumbed to the combined attacks of Spanish influenza and pneumonia. The deceased came from Scotland seven years ago and was 29 at the time of his death. He leaves a young widow and a family of five small children....In the old land he is survived by both his parents, to whom the deceased had longed to return before his call to the higher service.

Halifax Evening Mail, 4 October 1918, 6.

DEATH OF CAPTAIN ANGUS J. MCNEIL

Captain Angus J. McNeil, 6th battalion, R.C.G. regiment, late of the 95th regiment, died suddenly yesterday morning at ten o'clock after a few days illness with influenza at the Hamilton hospital, North Sydney....The officers and men of his company escorted his remains to the railway station at North Sydney last night, whence he was taken to his home at Iona, where the funeral will be held with military honors Wednesday morning.

Sydney Daily Post, 8 October 1918, 1.

TWO NEW DEATHS AND 85 NEW CASES GRIP YESTERDAY

Deaths Occur on Broadway and Tupper Street at Pier....Those who died were Mrs. John McIntyre, Broadway Street, Whitney Pier, and Fritz Herbert Best [FitzHenry Best], colored, 98 Tupper street....Mr. Best was 36 years old and was born in Barbados. His funeral will be held at 11 o'clock this morning from the family home. Burial will be in Hardwood Hill cemetery.

Sydney Daily Post, 10 October 1918, 1.

☞ There were eighty-five new cases in one day.

William Perkins, wireless operator on the steamer Wlelshmen [*Welshman*], died of influenza Saturday. He was 35 years old and a native of Burton, England. His funeral was held Monday from Beaton's undertaking parlor. Burial was in Hardwood Hill.

Sydney Daily Post, 15 October 1918, 5.

Joseph Anvonell, an Italian, died yesterday at his home 143 Laurier street, of influenza.

Sydney Daily Post, 15 October 1918, 1.

DEATHS AT GLACE BAY

Four deaths occurred from pneumonia in Glace Bay during the weekend, these being Seaman Frank Peddle, a native of Newfoundland. Hector McIntyre and Edward O'Leary, of Glace Bay, and Moses Long, on the Stirling. There are about 25 included in which there are a number of serious cases, in St. Joseph's hospital. Among those reported seriously ill is D. L. Macdonald, druggist. Another report is that while there are about 200 cases in the big town, there are very few serious cases. Marble Mountain, Orangedale and River Denys [all in Inverness County] are reported to be afflicted with the disease.

Sydney Daily Post, 16 October 1918, 3.

EIGHT MORE DEATHS IN SYDNEY

The Spanish Influenza Situation Is Growing Worse (Canadian Press Dispatch)

SYDNEY, October 15. Eight more death occurred here today, and the Spanish Influenza situation is reported steadily growing worse, owing to the reluctance of the city authorities to undertake the expense of fitting up an isolation hospital. No measures had been taken to isolate or quarantine persons suffering from the disease. Today the Board of Health took matters in its own hands and have wired Mark Workman, asking the use of a large residence belonging to the Dominion Steel Corporation, as an isolation hospital for severe cases. The great difficulty here is the lack of nurses. Seven nurses of the city hospital staff are down with the disease. Antigonish has promised nursing assistance. The situation is also reported growing worse elsewhere in this district. There were forty new cases in Glace Bay yesterday.

Halifax Morning Chronicle, 18 October 1918, 5.

INFLUENZA AT MARBLE MOUNTAIN

There are about 100 cases of influenza in Marble Mountain [Inverness County], it is reported, and a plea for outside medical assistance has been made. Medical Officer MacAuley [of Sydney] had been requested to go to the community, but he was unable to leave the city. The situation here has greatly improved over that pertaining two weeks ago although there are a number of serious cases of pneumonia. A Newfoundland paper stated that there are 300 cases of influenza here, but it is officially stated that when the epidemic was at its worst that there were not many more than 300 cases.

Sydney Daily Post, 21 October 1918, 5.

☞ This article seems to believe the worst was over. Nobody dreamed it would continue into 1920.

DEATHS FROM INFLUENZA

Emergency Hospital, Sydney: Howard Soyyeau [*sic*], French Cove, Richmond County.

Marine Hospital: Seaman John Franklin, England. City Hospital: No deaths. General Hospital, Glace Bay: John D'Arcy, Sydney.

Orangedale [Inverness County]: James E. McFarlane, station agent.

River Denys [Inverness County]: Mrs. McLeod, Big Brook....There are some bad cases in River Denys. Miss [*sic*] MacLeod, Big Brook, died....

There may be some cases in Grand Narrows, as they have asked for a doctor. Their nearest doctor is in Baddeck or Sydney.

Sydney Daily Post, 21 October 1918, 5

Difficulties in Searching Death Records

☞ There are often cases where no death record comes up while searching the HVS database because the name of the deceased has been garbled by all and sundry, including newspapers, people returning information for the death register, or transcribers. Howard Soyyeau, above, of French Cove, Richmond County, has a perplexing surname. He appears on Dr. Allan Marble's list as "Howard Sayyean." Using the HVS database, one must search only on 'S---, Howard', to get him. There are two death records for a Howard S---, which provide an even more bewildering variety of spellings: Sayyean, Sayyear, Sayylun, Sayyeau, Sayyeur.

The first record, in Book 30, Page 9, Number 50, has *Sayylun*, later crossed out, with *Sayyeau* written in in pencil. This Howard died at the Marine Hospital, October 20, 1918. A sailor, aged 21 and single, he was the son of Captain 'G. *Sayyean*' (or

Sayylan), born at 'Morrisburgh Cut', unidentified but somewhere in Nova Scotia, I assume, as there otherwise would be something to indicate location area. He was buried in North Sydney. His doctor was T. Mac Aulay; undertaker was B. I. (or B. R.) Lowden.

The second record, in Book 30, Page 41, Number 238, has "*Sayyeau*, Howard," aged 21, died October 19, 1918. He was single, a fireman (a stoker in the engine room of a steamship). His father is given as "Adolphe *Sayyeur*," and his place of birth "Forchu, N.S.," which is likely Cape Forchu, Yarmouth County. He died in Sydney's Hamilton hospital, of pneumonia. A Methodist, he was buried at "Lakeside" [*sic*], North Sydney. This return says the doctor was M. T. McLean and the undertaker was W. J. Dooley.

Are there two people here, same name, same age, same marital status, same length of illness, same cause of death, same burial site, and died October 19–20? Are all these matches in data merely coincidence? And how *does* one spell this name correctly?

The Canadian Census for 1911, Nova Scotia, Richmond County, St. Peters Subdistrict, Enumeration District 15, Page 10, lines 27–31, shows:

- Sayzeau, George W., age 34, was head of the family.
- Sayzeau, Dorothy, age 31, was his wife.
- Sayzeau, Jacob S., aged 63, lived with them, and was probably George's father.
- Sayzeau, Howard, age 13, their son [who would have been 20–21 in 1918].
- Sayzeau, William, age 10, second son.

This is the best guess for "Howard Soyyeau." Writing the y and the z in cursive, both, back then, would have tails, and could easily be mistaken for a double *y*. SAYZEAU.

Dr. MacAulay Puts His Foot Down

☞ By October 26, Sydney was suffering from a serious lack of influenza information, a lack of resolution, resources, and medical personnel. There were continuous conflicts—a lack of cooperation between City Council, the City Medical Officer, various other doctors with vested interests, closed businesses anxious about losing profits, with dazed reporters and concerned citizens not knowing what to think or do. There was a meeting of these when the board of health called a session. One has only to read the notes from the Board of Health meeting of September 26th to see the various factions floundering around, repeating their points of view ad nauseam. Just when all seemed settled, they'd all start up again.

Dr. J. F. MacAuley, city and district medical officer, finally had enough. He rose up, armed with common-sense science, and with an impressive mixture of exhaustion, politeness, and righteous wrath, he laid down the law. It was thunderously effective, and all those concerned sat mum and did what he told them. At least they sort of *said* they would. And then they'd all start arguing again.

"Pointed remarks were made at various stages of the meeting," said the reporter. The headlines for the following article in the *Sydney Daily Post* on the Monday of 28 October (p. 6) were so large no reader could have failed to note them. The newspaper reporter opened his article with a quick summation, and then adds the particulars of the unfolding drama. Read on:

 INFLUENZA BAN TO BE LIFTED WHEN ALL HOUSES IN THE CITY HAVING CASES ARE PLACARDED

City Medical Officer Claims His Advice Was Not Followed In Dealing With Epidemic—Physicians Did Not Report—May Be Prosecuted

Open air church services are allowed to be held, it was announced by Medical Officer MacAuley at noon.

The ban will be lifted some time in the future, but not tomorrow or Monday, and that is about all that is known about the influenza situation, officially or unofficially. It had been planned last night to hold a board of health meeting at 11 o'clock this morning, but when Ald. [Alderman] MacDonald did not turn up by 11:30 o'clock, the meeting was off.

When homes containing cases of influenza are placarded and those which contained cases during the past five days are fumigated to the satisfaction of the city medical officer, the board of health will hold a meeting and lift the ban on public gatherings. The decision was reached after a prolonged meeting of the board yesterday afternoon. Meeting at 2 o'clock the aldermen officially adjourned at 5 o'clock, but at 6 o'clock several were still in the city hall discussing the situation.

Pointed remarks were made at various stages of the meeting. At one stage Dr. McAulay [*sic*] asked whether the board was going to take the advice of outsiders. He had at the first meeting of the board advised placarding, but the advice of other doctors was taken and his suggestion was not carried out. Then ensued a discussion in which the doctor was upheld by several aldermen.

The board of health regulations are not being carried out, it was stated, and the blame was shuffled around a triangle. Dr. MacAulay blamed the board of health and the secretary and Ald. MacAdam then charged the doctor and cleared the board and secretary.

The action of the doctors in not reporting their cases was censured by the board and it was pointed out that they may be prosecuted. The allowing of sailors the freedom of the streets although deaths have occurred on board their ships was also condemned.

At one time, it looked as if the city churches would be opened on Sunday and theatres, pool rooms, lodgerooms [*sic*] on Monday, but the final decision was that the ban will be lifted at some time in the future.

The turning point, as it appeared to the *Post* reporter, was the statement of a city doctor.

The city and district medical officer, Dr. J. F. MacAuley, was in favour of a partial lifting of the lid under certain conditions, and Ald. MacAdam made a motion. Dr. Maculay [*sic*] stated that if houses were placarded and fumigated, and influenza patients were quarantined, he felt that theatres, churches, and all other gathering places but schools could be opened. Ald. McAdam included Dr. MacAuley's suggestions in his motion and Ald. McLeod stated that he would second the resolution provided that the recommendations were carried out.

Next, the *Post*'s reporter began to describe the actual meeting:

FULL BOARD ATTENDS

The meeting opened with the full board present: they being Chairman Steele, and Alds. MacDonald, McAdam, MacDougall and MacLeod. Mayor Fitzgerald, Deputy Mayor Morley and City Solicitor MacDonald were also present as spectators.

Ald. MacAdam, who had been delegated to interview the city doctors, since it had been apparently impossible to have the physicians [at an] interview [with] the city officials, reported that there were 70 new cases during the week. Thursday afternoon the following doctors gave him the following information: Dr. Rice, 10 new cases; Dr. Walsh 11 (7 of which were on Monday and the other 4 in one family); Drs John MacDonald, Lynch and Cowperthwaite two each; Friday: Drs. Egan, McIntyre, Curry, 0; Dr. Bruce a very few; Dr. Johnstone, 3 (a lot of whom are now well); Dr. E. N. McDonald, 14; Dr. Roy, 1; Dr. McRae, 6; Dr. MacAulay, 6; Dr. Nathanson, 7 (for Wednesday and Thursday). [This information is not in a usable form.]

The following were for lifting the lid: Drs. Rice, Walsh, John MacDonald, Lynch, Cowperthwaite, Egan, MacIntyre, Curry. He could not speak for the following doctors, Ald. MacAdam said.

City Clerk Curry stated that up to Thursday only six places could have officially been placarded, as only six names had been received. Ald. Steele said that one doctor told him he was too busy to sign the cards, and that Dr. Hattie [the provincial medical officer by whom the cards were required] was appointed by the government and he [himself] wasn't.

Underground [sneaky] work to have the ban lifted was indicated when Dr. MacAulay read a wire received by Provincial Medical Officer Hattie, from a local man, stating "Think conditions now safe. Please advise Dr. MacAulay to order ban lifted." The doctor said that Dr. Hattie had ordered that no person suffering from influenza may be removed from a ship without the authority of the city medical officer or the secretary of the board of health.

Then a spectator asked to be heard. He was himself a doctor.

Dr. Lynch visited the council chamber during the discussion, and he was asked by Ald. McAdam whether he could furnish the board with a list of places which should be fumigated or quarantined. The reply was that he could by going over his books, but the doctors wish an hour for themselves after their day's calls and anyway quarantining and placarding would be impracticable and unfair to the many who have already suffered from influenza.

"Conditions are improving," said Dr. Lynch. "Many colds are now being treated as Spanish flu and it would not be a square deal to placard the houses when severe cases of flu were not placarded. Two years ago we had much more serious epidemic of influenza and the churches were not closed."

Ald. McDougall then stood firmly for placarding and fumigating before lifting the ban and Dr. Lynch replied with the statement that placarding regulations had not been carried out in the past. Men living in homes where there were scarlet fever, scarletina and diphtheria went to work as usual, and Spanish influenza is not as bad as those diseases. Then came the statement that if placarding were the order, the doctors would state that their patients were suffering from a cold and not influenza. "We have to consider our patients," he said.

You can see what Dr. MacAuley was having to deal with. While one could posit, charitably, that Dr. Lynch hadn't yet taken in the unusual nature of this particular influenza, his stating that he and others wouldn't send in information because they couldn't be bothered, and Lynch's attempt to get his own way over the issue of placarding by saying he and others would then send the chief medical officer *false* information, seems to the mind of hindsight to be actionable, and to smack of what is now prosecuted as "Depraved Indifference." Dr. Lynch's views are appalling, short-sighted, ultimately disastrous.

Dr. MacAuley had had enough. He was "firm for fumigating and placarding," said the *Post* reporter.

"Quarantine regulations require the quarantining of persons for five days after contact and of patients for five days after convalescence," he said in reply to a question. "It is a short-lived germ after leaving the body as it is usually killed after two days of fresh air. The floors and walls of the room should be thoroughly scrubbed with a solution of bichloride or carbolic acid and they should be thoroughly aired and have sunlight for 24 hours."

Next he took on the various recalcitrant doctors, their opinions and excuses, and their failure to report data that was vitally necessary to tracking the flu and to grasping how actively destructive it was. Correct information kept people safe. He reminded the meeting that these doctors whose critiques had been made in writing or in person "gave their opinions gratis." Dr. MacAuley further pointed out that such persons who had given opinions on policy "have no responsibility for policy-making." He must have looked at the Board of Health commissioners and summed up: "You are the men responsible."

He then stated that they had no idea how many of the 2176 cases are convalescent; they have no idea of the number of unreported; they have no idea of the number of patients who have not called a doctor; they have no idea of the number of teachers laid up; they have no idea of the number of teachers who are boarding in houses where there is influenza [in regards to the proposed school reopenings—and no idea of the number of sick or infected-but-not-yet-actively-ill children there were]. "You are quite as much in the dark today as you were a week ago," he said. "It is the duty of the board of health to protect the health of the city. Conditions now do not warrant opening up unconditionally."

One would think that would have been enough to move them all to reason.

SUGGESTED PARTIAL OPENING

Dr. MacAuley then suggested that there should be a partial opening up under certain conditions. One was that if the schools were opened, the children should be inspected. Ald. MacAdam then made his motion but could not obtain a seconder. In making the motion the alderman said that it had been planned to reach foreigners during the Victory Loan campaign through the ministers and churches. In Boston, the lid had been lifted in three weeks [with disastrous results, it was later proven], the maximum time for every city. Sick people do not go to church. Ald. McDougall was of the firm opinion that houses should be quarantined as if the ban on theatres were raised all would go to them.

☞ It still hadn't sunk in how devastating and how extremely infectious this epidemic was. If you want to see how wrong he was, read the Guysborough County chapter herein of how a minister, sick but not yet showing, infected an entire congregation in Goshen, resulting in three deaths. He also infected the household hosting him.

The whole uproar started all over again.

THEATRE MANAGER PROTESTS

Later Mr....[some of this area of the column is illegible even under magnification] produced questions when he said that although the theatres are still closed there is still influenza in Sydney. "Where did the people get the disease," he asked. "They did not get it at the theatres. You are doing nothing to stamp it out, and it is getting down to a case of discrimination when although the theatres, in which influenza did not start, are quarantined, houses in which there is influenza are not. Is that common sense? Sailors from [ships?] containing influenza come in and [illegible in microfilm] and you cannot prevent them. Where does this disease come from?" he again asked, and chairman Steele replied that 14 or 15 doctors did not know. "It is in the air, I believe," he said.

Dr. MacAulay said that the public should have protection from houses just as much as from theatres. Every house in which there are or have been cases recently should be placarded, quarantined and fumigated. He reminded the board that he had suggested at the first meeting that houses should be placarded, and another lengthy discussion resulted. Mayor Fitzgerald and others said that the C.B.R. [Cape Breton Rail?] is living up to the regulations, during the day at least.

Ald. McLeod stated that the board should abide by the report of the city medical officer. He would second Ald. MacAdam's motion if they could find anyone to fumigate the houses. As it is, everything that has been done and every resolution passed might as well be written on the moon.

A discussion on whether the schools should be opened followed. Ald. Steel said that all towns and cities are looking toward Sydney, even Halifax. Ald. MacLeod then reiterated his statement that he would second the motion if he were certain that the placarding and fumigating would be carried out. He was apparently cautious owing to the lack of action on other resolutions passed by the board.

Sydney Daily Post, 28 October 1918, 6. (From Saturday afternoon edition.)

And so it went, round and round. Meanwhile, death continued to visit Cape Breton County.

This *exactly* illustrates the kind of situation described as disastrous by Dr. W. H. Hattie on September 30, 1918, as follows:

The various local boards of health are composed, in most instances, of laymen, who cannot be expected to take an active or well ordered part in activities which are so foreign to their other interests. While these boards may show evidence of an awakening when a dangerous infectious disease invades their districts, they do not always take efficient action, nor do they commonly realize that the most important function of a health organization is to *prevent* disease—that control of infection once it has obtained a footing is of less consequence to the community than the elimination of those conditions which invite the incidence of the communicable disease. Moreover a local board is apt to concern itself in its own district alone, and to overlook the interests of other communities. The communicable diseases find no barrier between different health sections, and the opportunity for their transmission is such that the development of a case at Cape Sable is not without interest to the people of Cape North.

Dr. W. H Hattie, Provincial Medical Officer, Annual Report of the Department of Public Health, Journals of the House of Assembly, Appendix 16, 1919.

 FLU EPIDEMIC AT ALDER POINT
Several People Succumb Before the Arrival of a Doctor
NORTH SYDNEY, Nov. 19. Spanish influenza is reported to be epidemic at Alder Point, and other places in the Bras D'Or district. At two homes in Alder Point on Sunday the patients had passed away before the arrival of the doctor. A number of new cases are reported in North Sydney during the past few days.
...Outbreak of Influenza at Sydney Mines
Eight Deaths Reported During the Last Forty-Eight Hours. A fresh outbreak of Spanish influenza is reported at Sydney Mines. Eight deaths occurred Saturday and Sunday and the health authorities have decided on drastic action....An urgent request has been sent to Halifax for doctors and nurses.

Sydney Daily Post, 2 December 1918, 1.

DEATHS FROM FLU AT NORTH SYDNEY
The death of Nicholas Bonini, oldest son of Mr. and Mrs. Sylvester Bonini, Queen Street, occurred Saturday morning after a nine days' illness of influenza and pneumonia. The deceased was 28 years of age and for some time past carried on business as a barber on Queen street....Another death occurred from influenza pneumonia on Saturday when Miss Sadie MacDougall of Margaree passed away at the Hamilton Hospital. Miss MacDougall came to North Sydney from Inverness only a little over a month ago, and was employed at the Western Union cable office. Her remains were sent home last night for burial.

Several departments of St. Joseph's school were closed this morning on account of the illness of a number of the sisters.

Sydney Daily Post, 31 December 1918, 1.

☞ Sadie MacDougall was not found on the HVS search engine, but the record for a "Saidie McDougall" shows a telegraph operator from Margaree Falls, who lived

Death record for Saidie McDougall, born in Margaree Forks, working in Sydney as a telegraph operator, died of influenza/pneumonia, as did these other North Sydney folk. (*Nova Scotia Archives*)

on King Street, North Sydney. She died of influenza on November 9, after an illness of two weeks. Her father's name was Donald. She was buried in the "RC" cemetery, Margaree Forks.

HVS, Cape Breton County Death Register, 1918, Book 30, Page 47, Number 273.

☞ Saidie McDougall (275), was the first person entered on page 47 of the 1918 death register. The other five death entries following from North Sydney, for a period between November 10 and December 5. All died from influenza and pneumonia.

- Nicholas Bonini (276), 28, a barber, lived on Queen Street. Ill a week, d. November 30.
- Eliza Amey (277), aged 4, Minto Street. Ill a week, d. December 2. Her mother, Mrs. Philip Amey, died a day later, but lacks an entry.

- Vivian Jane Hutchins (278), 3 years, 7 months; Ingraham Street. Ill 11 days, d. December 3.
- Michael F. McNeil (279), 28, King Street, C.G. Railway section man. Ill one week, d. December 3.
- Mary Bathurson, 68, Green Hotel, Blowers Street; born in PEI, wife of John, ill a week, d. December 5.

HVS, Cape Breton County Death Register, 1918, Book 30, Page 47,
Numbers 275-280.

☞ Dr. Allan Marble wrote on his newspaper-articles list, after his last entry for the 1918 *Sydney Record* material, that he had found no influenza deaths in Cape Breton County "before 24 September 1918" in this paper. He only recorded the one item below for 1919: "*Sydney Record*, mfn# 1,970: 2 January 1919, p. 2. Frank Hulmden died at Sydney Mines on 18 January, aged 29." The original death record gives this man's name as Holmden. He was an accountant, born in England, aged 29.

HVS, Cape Breton County Death Register, 1919, Book 30, Page 184, Number 850.

☞ Dr. Marble finished his notes by writing that, for the year 1919, "Very few obituaries included in paper." That concluded Dr. Marble's extracts from the 1919 *Record*. Next, he lists articles from the *Sydney Daily Post*. After the end of this paper's 1918 articles, Dr. Marble notes a few miscellaneous items related to the flu, but never expands on these:

Sydney Daily Post, mfm 1,370:

• 24 January 1920, p. 11.	No influenza in Sydney or the province.
• 31 January, 1920, p. 13.	4,706 new cases of flue reported in New York on Wednesday.
• 4 February, 1920, p. 1.	No widespread epidemic of flu in any province.
• 5 February, 1920, p. 1.	Alex McKinnon of Nova Scotia died of influenza at Cobalt, Ontario on 4 Feb. Influenza is spreading rapidly in Ontario.
• [5] February, 1920, p. 8.	Montreal has 96 flu cases, but it is a mild disease.
• 6 February 1920, p. 1.	Flu epidemic serious in Toronto.
• 7 February 1920, p. 1.	Three cases of influenza in Sydney [NS].
• 13 February, 1920, p. 3.	Much influenza in Toronto. 90 deaths in one day.
• 14 February, 1920, p. 3.	Ontario scourged by flu. A dearth of nurses.

- 14 February, 1920, p. 11.

  Social service nurse app'ted in Cape Breton to provide nursing to returned soldiers. [Only one for all of Cape Breton!]

- 16 February, 1920, p. 1.

  Headline–Sydney Prepares for Influenza Epidemic. Vaccine and an emergency hospital to be obtained.

- 19 February 1920, p. 9.

  11,160 cases reported in Ontario so far in month of February – 539 deaths. It is said to be on the wane.

- 20 February 1920, p. 1.

  Thirty cases of influenza have been noted in the Sydney area.

- February 1920, p. 1.

  50 cases in Sydney, since first outbreak.

- 23 February 1920, p. 1

  About 30 cases at Louisbourg.

- 24 February 1920, p. 3

  No deaths from flu in Sydney yet.

- 25 February 1920, p. 1

  Influenza situation in Sydney becoming serious.

- 1 March, 1920, p. 1

  Flu situation in Sydney much improved. New Waterford wants a hospital. Dominion Coal has promised $35,000 in cash and workmen will be asked to contribute $13 per man per year, for the next 15 years. Finished to 6 March 1920."

Allan Marble, unpublished list of Nova Scotia newspapers, 1918-20. Used by permission.

☞ Since Dr. Marble records no obituaries for any of the 1920 flu victims, here are profiles of four of the fifty people to succumb to the Great Influenza in Cape Breton County that year, chosen at random.

☞ "Anastasia Shea, 40, d. 18 March 1920, Port Morien, housewife." She was born in Nova Scotia in 1880, to Thomas Hawley and his wife Anastasia Pendegrast. Described as "Irish," she married William Hawley of Port Morien, a coal miner. Anastasia was pregnant when she fell ill from influenza on March 11, which became pneumonia at some point in the next seven days. On March 18, she went into labour, probably precipitated by the disease. She died at 8.00 p.m. that same day. Cause of death was given as "Heart Failure from Influenza & Pneumonia." Secondary cause of death: "Confined, March 18th." ("Confined" or "In her confinement" was a euphemism for a woman's labour and delivery of a baby.) Nothing was said about the child, who may have not been delivered. There is no 1920 birth or death certificate for a child of William and Anastasia Shea on record. A. K. Roy was her doctor. D. F. MacAulay, the undertaker, buried her body the next day, somewhere in Port Morien.

Anastasia and William had produced at least four other children: Kathleen Margaret, born 20 February 1908; Helen Jean, born 13 December 1909, died 22 January 1911 of scarlet fever and toxaemia; William Newman, born 17 November 1911; and Rose Mary, born on March 6, 1914.

> HVS, Cape Breton County, 1920, Book 56, Page 629. There are three separate choices for Anastasia in the HVS search engine, but they all refer you to the one record, on page 629: Annastasia Shea, Anastatia Shea, both in Port Morien, and a third Anastasia Shea in Sydney—all on page 629.

☞ Information on the three children: HVS, Cape Breton County, Birth Registers: search 1908 for Kathleen Margaret Shea, 1909 for Helen Jean Shea, 1911 for William Newman Shea, and 1914 for Rose Mary Shea. Cape Breton County, Death Registers: search 1911 for Helen Jean Shea.

☞ "John T. Peach, 59, d. 20 March 1920, Port Morien, farmer." He resided at Birch Gardens, Port Morien, and was a farmer for most of his life. He died of influenza and pneumonia, after a short illness of about seven days, on March 20 at 1 P.M. His father's name was William James Peach, his mother's Margaret Wadden Peach. A brother, Archie Peach, was the informant for the death certificate. John T. Peach was buried two days later, somewhere in Port Morien. The death record doesn't say what cemetery. The undertaker was D. F. MacAulay.

> HVS, Cape Breton County Death Register, 1920, Book 56, Page 630.

☞ "Mrs. Mary Jessome, 35, d. 18 March 1920, Little Bras D'Or." This woman's information was given for the death record by her brother-in-law, Thomas Jessome. Perhaps her husband was ill, or away; his name and occupation are not given. Mary wasn't a widow; the record lists her as married. Thomas says for the record that he doesn't know her date of birth, but that she had worked as a housewife from 1910 to 1920, and had been living at her present residence in Little Bras d'Or for five years. He remembered that her father's name had been John McNeil, and that her mother was Mary Connell McNeil. The doctor, whose name, where he signed the record, is illegible, stated that the cause of death was "Influenza—condition aggravated by Labor." Nothing was said about the baby, born or unborn. Mary Jessome was buried in Little Bras d'Or by undertakers J. N. Francis & Sons, Sydney Mines.

> HVS, Cape Breton County Death Register, 1920, Book 56, Page 641.

☞ Cape Breton County lost at least 293 people in the last four months of 1918, between 6 September and December 24. A further 42 died between January 1 and March 31, 1919, and in the resurgence of the influenza in 1920, 50 more souls perished.

And, as you can see, according to Dr. Marble, there were almost no obituaries in the newspapers after 1919, even though some fifty people had died of influenza.

CAPE BRETON COUNTY, VITAL STATISTICS, DEATH REGISTER, BOOKS 29, 30, 56, 57

1918

1. Arthur H. Garlock, 18, d. 23 September 1918, Sydney; seaman, Clinton, Iowa; U.S.S. *Chattanooga*.

2. Hannah Harloff, 4 years 6 months, d. 6 September 1918, North Sydney.

3. John Crilly, 21, d. 26 September 1918, North Sydney, U.S. Navy [*airman*].

4. William J. Campbell, 14, d. 30 September 1918, North Sydney, student.

5. William Theophilus Schaffert, 30, d. 30 September 1918, North Sydney, U. S. Navy.

6. Peter J. McNeil, 5, d. 3 September 1918, Glace Bay.

7. James McKeigen, 8, d. 30 September 1918, Glace Bay.

8. Sarah Annie McPhee, 42, d. 9 October 1918, Dominion.

9. Gertrude Curry, 28, d. 30 August 1918, Port Morien, housewife.

10. James Walsh, 50, d. 18 September 1918, New Waterford, carpenter.

11. George Wareham, 41, d. 25 September 1918, New Waterford, miner.

12. Mary Fraser, 21, d. 23 September 1918, New Waterford, housework.

13. Mary Jessie McDougall, 10, d. 27 September 1918, New Waterford, student.

14. Jean Wilson Cummings, 1 month, d. 29 September 1918, New Waterford.

15. Marie Velenori, 1 year, d. 30 September 1918, New Waterford.

16. John Findlayson, 29, d. 29 September 1918, New Waterford, miner.

17. Christina McLeod, 23, d. 3 October 1918, Sydney, housemaid.

18. James Clark, 26, d. 2 October 1918, Sydney, soldier.

19. Lemuel Davis, 26, d. 4 October 1918, Marine Hospital, Sydney, druggist.

20. Henry Wilson, 34, d. 4 October 1918, Sydney, labourer.

21. Annie Brower, 19, d. 4 October 1918, Sydney, maid at hotel.

22. Charles Stephens, 50, d. 5 October 1918, Sydney, carpenter.

23. Mary McGrath, 34, d. 5 October 1918, Sydney, housewife.

24. Edgar Clancy, 31, d. 7 October 1918, Sydney, steel company worker.

25. FitzHerbert Best, 36, d. 8 October 1918, Sydney, labourer.

26. Christina McIntyre, 32, d. 9 October 1918, Sydney.

27. J. McLeod (male), 40, d. 24 October 1918, Marine Hospital, Sydney, 4th engineer on a steamship.

28. Robert Auntivine, 21, d. 24 October 1918, Marine Hospital, Sydney, hose tender [*sic; original written "hawse" (or house or horse, but not hose) tender, S.S. Corinthian. Book 30, Page 5, Number 26.*]

29. Richard Butcher, 28, d. 25 October 1918, Sydney, stoker on a steamship.

30. Lt. G. Lake, 38, d. 25 October 1918, Sydney, HMSC *Shearwater*.

31. Donald Matheson, 1 year 6 months; d. 26 October 1918, Sydney.

32. Catherine Petrie, 14, d. 28 October 1918, Sydney, student.

33. John H. Doyle, 54, d. 28 October 1918, Sydney.

34. Alex Le Flenn, 21, d. 29 October 1918, Sydney. French [*citizen*].

35. Margaret O'Handley, 73, d. 30 October 1918, Sydney.

36. Kate Ann McAskill, 36, d. 31 October 1918, Sydney.

37. Alexander Matheson, 18, d. 31 October 1918, Emergency Hospital, Sydney.

38. Howard Saiyyean [*Sayzeau*], 21, d. 20 October 1918, Marine Hospital, Sydney, sailor.

39. Leslie Campbell, 18, d. 21 October 1918, Sydney, HMCS *Shearwater* at Sydney.

40. John J. McDougall, 28, d. 22 October 1918, Quarantine Hospital, Sydney, brakeman.

41. William Murphy, 29, d. 22 October 1918, Sydney, farmer and pilot.

42. Margaret Campbell, 60, d. 22 October 1918, Sydney, dressmaker.

43. Samuel Morrison, 40, d. 22 October 1918, Sydney, machinist.

44. David Finn, 19, d. 23 October 1918, Marine Hospital, Sydney, sailor.

45. George Howard, 31, d. 23 October 1918, Marine Hospital, Sydney, greaser.

46. Annie McNeil, 28, d. 16 October 1918, Sydney, housewife.

47. Mary Johnstone, 33, d. 16 October 1918, Sydney, housewife.

48. R. McCreadie, 31, d. 16 October 1918, Marine Hospital, Sydney.

49. Mary Johnstone, 7 months, d. 17 October 1918, Sydney.

50. Albertina Dentens, 29, d. 17 October 1918, Sydney, housewife.

51. J. Gielist, 40, d. 18 October 1918, Sydney, labourer.

52. Margaret Greaves, 52, d. 18 October 1918, Royal Hotel, Sydney.

53. John Lairsey, 1 year 10 months, d. 19 October 1918, Sydney.

54. John Frankland, 42, d. 20 October 1918, Marine Hospital, George Street, Sydney, chief gunner.

55. Myrtle Neville, 16 months, d. 10 October 1918, Sydney.

56. S. Biggs, 29, d. 10 October 1918, Sydney, Marine Hospital, sailor. [*Book 30, Page 13, Number 27 (later changed to 75), records that he was born in Sussex, England; was Church of England, and was buried at Hardwood Hills, Sydney.*]

57. John R. Martin, 24, d. 10 October 1918, Moxam Hospital, King's Road, Sydney, soldier. [*Book 30, Page 13, Number 28 (number crossed out later and changed to 76).*]

58. Josephine Boudrout, 32, d. 11 October 1918, Sydney, housewife. [*Book 30, Page 13, Number 29 (number crossed out later and changed to 77). HVS Search Engine has her as "Boudreau."*]

59. Clifford Perkins, 38, d. 11 October 1918, Sydney, wireless operator, S.S. *Welshman*.

60. John McDonald, 29, d. 12 October 1918, Sydney.

61. Johanna McIntyre, 9 months, d. 12 October 1918, Sydney.

62. David Pottie, 32, d. 14 October 1918, Sydney, fireman, S.S. *Kovicden* at Sydney.

63. Ronald Fletcher, 7 months, d. 14 October 1918, Sydney.

64. Joseph Anvonell, 45, d. 14 October 1918, Sydney, labourer.

65. Jean McDonald, 30, d. 14 October 1918, Sydney, housewife.

66. Raymond Frost, 20, d. 15 October 1918, Atlantic Hotel, Sydney, steel worker.

67. John Gurts, 36, d. 15 October 1918, Marine Hospital, Sydney, fireman. [*Book 30, Page 16, Number 45 (number crossed out later and changed to 93), records he was born in "Holland," was married, a Roman Catholic, and was buried at Calvary Cemetery.*]

68. Barbara Curtis, 19, d. 16 October 1918, Sydney, housewife.

69. Dan McNeil, 17, d. 4 December 1918, Sydney, labourer.

70. Duncan Meikle, 35, d. 5 December 1918, Sydney, commission merchant.

71. William Warren, 38, d. 8 December 1918, Sydney, steelworker.

72. Margaret McInnis, 18, d. 9 December 1918, Sydney.

73. Laura Cockell, 28, d. 11 December 1918, Sydney, housewife.

74. Ala Nyjoke, 1 year, d. 11 December 1918, Sydney.

75. Dan Campbell, 20, d. 23 November 1918, Sydney, teamster.

76. Emma Kippin, 32, d. 25 November 1918, Sydney.

77. Annie McQueen, 22, d. 25 November 1918, Sydney, housewife.

78. Mary McMillan, 26, d. 26 November 1918, Sydney.

79. Alice Ryan, 30, d. 26 November 1918, Sydney, bookkeeper.

80. George Carlin, 26, d. 29 November 1918, Sydney, electrical worker.

81. Harry Purdy, 27, d. 18 November 1918, Sydney, moulder.

82. Mary McDougall, 18, d. 19 November 1918, Sydney, bookkeeper.

83. Edward Wall, 24, d. 1 November 1918, Sydney, wireless operator.

84. Carl Olsen, 28, d. 1 November 1918, Sydney, sailor.

85. George Boutilier, 22, d. 4 November 1918, Sydney, returned soldier.

86. Ronald Johnston, 35, d. 8 November 1918, Sydney, steel worker.

87. Annie Robertson, 4, d. 12 December 1918, Sydney.

88. Fannie Miller, 45, d. 12 December 1918, Sydney, housewife.

89. Dan McKeigan, 33, d. 13 December 1918, Sydney, steel worker.

90. Effie Morgan, 35, d. 16 December 1918, Sydney.

91. Mabel McRae, 32, d. 16 December 1918, Sydney, housewife.

92. Eleanor Gordon, 6, d. 17 December 1918, Sydney.

93. Lillian Good, 35, d. 22 December 1918, Sydney, housewife.

94. William Hall, 38, d. 24 December 1918, Sydney, labourer.

95. Rev. James Wiltshire, 28, d. 25 December 1918, Sydney, clergy.

96. George Dunning, 52, d. 24 December 1918, Sydney, wire splicer.

97. John Edward, 46, d. 28 December 1918, Sydney, steel worker.

98. Ignac Podowaka, 27, d. 20 December 1918, Sydney, steel worker.

99. Catherine McRae, 87, d. 20 October 1918, Sydney Forks.

100. Arabella McKenzie, 28, d. 16 November, Sydney River, housewife.

101. Harry Gordon, 18, d. 5 October 1918, North Sydney, machinist.

102. Angus McNeil, 58, d. 7 October 1918, North Sydney, Captain, Army.

103. Harriet Lovell, 28, d. 9 October 1918, North Sydney, housewife.

104. Emma Green, 19, d. 19 October 1918, Lorne Street, North Sydney, house-maid. [*HVS Search Engine lists her as "Emona Green." Emma Green was born in Newfoundland. Book 30, Page 39, Number 231.*]

105. Margaret Nicholson, 34, d. 11 October 1918, North Sydney, housekeeper.

106. Hector McLean, 24, d. 13 October 1918, North Sydney, soldier.

107. Byron Dickson, 38, d. 14 October 1918, North Sydney, marine engineer.

108. Thomas Brennan, 31, d. 15 October 1918, North Sydney, aviator.

109. Carmen Brewer, 20 d. 20 October 1918, North Sydney, telegrapher.

110. Priscilla Gardiner, 38, d. 24 October 1918, North Sydney, housewife.

111. Sarah Skinner, 30, d. 26 October 1918, North Sydney, housework.

112. Norman Squires, 4, d. 27 October 1918, North Sydney.

113. Eliza Eastman, 34, d. 27 October 1918, North Sydney, housewife.

114. Frank Hiller, 50, d. 2 November 1918, North Sydney, railway section man.

115. Ann Cameron, 60, d. 2 November 1918, North Sydney, housewife.

116. John LeMoine, 28, d. 14 November 1918, North Sydney, merchant.

117. Clarence Smith, 16, d. 23 November 1918, North Sydney, druggist clerk.

118. Saidie McDougall, 21, d. 29 November 1918, North Sydney, telegraph operator.

119. Nicholas Bonini, 28, d. 30 November 1918, North Sydney, barber.

120. Eliza Amey, 4, d. 2 November 1918, North Sydney.

121. Vivian Hutchins, 3, d. 2 December 1918, North Sydney.

122. Michael McNeil, 28, d. 3 December 1918, North Sydney, railway section man.

123. Mary Bathurson, 63, d. 5 December 1918, North Sydney, housewife.

124. Mary Rudderham, 68, d. 7 December 1918, North Sydney, housewife.

125. Robert Bonnar, 40, d. 8 December 1918, North Sydney, labourer.

126. Robert Peeler, 29, d. 9 December 1918, North Sydney, seaman.

127. Annie Young, 34, d. 13 December 1918, North Sydney, domestic.

128. John Richards, 69, d. 15 December 1918, North Sydney, labourer.

129. Alonzo Degrish, 30, d. 20 December 1918, North Sydney, seaman.

130. Annie Googoo, 35, d. 27 October 1918, Georges River, housewife.

131. William McDaniels, 27, d. 7 November 1918, Georges River, labourer.

132. Charles Googoo, 30, d. 9 November 1918, Upper North Sydney, labourer.

133. Jane C. Almon, 30, d. 15 November, Georges River, housewife.

134. Martin Gaddon, 12, 14 November 1918, Georges River, student.

135. Maria Hodges, 26, d. 20 November 1918, Georges River, housemaid.

136. Margaret McArthur, 59, d. 5 December 1918, Sydney Mines, housewife.

137. John McLean, 22, 5 December 1918, Georges River, labourer.

138. Alexander Ronayze, 17, d. 5 December 1918, Sydney Mines, steel worker. [*His death record gives his surname as Ronayze, but his father Hugh's surname as Roneyze; Book 30, Page 55; Number 323.*]

139. Daniel McPhee, 36, d. 5 December 1918, Sydney Mines, coal miner.

140. John Ronayze, 29, d. 8 December 1918, Sydney Mines, steelworker.

141. Beatrice McLean, 37, d. 8 December 1918, Sydney Mines, housewife.

142. Malcolm McDonald, no age given, d. 8 December 1918, Little Bras D'Or, [*sic*] engineer.

143. M. W. Stewart, male, 35, d. 9 December 1918, Sydney Mines, accountant.

144. Francis Quinn, male, 17, d. 10 December 1918, Sydney Mines, schoolboy.

145. Annie McDonald, 39, d. 11 December 1918, Sydney Mines, housewife.

[*At 146 on the list there is a second entry for Annie Young (see 127), noticed by Dr. Marble on his original list. The numbering is amended in this present list, omitting the repeat entry.*]

146. Eliza Beddow, 19, d. 16 December 1918, Sydney Mines.

147. Catherine M. Boyde, 20, d. 26 November 1918, Sydney Mines, housewife.

148. John J. McLean, 35, d. 26 November 1918, Sydney Mines, locomotive engineer.

149. Mary Cox, 37, d. 27 November 1918, North Sydney, housewife.

150. Edna Barrington, 30, d. 29 November 1918, Sydney Mines, housewife.

151. William Cann, 31, d. 3 December 1918, Sydney Mines, coal miner.

152. Metro Stialchuk, 53, d. 30 October 1918, Sydney Mines, labourer.

153. Charles Holm 55, d. 30 October 1918, Sydney Mines, labourer.

154. Sarah Brewer, 5, d. 3 November 1918, Sydney Mines.

155. Lillian Metcalf, 41, d. 8 November1918, Sydney Mines, housewife.

156. Mrs. M. R. McDonald, 30, d. 15 November 1918, Sydney Mines, housewife.

157. Alfred Lean, 50, d. 19 November 1918, Florence.

158. Mary McKenzie, 24, d. 28 December 1918, Sydney Mines, clerk.

159. Elizabeth Gilbert, 25, d. 27 November 1918, Sydney Mines, housewife.

160. James Brown, 32, d. 18 November 1918, Florence, coal miner.

161. Mary McDonald, 5, d. 18 December 1918, Sydney Mines.

162. Angus Morrison, 19, d. 20 December 1918, Leitches Creek, farmer.

163. Anthony Mososka, 70, d. 25 December 1918, Sydney Mines, labourer.

164. Malcolm Ferguson, 50, d. 10 October 1918, Sydney Mines, electrician.

165. Clarence Bennett, 16, d. 14 October 1918, Sydney Mines, labourer.

166. Mary Keepens, 38, d. 16 October 1918, Little Bras D'Or [sic], housewife.

167. Albert Gooding, 26, d. 21 October 1918, Sydney Mines, steel worker.

168. Mary Long, 26, d. 28 October 1918, Little Bras D'Or [sic], housewife.

169. John Gates, 31, d. 1 December 1918, Glace Bay, miner.

170. Lena Forbes, 20, d. 2 December 1918, Louisbourg, housemaid.

171. Charles Carter, 21, d. 29 November 1918, Glace Bay, soldier.

172. Samile Wareham, 31, d. 1 December 1918, Glace Bay, miner.

173. George Carnell, 62, d. 1 December 1918, Glace Bay, painter.

174. Cyril Rice, 38, d. 1 December 1918, Glace Bay, miner.

175. Joseph Saccary, 18, d. 5 December 1918, Glace Bay, miner.

176. Alex Gillis, 2, d. 4 December 1918, Glace Bay.

177. Mary Campbell, 22, d. 7 December 1918, Glace Bay, housegirl.

178. Francis Chiasson, 2, d. 5 December 1918, Glace Bay.

179. James Corbett, 49, d. 9 December 1918, Dominion, trader. [*Identified as a pool room worker in a second record of his death, Number 228 on Dr. Marble's list.*]

180. Jessie Gilmet, 26, d. 10 December 1918, Glace Bay.

181. Harry Brooks, 28, d. 19 October 1918, Glace Bay, taxi driver.

182. Harriet McDonald, 3, d. 21 October 1918, Glace Bay.

183. John D'Arcy, 30, d. 20 October 1918, Sydney, accountant.

184. Mrs. Susanna Morgan, 36, d. 21 October 1918, Glace Bay, "wife."

185. Mrs. Ellen Livingstone, 38, d. 21 October 1918, Glace Bay.

186. Charles Hawley, 86, d. 23 October 1918, Ingonish, fisherman.

187. Catherine McRitchie, 18, d. 28 October 1918, St. Ann's.

188. Beatrice Brooks, 19, d. 27 October 1918, Glace Bay, housewife.

189. Mrs. Veronica O'Neil, 36, d. 27 October 1918, Glace Bay, housewife.

190. Mrs. Emma McPherson, 50, d. 28 October 1918, New Aberdeen, housekeeper.

191. Bian [sic] Moffatt, (male) 25, d. 31 October 1918, Dominion, clerk.

192. Mary Hayes, 19, d. 31 October 1918, Glace Bay, housewife.

193. James McFarland, 6, d. 6 November 1918, Glace Bay.

194. Rev. Ronald McDonald, 30, d. 3 November 1918, Glace Bay, clergy.

195. Murdoch McPherson, 33, d. 1 November 1918, Glace Bay, no occupation given.

196. Mary Cameron, 36, d. 12 December 1918, Dominion, housewife.

197. Harry Miller, 36, d. 13 December 1918, New Aberdeen, miner.

198. Mrs. Catherine Baker, 41, d. 14 December 1918, Glace Bay, housewife.

199. José Garcia, 5, d. 17 December 1918, Glace Bay.

200. Heather [*Hector N.*] Warren, 20, d. 17 December 1918, Glace Bay, miner. [*Book 30, Page 79, Number 457.*]

201. Jacob Bradbury, 9 months, d. 18 December 1918, Glace Bay.

202. William Wagner, 36, d. 18 December 1918, Dominion, miner.

203. Alice McDonald, 10, d. 19 December 1918, Glace Bay.

204. Mary McNeil, 3, d. 20 December 1918, Glace Bay.

205. Elizabeth Gilday, 4, d. 20 December 1918, Glace Bay.

206. Mary Chiasson, 13 months, d. 21 December 1918, Glace Bay.

207. Zaccho Kerniner, 34, d. 21 December 1918, Glace Bay, miner.

208. John Maxwell, 26, d. 20 December 1918, Glace Bay, clerk.

209. Elsie Chiasson, 31, d. 13 December 1918, Reserve Mines.

210. Clement Gilday, 3, d. 22 December 1918, Glace Bay.

211. Anthony McLeod, 11 months, d. 27 December 1918, Glace Bay.

212. Mrs. Nellie Mobley, 29, d. 29 December 1918, Glace Bay, housewife.

213. Henry Martell, 19, d. 8 October 1918 [*in Sydney, residence in*] Rockdale, Richmond County, soldier.

214. Jean Boudville (female), 22, d. 6 October 1918, Reserve Mines.

215. Kathleen Attwood, 3, d. 12 October 1918, Glace Bay.

216. Morris Long, 45, d. 13 October 1918, Glace Bay, merchant.

217. Francis Peddle, 34, d. 14 October 1918, Glace Bay, sailor.

218. Hector McIntyre, 30, d. 12 October 1918, Glace Bay, trader.

219. Mrs. Isabel Moffatt, 34, d. 16 October 1918, Glace Bay, housewife.

220. Augustus Peck, 32, d. 20 November 1918, Glace Bay, soldier.

221. Emma Anthony, 27, d. 27 November 1918, Glace Bay.

222. Margaret McDonald, 59, d. 29 November 1918, Glace Bay.

223. Mrs. Mary O'Toole, 30, d. 8 November 1918, Glace Bay, housewife.

224. Mabel McLean, 4, d. 10 November 1918, Glace Bay.

225. John Lewis, 50, d. 14 November 1918, Glace Bay, miner.

226. Roberta Norman, 27, d. 13 November 1918, Glace Bay, housewife.

[*The next entry (James Corbett, Number 180) was a repeat of an earlier record, and thus has been eliminated from this present list. Dr. Marble's list notes this is a second record, but keeps the entry.*]

227. Baby Wagner, 16 months, d. 11 December 1918, Dominion.

228. Christena [*sic*] McVarish, 22, d. 22 December 1918, Dominion, tailoress.

229. Veronica Boudreau, 11 months, d. 12 December 1918, Dominion.

230. Mary Cameron, 36, d. 12 December 1918, Dominion, housemaker.

231. Baby Thompson, 13 months, d. 25 December 1918, Dominion.

232. Tressa Simmons, 27 days, d. 12 December 1918, Dominion.

233. George Lahey, 8 months, d. 29 October 1918, Main-a-Dieu.

234. Frank Blanchford, 27, d. 17 October 1918, Marine Hospital, Louisbourg.

235. Earl Corkum, 26, d. 22 October 1918, Marine Hospital, Louisbourg, cook, S.S. *Canadian*.

236. John Hureau, 19, d. 26 December 1918, Arichat. [*This fisherman from Arichat died "on board a vessel" in Cape Breton County waters, thus appears in that county's death register, Book 30, Page 99, Number 549. He resided in Arichat, had been born in Cape Auguet, Richmond County, was a fisherman there, so apparently after his body was sent home for burial, he was also entered in the Richmond County register by error (Book 47, Page 460, Number 985). The HVS Search Engine gives his name as Hurean, to add to the confusion.*]

237. Dennis O'Day, 15, d. 14 December 1918, Port Morien.

238. Annie MacQueen, 19, d. 10 November 1918, New Waterford, clerk.

239. Thomas Dickson, 10, d. 11 November 1918, New Waterford, student.

240. Mary Vallie, 21, d. 24 November 1918, New Waterford, housewife.

241. Dan MacEachern, 7, d. 2 October 1918, New Waterford, student.

242. Harry Brown, 26, d. 29 October 1918, New Waterford, miner

243. Annie Campbell, 8, d. 5 November 1918, New Waterford, student.

244. Margaret Martell, 25, d. 4 December 1918, New Waterford, housewife.

245. Bessie Gillingham, 19, d. 3 December 1918, New Waterford, housewife.

246. Mary MacIsaac, 27, d. 4 December 1918, New Waterford, housewife.

247. Elizabeth Hannan, 4, d. 6 December 1918, New Waterford.

248. Angus Gillis, 47, d. 6 December 1918, New Waterford, carpenter.

249. Andrew Penny, 23, d. 9 December 1918, New Waterford, miner.

250. Peter Campbell, 27, d. 10 December 1918, New Waterford, labourer.

251. Margaret McNeil, 14, d. 12 December 1918, New Waterford, student.

252. Ernest Tugman, 21, d. 14 December 1918, New Waterford, soldier.

253. Therese Martin, 3, d. 15 December 1918, New Waterford.

254. Eliza Beddan [*Eliza A. Beddow*], 19, d. 18 December 1918, New Waterford, housemaid. [*HVS, Book 30, Page 109, Number 590, shows she was Anglican, born in England, and that her father's name was Joseph Beddow. There is a second record in the register for her, as Eliza A. Beddow, in which all particulars are the same, except her residence is shown as Fraser Avenue, Sydney Mines: Book 30, Page 58, Number 339. It has been eliminated from this list as a duplicate.*]

255. Lydia MacDonald, 2, d. 17 December 1918, New Waterford.

256. Genevieve O'Hara, 4, d. 17 December 1918, New Waterford.

257. Ellen Hannigan, 32, d. 19 December 1918, New Waterford, housewife.

258. Mary MacAulay, 32, d. 30 December 1918, New Waterford, housewife.

259. William Murphy, 26, d. 23 October 1918, South Bar, labourer.

260. Mrs. Hallary [*Hillary*] Brown, 28, d. 23 October 1918, New Victoria, housewife. [*Husband's name: Hillary. Book 30, Page 111, Number 600.*]

261. Ignatius Kelly, 11 months, d. 26 October 1918, Lingan.

262. James MacGillivray, 70, d. 29 November 1918, New Victoria, pilot.

263. Tèsere Malguen, 38, d. 5 December 1918, New Waterford, miner.

264. Orville MacGillivray, 28, d. 7 December 1918, New Waterford, clerk.

265. Margaret Petrie, 72, d. 18 December 1918, New Victoria, housework.

266. Charles Devos, 24, d. 19 November 1918, Little Bras D'Or [*sic*], mechanic.

267. Albert McGrath, 19, d. 16 November 1918, Boularderie, miner.

268. William Devos, 63, d. 20 November 1918, Little Bras D'Or [sic], farmer.

269. Walter White, 2, d. 12 October 1918, Little Bras D'Or [sic].

270. Mary Arsenault, 3 hours old, d. 1 November 1918, Little Bras D'Or [sic].

[There was a numbering error here, on Dr. Marble's list; Walter White and Mary had the same number but this has been corrected.]

271. Mrs. Annie Turbide, 31, d. 16 November 1918, Alder Point, housewife.

272. Simon Le Blance [sic], 4 months, d. 28 October 1918, Little Bras D'Or [sic].

273. Mary Le Goff, 2 months, d. 21 November 1918, Alder Point.

274. James A. Powers, 26, d. 14 November 1918, Alder Point, miner.

275. Michael Gillis, 31, d. 12 December 1918, Florence, miner.

276. Elizabeth Vigneau, 66, d. 25 November 1918, Alder Point.

277. Lillian Pero, 12, d. 12 November 1918, Alder Point, student.

278. Hubert Pero, 14, d. 25 November 1918, Alder Point.

279. Emmaline McLennan, 5, d. 12 November 1918, Alder Point.

280. Helen Theriault, 18 months, d. 27 October 1918, Alder Point.

281. Elizabeth Long, 20, d. 19 November 1918, Little Bras D'Or, housewife.

282. Margaret Shephard, 29, d. 18 October 1918, Florence, housewife.

283. Rebecca Bond, 64, d. 2 October 1918, Little Bras D'Or [sic], housewife.

284. Ethel Brown, 2, d. 11 November 1918, Florence.

285. Stephen McNeil, 19, d. 25 December 1918, Shenacadie, farmer.

286. Lizzie McNeil, 22, d. 9 December 1918, Ben Eoin, housework.

287. Elizabeth Chaisson, 31, d. 14 December 1918, Reserve Mines, housewife.

288. Wreathe O'Brien, 3 months, d. 7 December 1918, Gardiner Mines.

289. Sarah Gillis, 1, d. 24 December 1918, Reserve Mines.

290. John Olive, 1, d. 12 January 1919, Reserve Mines.

291. C. McDonald, 45, d. 14 December 1918, Reserve Mines, miner.

292. John McDonald, 8 months, d. 10 December 1918, Dominion.

293. Walter McLeod, 17, d. 24 December 1918, Glace Bay, miner.

1919

294. William Rideout, 5, d. 19 March 1919, North Sydney.

295. Edith Luffman, 6 months, d. 27 March 1919, North Sydney.

296. Lowrie Christie, male, 51, d. 29 March 1919, North Sydney, merchant.

297. Edward Farrell, 9, d. 1 January 1919, N. Sydney, student.

298. Mrs. Wesley Pike, 50, d. 13 March 1919, North Sydney, housewife.

299. Walter Yorke, 10 months, d. 14 March 1919, North Sydney.

300. Frank Holmdees, 29, e. 20 January 1919, Sydney Mines, accountant.

301. Marjorie Chorme, 3, d. 23 January 1919, Sydney Mines.

302. Willis Herald, 48, d. 25 March 1919, Sydney Mines, coal miner.

303. Thomas Porter, 27, d. 25 March 1919, Sydney Mines, labourer.

304. Maria McRae, 76, d. 28 March 1919, Sydney Mines, housewife.

305. Janet Hunter, 29, d. 8 February 1919, Sydney Mines, housewife.

306. Nellie Henderson, 27, d. 13 March 1919, Sydney Mines, housewife.

307. John Henderson, 33, d. 30 March 1919, Sydney Mines, cook.

308. James McLellan, 15, d. 17 February 1919, Glace Bay.

309. Dan McDonald, 35, d. 1 January 1919, Dominion, miner.

310. Mary McDonald, 14, d. 24 December 1918, Glace Bay.

311. Clarence G. Wadden, 3, d. 2 January 1919, Glace Bay.

312. Mrs. Katie MacKie, 30, d. 3 January 1919, Glace Bay.

313. Lydia Paddock, 37, d. 7 January 1919, Glace Bay.

314. Clarence Peters, 4, d. 4 January 1919, Glace Bay.

315. William McDonald, 29, d. 9 January 1919, Glace Bay, machinist.

316. Eileen Vokey, 6 months, d. 12 January 1919, Glace Bay.

317. Rosa Caccebetto, 31, d. 5 March 1919, Dominion, housewife.

318. Sarah Matheson, 70, d. 18 January 1919, Louisbourg, housewife.

319. Charles Lahey, 22, d. 16 March 1919, Main-a-Dieu, fisherman.

320. Catherine MacDonald, 16, d. 7 November 1918, Catalone, student. [Not in HVS database.]

321. Desire Norlea, male, 38, d. 5 December 1918, New Waterford, miner. [Not in HVS database.]

322. Stanley Burke, 11 months, d. 13 January 1919, Lingan.

323. N. A. Young, 5 months, d. 13 March 1919, Little Bras D'Or [sic].

324. Elizabeth Campbell, 75, d. 2 March 1919, Little Bras D'Or [sic], housewife.

325. Elizabeth McInnis, 72, d. 26 March 1919, Balls Creek, housewife.

326. Mary Patterson, 4, d. 23 January 1919, Benacadie.

327. Katie Stewart, 27, d. 10 January 1919, Gabarus, housewife.

328. James Stacey, 38, d. 19 January 1919, Gabarus, fisherman.

329. Dan McDonald, 20, d. 5 April 1919, Mira, farmer.

"To the end of March 1919." [A. Marble note.]

1920

330. Murdena MacLean, 39, d. 10 January 1920, Sydney Mines.

331. William K. McDonald, 45, d. 23 January 1920, Glace Bay, clerk. [Cause of death: "Epidemic Influenza." Book 56, Page 353.]

332. Sarah MacLennan, 68, d. 18 January 1920, Florence.

333. Pete McAskill, 17, d. 29 January 1920, Ben Eoin, labourer.

334. Lucie Sollazzo, 32, d. 18 February 1920, Sydney.

335. Daniel McDonald, 28, d. 25 February 1920, Sydney, street car employee.

336. Adelaide Lewis, 67, d. 17 February 1920, Sydney, housework.

337. Lloyd F. MacKeigan, 15 months, d. 19 February 1920, Sydney Mines.

338. John Pembroke, 32, d. 17 February 1920, Glace Bay, lumberman.

339. Percy L. Frizzell, 31, d. 21 February 1920, Glace Bay, engineer.

340. Elizabeth Angevin, 75, d. 1 March 1920, Sydney, housekeeper.

341. Christy McIntyre, 24, d. 2 March 1920, Sydney, housework.

342. Mary Pancks, 1 year 6 months, d. 8 March 1920, Sydney.

343. Alfred Watkins, 5, d. 8 March 1920, Sydney.

344. Minnie Coombs, 24, d. 8 March 1920, Sydney, housewife.

345. Thomas F. Haley, 2 months, d. 8 March 1920, Sydney.

346. Ida May Gosse, 1 year 6 months, d. 10 March 1920, Sydney.

347. Sarah McLeod, 24, d. 11 March 1920, Sydney, housekeeper.

348. Edward Gould, 39, 12 March 1920, Sydney, chauffeur.

349. Violet Collie, 16 months, d. 12 March 1920, Sydney.

350. Fannie Fidgen, 40, d. 12 March 1920, Sydney, housewife.

351. Daniel Brown, 19, d. 13 March 1920, Mira Road, farmer.

352. Michael Walsh, 1 month, d. 16 March 1920, Sydney.

353. Annie L. Cochran, 53, d. 16 March 1920, Sydney, housekeeper.

354. Mary Delandey, 30, d. 24 March 1920, Sydney.

355. Sernan [*Sennan*] McDonald, 34, d. 13 March 1920, North Sydney, timekeeper. [*1920, Book 56, Page 587*].

356. Maud Horwood, 36, d. 14 March 1920, North Sydney, housework.

357. Patricia Young, 12 days, d. 17 March 1920, North Sydney.

358. Annie Tremblet, 26, d. 30 March 1920, Sydney Mines, housewife.

359. Patrick Sullivan, 75, d. 30 March 1920, Sydney Mines, labourer.

360. Neil McIsaac, 27, d. 17 March 1920, Glace Bay, miner.

361. Effie A. McDonald, 26, d. 22 March 1920, Glace Bay, housework.

362. John E. McCormick, 51, d. 12 March 1920, Dominion, miner.

363. Unidentified Infant, 3 months, d. 15 March 1920, Port Morien.

364. Anastasia Shea, 40, d. 18 March 1920, Port Morien, housewife.

365. John T. Pench, 59, d. March 1920, Port Morien, farmer.

366. Mrs. Mary Jessome, 35, d. 18 March 1920, Little Bras D'Or [*sic*].

367. Elmore D. Coakley, 17, d. 31 March 1920, Florence.

368. Mrs. Annie McLennan, 26, d. 18 March 1920, Benacadie, farmer.

369. Murdena McDonald, 19, d. 4 April 1920, Victoria Mines, teacher.

370. Francis McGillivray, 43, d. 25 April 1920, [*no location*], rail straightener. [*1920, Book 57, Page 21, has "Francis M. McGillivray, 73 Esplanade, Sydney." HVS Search Engine has him as McGillvray.*]

371. Michael McKinnon, 67, d. 19 April 1920, North Sydney, farmer.

372. Josie McNeil, 17 months, d. 1 April 1920, Sydney Mines.

373. Mrs. Maud Cameron, 28, d. 1 April 1920, Sydney Mines, housewife.

374. William Martin, 35, d. 8 April 1920, Sydney Mines, fireman.

375. Alice M. Sheppard, 16, d. 8 April 1920, Glace Bay, housework.

376. Norman McIntyre, 20, d. 26 April 1920, Glace Bay, watchman.

Chapter V

COLCHESTER COUNTY

IN COLCHESTER COUNTY, there were at least fifty confirmed deaths from the Great Influenza; forty-six between 1918 and 1919, plus five more deaths in 1920.

The Colchester Historeum has made a collection of obituaries from local newspapers. Archivist Ashley Sutherland kindly sent those from 1918 through 1920, with the influenza deaths marked. As you read through them, keep in mind that they are given chronologically by date of death, not by date of publication. And please note that beginning sometime in October 1918, the *Truro Daily News* began exhibiting some very strange spelling habits: deth, ded, helth offiser, etc. These are transcribed exactly as typeset.

"25th September, p. 1—First mention of Spanish Influenza, and many deaths in New York and of soldiers in military camps," wrote Dr. Allan Marble, making a list of articles found in the *Truro Daily News* about the pandemic. A report of September 30 (p. 4) noted that 149 people had died in Boston during a single 24-hour period, and that "There have been 5 deaths in Sydney and North Sydney last week. 1,200 cases in New Waterford." This same page also carried the first account of influenza deaths with a connection to a Colchester County family, as follows.

A FORMER TRURO FAMILY IN GRIEF

Word has been received by Mrs. Charles Biswanger, Prince Street, East Truro, that her two nieces, Mrs. W. E. Wilson and her sister, Miss Muriel Biswanger, of Dorchester, Mass., had died on Sept. 18th and 25th from the dread "Influenza" which is so prevalent in the New England States at present.

Truro Daily News, 30 September 1918, 4. Courtesy the Colchester Historeum.

By October 2, the newspaper was publishing material from the public health office; the one in this issue had a description of influenza symptoms. On October 7, there was an account of all the "Truro nurses going to Boston to provide nursing services during the Spanish Influenza" (p. 6). Truro itself was mobilizing (p. 8): "Truro Board of Health takes action. It was decided to prepare the Willow Street Hospital for patients...A few cases have appeared in Truro, and they are severely quarantined." The Great Pandemic had arrived in the city. By October 9, however, the paper announced that only six cases had been reported (p. 1). Things began to seem manageable, but sadly, things were not.

FLU IN TRURO
Helth Offiser [*sic*] reports. 6 New Cases in Truro, with three more deths [*sic*], children, at the Indian Reservation.

Do not go into crowds.

Do not get in Drafts.

Keep your homes aired, thoroly [*sic*] aired.

Truro Daily News, 17 October 1918, 4.

☞ The HVS Death Register for Colchester County, 1918, gives the names of those three Mi'kmaw children above, as well as another one who had succumbed prior to this date. They were the first to die on the Millbrook Reserve, but sadly, they were not the last.

☞ Peter Cope, aged 6 weeks, Indian Reserve [Millbrook, Truro District]; died October 11, Spanish Influenza and Pneumonia, ill 1 week. Listed as "Indian" in death register. His father was Alex Cope. He was born and died on the Indian Reserve and there was buried. No undertaker was used. Doctor was H. V. Kent. The return was made by Joseph Gould, October 11. This child died on October 11, but wasn't entered in the register until after the other children who died October 16–17, below.

HVS Death Register, Colchester County, Year 1918, Book 32, Page 88, Number 331.

☞ Sarah Glode, aged 5, Indian Reserve [Millbrook, Truro District]; died October 16, 1918, Influenza and Pneumonia, ill 1 week. Listed as "Indian" in death register. Her father was James Glode. A Roman Catholic, she lived and died on the Reserve, and then was buried there. Death caused by Influenza/Pneumonia Broncho. The doctor's name was H. V. Kent, the undertaker was J. C. B. Olive. Person returning the information: Joseph Gould, October 17, 1918.

HVS Death Register, Colchester County, Book 32, Page 87, Number 323.

☞ Catherine Elizabeth Glode, 17 months, Indian Reserve [Millbrook, Truro District]; died October 16, 1918, Influenza and Pneumonia, ill 6 days. Listed as "Indian" in death register. Her father was James Glode. A Roman Catholic, she lived and died on the Reserve, and then was buried there. Death caused by Influenza/Pneumonia Broncho. The doctor's name was H. V. Kent, the undertaker was J. C. B. Olive. Person returning the information: Joseph Gould, October 17, 1918.

HVS Death Register, Colchester County, Year 1918, Book 32, Page 87, Number 324.

Adelaide Thomas, aged 2 years, Indian Reserve [Millbrook, Truro District]; died October 17, 1918, Influenza and Pneumonia, ill 6 days. Listed as "Indian" in death register, Adelaide was born on the Indian Reserve, Truro. Her father was Michael Thomas. She was 2 and a half years old when she died. The doctor's name was H. V. Kent, the undertaker was J. C. B. Olive. Person returning the information: Joseph Gould, October 17, 1918.

HVS Death Register, Colchester County, Year 1918, Book 32, Page 87, Number 325.

 INFLUENZA IN TRURO
2 New Cases on 18th.
2 New Cases on 19th.
1 Deth J. N. Hunt of Digby Co. [died in Truro, October 18].

Truro Daily News, 19 October 1918, 4.

 The HVS, Colchester County Death Register, 1918, Book 32, Page 118, Number 469, shows that Jacob Nelson Hunt of Smiths Cove, Digby County, died in Truro on October 18, with cause of death listed as "Pneumonia—Lobar." He had been ill for sixteen days. His body was returned to Smiths Cove for burial. He was a Baptist. Dr. Dunbar attended; J. C. B. Olive was the undertaker who prepared him for the return to Digby County. (The registrar at this time was A. B. Fletcher.)

 Oct. 28. The remains of Mr. Lyle Carrol [Carroll] arrived here on the 21st [death date unknown, but prior to October 21] from Montreal. Mr. Carrol was the son of William Carroll, Lornvale, and had been married only six months ago. His death was due to pneumonia as a result of Influenza. A large funeral cortege met the remains at the Station, and proceeded to the Cemetery. The sorrowing wife accompanied the remains home.

Truro Daily News, 31 October 1918, 2.

 See below for a second notice one week later.

 DIED IN TORONTO
Lyall Carroll, of Londonderry died quite suddenly of Influenza at Toronto last week [date unknown, but prior to October 21]. The remains were taken to his old home for burial. He leaves a wife, a bride of a few months, formerly Miss Violet Cox, also of Londonderry, but who resided in New Glasgow, for a time.

Truro Daily News, 7 November 1918, 10.

THE LATE MRS. GORDON SCOTT

[Extracted from] *Herald Democrat*, Leadville, Colorado, Oct. 23.
It was a sad concourse of friends who gathered at 3.30 yesterday afternoon at the home of Gordon R. Scott to attend funeral services for his late wife, whose death Saturday of pneumonia, when she was in the prime of life, 24 years old, was one of the saddest which has occurred since the present serious epidemic began. Because of the epidemic, the funeral services were private and under the board of health's ruling only members of the household and relatives were permitted to gather indoors, but a large number of friends stood on the lawn while the services were carried out within the house, and at their conclusion drove to the A.O.U.W cemetery in carriages behind the hearse....Mr. Scott is a well-known mining leaser.
Truro Daily News. 9 November 1918, 10.

☞ Mrs. Scott died of pneumonia, but arising out of an influenza epidemic, according to this report. This is evidence of how influenza/pneumonia deaths often were reported solely as pneumonia deaths, both in Canada and the United States. It is not known what Mr. Scott's connection with Colchester County was. His wife was from Colorado. Mrs. Scott died circa October 21.

NOTES FROM GREAT VILLAGE

The terrible epidemic of Influenza that has visited our land has also touched our Village, but we are glad, to note all cases have recovered excepting Miss Viola Copp, whose young life was full of promise, developed pneumonia and after one week's illness passed from her earthly to her Heavenly Home. Although all that was done that could be done to save her by loving hands good nurses and Doctors, passed from our midst on Tuesday A.M. Oct. 22nd.
Truro Daily News, 8 November 1918, 8. Courtesy the Colchester Historeum, Truro. HVS, 1918, Book 32, Page 105, Number 396. Viola May Copp, daughter of George Copp, died of Influenza/Pneumonia, ill 10 days.

MISS B. FRASER DIED TUESDAY AT SHAWINIGAN FALLS

Miss Beatrice Fraser, for nine years a teacher of piano on the staff of the Mount Allison Conservatory of Music, passed away at Shawinigan Falls, P.Q., on Tuesday morning the 22nd, a victim of pneumonia. She had been ill a fornight [*sic*] before her demise, with the prevailing influenza.

After resigning her connection with the Ladies' College staff last spring she accepted a clerical position in the employ of one of the manufacturing concerns located about the great power plant at Shawinigan Falls. Miss Fraser was a most popular and successful teacher. She was a graduate of the Mount Allison Conservatory of Music. Pupil of Mrs. Allan Lewis Seymour, and Dr. Percy

Goetschius, at the Institue of Musical Arts, New York, and of Wager Swayne, Paris. [*sic*]

In addition to her thorough musical education, she had unusual skill in interesting her pupils. She was appreciated by her pupils and fellow teachers, not only for her high character and sterling integrity but was beloved by a wide range of friends for her unselfish interest in others and her rare intellectual and social charm. [Taken from the] *Sackville Tribune,* Oct. 24.

Truro Daily News, 26 October 1918, 5. Courtesy the Colchester Historeum, Truro.

SAD NEWS OF THE DETH [*sic*] OF MISS BEATRICE FRASER

Friends were indeed shockt [*sic*] yesterday, when they heard the sad news of the quite sudden deth at Shawinigan Falls, Quebec, of Miss Beatrice (Betty) Fraser from the prevailing epidemic, Spanish Influenza. Miss Fraser for some time has been on the Staff of this big Company [*sic*] that has important electro-Chemical industries connected with the War. No more popular girl every [*sic*] lived than the deeply lamented Beatrice Fraser.

She was an expert musician and for some time was on the Staff of the Consertory [*sic*] of Music at the Mount Allison Ladies College.

In the immediate family there survive in Halifax, the Mother, Mrs. R. D. Fraser, and three sisters, Miss Mary Fraser, Miss Flo Fraser, Matron at Military Hospital, and Edith, Mrs. Kent, wife of Capt. Harry A. Kent, overseas; and three brothers, William S. Fraser, in Cable Office in Ma illa [Manilla]; Dr. Lewis, F., Fraser [*sic*], of C.M.C., France, and Gunner Leveson Fraser, Canadian Siege Battery, France.

The remains will arrive in Truro by No 4, Express Maritime tomorrow, Thursday at 1,25 p.m. and the funeral will take place from St. Johns Church immediately on arrival of this Express.

Truro Daily News, 23 October 1918, 4. Transcribed exactly as printed. Courtesy the Colchester Historeum, Truro.

YOU MUST COMPLY WITH THE LAW

Lawas [*sic*] are made in the interest, and for the protection of the people at large. Our Board of Helth on account of the prevalence of Influenza, ordered all eating p.aces [*sic*] and Café's to be closed at 10 o'clock p.m. One establishment disregarded this by-law and the result was a fine in Stipendiary Crowe's Court of $15 or 30 days in jail. The fine was paid.

Truro Daily News, 23 October 1918, 4. Transcribed as printed. Courtesy the Colchester Historeum, Truro.

INDIANS AND THE 'FLU'
A meeting of the Board of Health was held at the Civic Building last night to decide as to the Policy of taking care of Indians stricken with influenza, at the Truro Emergency Hospital. In view of the Indians being wards of the Dominion Government, with a government appointed and paid Medical Practitioner to tend them in sickness, and a Government Agent, located here, whose government specified duties are to care for them in need and sickness, the costs for which are authorized by the Government, and as the Property of the Present Hospital Staff is to its limit, it was decided to not admit Indians to the Hospital. Miss McIntosh, trained Nurse of New Annan, is in Charge of the Hospital and with Miss Lynds, of Truro, assistant.

Truro Daily News, 23 October 1918, 3. Courtesy the Colchester Historeum, Truro.

INFLUENZA IN TRURO
We have but one new case to report yesterday and no new cases up to noon today. The obliging Helth Offiser [*sic*] keeps the public informd of this epidemic, as fast as the cases are reported to him, and we hope there is no delay in these daily report. When the public are taken into the confidence of the Helth authorities, when any epidemic is raging, we invariably find that the strict Helth Regulations, are better heeded. Let us know fully about this Inflluenza [*sic*] and the success that is being met with in combatting the disease.

Truro Daily News, 23 October 1918, 4. Transcribed exactly as printed. Courtesy the Colchester Historeum, Truro.

ANOTHER TRURO DEATH FROM INFLUENZA.... 88 CASES SO FAR IN THE TOWN
TRURO, October 26...At the Indian reserve, three miles south of here, there have been four deaths. The situation there has been much improved lately, there having been no new cases for three days.

Halifax Evening Mail, 28 October 1918, 1.

☞ The Nova Scotia Department of Public Health bulletin below was published in one form or another, completely or partially, all across the province. The first part appears in the Annapolis County chapter. The following is another excerpt published in the *Truro Daily News.*

EPIDEMIC INFLUENZA
(Issued by the Department of the Public Health, Nova Scotia).
It cannot be too strongly urged that safety lies particularly in avoiding close association with those who are ill, and, as many cases are mild and strongly

resemble ordinary colds, those who have colds should be kept at a distance. The infective agent is given off in the discharges from throat and nose, and in the fine spray which is ejected in the acts of coughing, sneezing and loud talking. Such sprays is [sic] ejected to a distance of from four to five feet. Keep out of its range.

Truro Daily News, 23 October 1918. Courtesy the Colchester Historeum, Truro.

SAMUEL L. WALKER DIED IN LOS ANGELES, OCTOBER 24

The deth [sic] occurred at Los Angeles, California, on October 24 of Samuel L. Walker, youngest son of Catherine M. Walker and the late Fred Walker. The deceased was formerly a native of Gay's River, but has resided in California for the past ten years. Following an attack of Influenza pneumonia developed and he died in a hospital. This young man was but 29 years of age, and leaves a sorrowing wife, who was very ill at home, with the same disease at the time of her husband's death; also three children to mourn their loss.

Truro Daily News, 22 November 1918, page 2. Courtesy the Colchester Historeum, Truro.

SAD NEWS OF THE DETH [sic] OF MISS MAGGIE MCCULLOCH

Friends were indeed shockt [sic] yesterday morning, when they heard the sad news of the sudden deth, at North Noel Road, of Miss Maggie McCulloch, from pneumonia, after Spanish Influenza. She had been at her sister's at East Noel Road [Mrs. Daniel Page], returning home on Friday morning, and passed away Friday night at 11 o'clock [25 October], at the age of sixteen....Miss McCulloch leaves to mourn a sorrowing father and mother, six brothers and five sisters. The brothers are Stephen, Alonzo, Harry, Everett, Milton and William; the sisters are Mrs. Mabel Weeks, and Blanche and Susie at home; Mrs. Robert Page of Rawdon, who came Sunday to attend her sister's funeral, and Mrs. Daniel Page, East Noel Road, who was sick and couldn't attend her sister's funeral. [Perhaps she had influenza as well.]

Because of the Board of Helth [sic] ruling, only the immediate family were permitted to attend the services in the house, but many neighbors and friends were present, remaining in the open air near by, to pay their last tribute of respect to the departed one. The funeral service was conducted by the Rev. Mr. Milligan of Kennetcook.

Truro Daily News, 30 October 1918, 3. Courtesy the Colchester Historeum, Truro.

C.G.R. FIREMAN JOSEPH WORK DIED OCTOBER 26TH 1918, TRURO N.S.

At the Hospital, Truro, N.S., there occurred October 27th [sic], the death of C.G.R. Fireman Joseph Work [Works], son of Mr. and Mrs. James Work [Works],

Harmony Road, Col. Co., N. S. The deceased was ill eleven days suffering with pneumonia.

Truro Daily News, 28 October 1918, 8. Courtesy the Colchester Historeum, Truro.

 Note the two different death dates in the same article. HVS, 1918, Book 32, Page 92, Number 349 has his death date as October 26. He lived on Queen Street, Truro; his father was James. This man has two records, both in the Colchester County Register, the second, on Page 93, Number 357, is an error: "Same as 349," it says, but with less information. In both records, the family name is "Works," not "Work." So: his name was Joseph Works, father James Works. It's not clear whether influenza contributed to his death, but it seems likely.

LIFE LOST AS NOBLY AS IF ON BATTLE FIELD
Halifax, N.Y. [*sic*] Oct. 29

Mayor Hawkins [of Halifax] has received word of the death at Brockton, Mass., of Miss Nellie A Gray [prior to October 29], of this city [Truro] who was one of the party of nurses sent from here to help in the fight against the Spanish influenza epidemic in Massachusetts. Miss Gray, who had planned to return to her home this week, contracted influenza when sewing at a field tent hospital near Brockton.

Truro Daily News, 31 October 1918, 3. Courtesy the Colchester Historeum, Truro.

DEEP AFFLICTION IN A BROOKSIDE FAMILY

A few days ago, Mrs. Angus McKenie [McKenzie], Brookside, was called to the bedside of her daughter, Mrs. McGinty at Moncton. Yesterday word was received that Mrs. McGinty had passed away, and that her husband was very low with Spanish Influenza. Nine children are left to mourn a kind mother. The eldest is but fifteen years, and we are informed many of the children are sick with Influenza.

Mrs. McKenzie has been a mother in Israel to any sick in her own community, and it is to be hoped she will remain immune to this epidemic while ministering to the necessities of this stricken Moncton household, with whom we sympathize.

Truro Daily News, 28 October 1918, 2. Courtesy the Colchester Historeum, Truro.

 Sadly, Mrs. McKenzie came home from New Brunswick infected; the illness then manifested, and she died of influenza only two days after this article appeared.

MRS. ANGUS MACKENZIE, BROOKSIDE, DIES IN EMERGENCY HOSPITAL

The sad news has come to relativs [*sic*] and other friends, that Mrs. Angus MacKenzie of Brookside had died at eight o'clock on the Morning of Oct. 30 at the Emergency Hospital, Willow Street, Truro of pneumonia.

Mrs. MacKenzie had been to Moncton nursing her daughter, Mrs. Owen NcGinnity [McGinty], who later died of Influenza leaving nine small children, and shortly after she arrived at her Brookside home was taken ill, on October 26th, later was taken to Hospital, where she past away after four day's illness.

Truro Daily News, 30 October 1918, 4. Courtesy the Colchester Historeum, Truro.

THE DETH [*sic*] OF CECIL LINGARD

There died October 31, at the Emergency Hospital of Pneumonia, following Flu, Cecil Lingard, aged 17 years. He has been ill for some few days, and was taken sick at his rooms at the Carleton House, Havelock Street. He was a native of Tennecape, Hants County, to which the body was sent for interment.

Truro Daily News, 31 October 1918, 4. Courtesy the Colchester Historeum, Truro.

CHARLES E. GROVES, BORN IN CENTRAL ONSLOW, DIED IN HAVERHILL, MASS

Friends and relatives of Mrs. Annie Lennon will be grieved to hear of the death of her oldest son, Chas. E. Groves in Haverhill, Mass. of influenza, on Nov. 1st, 1918. He was born in Central Onslow, Col. Co. in 1892, and was the son of the late Geo. W. Groves, who died 24 years ago. His mother is a native of Stewiake [*sic*], N.S.

Truro Daily News, 13 November 1918, 1. Courtesy the Colchester Historeum, Truro.

MORRISON. At Cranbrook, B.C. of Spanish Influenza, November 2, Clarence Fletcher Morrison, aged 26 years, formerly of Glenholme, Col. Co.

Truro Daily News, 13 November 1918, 8. Courtesy the Colchester Historeum, Truro.

THE SUDDEN PASSING OF MRS. J. B. LYNN

Exceedingly sad was the word from Ainslie Hospital [Truro] on Sunday morning [November 3] that Eva L. Lynn, wife of J. B. Lynn, had died from pneumonia—after an illness of but seven days....Mrs. Lynn was suffering from influenza that was followed by a sharp attack of pneumonia which is so fatal in this epidemic that is still prevalent over our whole country.

Truro Daily News, 4 November 1918, 4. Courtesy the Colchester Historeum, Truro. HVS, Colchester County, 1918, Book 32, Page 85, Number 309.

Eva Lynn, 24, was born in Brockhurst, Ontario, and died on November 3. Her death record shows the name "Lynn, Ida L." The first name has been crossed out and replaced with only "Eva." The HVS search engine gives her name as "Eva L." Lynn. Despite the newspaper article stating she died of influenza-precipitated pneumonia (see above), cause of death is given merely as "Pneumonia." Not only that, but an adjoining death record (Number 310, later crossed out as a stillbirth), following hers, shows that a male infant of Mr. J. D. Lynn's was stillborn on the same day, November 3. The death is entered merely as "Lynn, infant of J. D." So Mrs. Lynn was in labour when she died, but this is not mentioned on the death certificate, either. Her son never drew his first breath. Mrs. Lynn should be counted as an influenza victim, and perhaps her baby should as well.

Mrs. Angus McKinnon. At the Emergency hospital Willow Street, Nov. 5th, of pneumonia, following Spanish Influenza. Bertha, wife of Angus McKinnon of Queen Street, East, passed away.

> *Truro Daily News*, 5 November 1918, 8. Courtesy the Colchester Historeum, Truro. HVS, 1918, Book 32, Page 85, Number 312. Bertha M. Fisher McKinnon was born in 1858 in Upper Stewiacke.

Catherine Paul, aged 11 years, 8 months, born on and resided at the Indian Reserve [Millbrook, Truro District]; died November 5, 1918, Influenza, length of illness not given. Her father was "J. D. Paul" [John Denny Paul?] The doctor was H. V. Kent. The family were Roman Catholic, and the child was buried somewhere in Truro. Her return was made by Joseph Gould, 6 November.

> HVS Death Register, Colchester County, 1918, Book 32, Page 85, Number 313.

Mrs. David Davis and her two sons, of Five Islands, Colchester County, all came down with influenza. She was 32. Her older boy, Cecil Raymond, was 2 years and 7 months old and her younger son, Bernard, had only just been born. On November 5, 1918, they all died of it. Bernard had lived only two days.

> HVS, 1918, Book 32, Page 208, Numbers 414, 415, and 416.

Pregnant women were the people most at risk from this Influenza.

MRS. J. A. WRIGHT DIED IN VANCOUVER, B.C. NOVEMBER 6
The death occurred Nov. 6 at the family residence, 926 Cotton drive, of Margaret Wright, beloved wife of J. A. Wright, in her 32nd year. Deceased leaves besides her husband, four children, youngest only ten days old....Maggie Annand was born at Pine Grove, Gays River, and came West with the rest of the family when only a little girl. Since her marriage, her husband, home and children absorbed her fully and it looked as if there were still many years of the same happy life, until the Spanish Influenza claimed her as a victim.

> *Truro Daily News*, 20 November 1918, 1. Courtesy the Colchester Historeum, Truro.

THE DEATH OF MRS. ARCHIBALD PHINNEY

fAfter [*sic*] an illness of four weeks from Influenza, there past away at the home residence Lyman Street, Truro, on November 7, Emma A. the beloved wife of Mr. Archibald Phinney, aged 39 years....The funeral will be held Sunday at 2.30 from the home residence.

Truro Daily News, 8 November 1918, 5. Courtesy the Colchester Historeum, Truro.

THE LATE ELISHA R. MILLS, DIED NOV. 10

A Hero of Many Fights Gone to His Rest.

The sad news reached Truro, on the 11th, of the deth at Pugwash, of Elisha R. Mills, son of Mr. and Mrs. McLeod Mills, Victoria Street, Truro, the deth [*sic*] having occurred on Sunday, Nov. 10th..

Truro Daily News, 12 November 1918, 5. Courtesy the Colchester Historeum, Truro. (See Cumberland County chapter for further information.)

DEATH OF WILBERT B. MACDONALD IN TRURO, N.S., NOVEMBER 17TH 1918

The death of Wilbert B. MacDonald aged 22 years at the Willow Street Emergency Hospital, Truro, N.S. on Sunday, November 17th, His deth [*sic*] was due to double pneumonia, following an attack of Influenza. Mr. MacDonald was born in Truro, but has lived in Halifax since 1901. When the war broke out he volunteered in the 63rd Regiment, and rendered excellent service in the Fortress Intelligent [*sic*] Department. He has been in Truro about a year, and was in the employ of the Canadian Government Railway. His father Isaac was connected with the Gents. Furnishing Department of Blanchard Bentley and Co. His mother, (formerly Miss May Bates) moved to Philadelphia about two years ago. She arrived in Truro late Friday night and was with him at the time of his death. He is survived by his parents and one younger brother, Lawrence, who is now in France, with the 17th Reserve Battalion.

Truro Daily News, 18 November 1918, 4. Transcribed exactly as published, including punctuation. Courtesy the Colchester Historeum, Truro.

DEATHS....

Forty cases of Influenza at Londonderry Mines.

Truro Daily News, 25 November 1918, 4. Courtesy the Colchester Historeum, Truro.

THE NEWS FROM LONDONDERRY

Mrs. Moore, an aged resident, died on the 18th and was buried on the 20th. Mrs. Moore, who lived [with] her son, Roger, had been in failing health recently, contracted Influenza, and died quite suddenly....

DEATHS   103

District No. 7   Londonderry N.S. County of Colchester

No. 391   No. 392   No. 393

Death records for Sarah Moore, Hilda Esau, and Barbara Patriquin, Londonderry. *(Nova Scotia Archives)*

Pte. Graham and two little sons, of Halifax, spent a few days last week at the home of his father-in-law, Mr. Dan Gibbs, Lornvale. Pte. Graham's wife was a recent victim of Influenza, at Halifax.

There are about 40 cases of 'flu' in town. Mr. and Mrs. Henry Tattrie, two sons and little daughter, Mabel, are down with it [see below, Chester Tattrie].

Mrs. Delay and four children are also among the number of those afflicted by the disease.

Dr. R. O. Shatford is kept busy with his patients here and in the surrounding vicinity....

Don Soy, son of I. J. Soy, is quite ill with pneumonia.

Chester, the young son of Mr. and Mrs. H. Tattrie, is reported very low with pneumonia following Influenza.

Members of the families of John Patriquin are reported to be laid up with the prevailing epidemic.

Truro Daily News, 27 November 1918, 3. Courtesy the Colchester Historeum, Truro.

Londonderry death records (HVS, 1918, Book 32, Page 391-393) show intriguing causes of death. The "Mrs. Moore," dead of influenza in the previous article, was Sarah Jane Moore (391), a widow, who died on 18 November. Her cause of death is given here as "Bronchitis and Heart Failure," even though the newspaper is quite specific that she had contracted influenza. A schoolgirl, David Esau's daughter Hilda (392), not mentioned by name in the previous article, died December 1, and her cause of death is given as "Influenza/Meningitis." John Patriquin's wife, Barbara Patriquin (393), died of "Influenza and Pneumonia" on December 1st.

All three people had the same physician, Dr. R. O. Shatford, M.D., who, if the newspaper article is correct, diagnosed these three Influenza deaths, all presenting differently, as bronchitis/heart failure, influenza/meningitis, and influenza/pneumonia. This is a good example of how variously the disease could present itself—if it can cause a doctor to diagnose it three separate ways, and in the middle of Londonderry's epidemic status.

DETH [*sic*] OF FRANK MACAULAY AT TRURO NOV. 23RD

The deth [*sic*] of Frank MacAuley, aged 32 years, occurred at the Emergency Hospital, Willow Street, on November 23rd. His home was in East Noel, Hants Co. where the remains were forwarded Monday afternoon for burial. Mr. MacAuley was attack with "Flu" which later develop into pneumonia.

Truro Daily News, 25 November 1918, 4. Transcribed exactly as printed. Courtesy the Colchester Historeum, Truro.

INFLUENZA EPIDEMIC AT LONDONDERRY

Truro, November 30. Influenza is said to be epidemic at Londonderry where forty cases are reported. In the rest of the county the disease is pretty well stamped out. No new cases were reported in Truro today or yesterday. What influenza there is here appears to be of a mild type and there have been no deaths for some time. The provincial normal college will re-open on Monday and the Nova Scotia agricultural college will begin sessions on Tuesday.

Halifax Evening Mail, 2 December 1918, 4. Courtesy the Colchester Historeum, Truro.

DEATH OF HARRY MACKAY ONSLOW N.S. DECEMBER 9TH

The death of Harry Mackay, occurred at his home in Onslow N.S. on December 9th. Aged 33 years and 4 months. His death was due to Influenza, after a weeks illness. He is survived by his wife, formerly Miss Ella McNutt, and two children, Elizabeth and Roy.

Truro Daily News, 10 December 1918, 3. Transcribed exactly as printed, including punctuation. Courtesy the Colchester Historeum, Truro.

BRUCE. Hilden, Col. Co. N.S. December 10th, Mrs. James Bruce, aged 47 years, Death due to Influenza.

Truro Daily News, 11 December 1918, 4. Transcribed exactly as printed, including punctuation. Courtesy the Colchester Historeum, Truro.

DEATH OF MR. DANIEL J. WALSH, DECEMBER 4TH

The death of Daniel J. Walsh, Waddell Street, occurred at the Emergency Hospital, Willow Street, December 4th, at one o'clock in the afternoon. His death was due to pneumonia, following an attack of Influenza, after an illness of a few days. He was thirty-eight years of age, and a native of Newfoundland, coming to Truro about two years ago. He is survived by his wife (formerly Miss Ida Langille, Truro) and one brother, James, in Newfoundland.

Truro Daily News, 5 December 1918, 7. Courtesy the Colchester Historeum, Truro.

 SUDDEN AND SAD

Very sad indeed, was the sudden death from Influenza, of one of our most beloved young girls. Miss Lola Thompson was working in Trenton [Pictou County] at the time [December 6, 1918]. Lola was much loved and respected by all who knew her and her sudden death caused deep sorrow to her many friends. Mr. and Mrs. Malcolm Thompson and family have the sincere sympathy of the community in their sorrow. ["Central New Annan, Col. Co.," says a note added to this photocopy of her death notice.]

Truro Daily News, 3 January 1919. Courtesy the Colchester Historeum, Truro.

The HVS, Pictou County Death Register, 1918, Book 45, Page 370, Number 1303, shows her name as "Leola" Thompson on the original record, and as "Liola" Thompson in the HVS search engine. She was 20, and working in Trenton as a stenographer. On 6 December 1918, she died there of influenza, having been ill only two days. She was buried in New Annan.

 OBITUARY. Miss Estella Mabel Higgins. On December 4th, there passed away at the home of her parents, Mr. and Mrs. Albert Higgins of Belmont, their daughter Estella Mabel, at the early age of 26 years. Miss Higgins had returned home from her school in Canard to spend her Christmas vacation with her parents. An epidemic of influenza that was sweeping over Belmont reached her father's family and laid all low excepting the father....The best medical skill and the most faithful services of a trained nurse failed to arrest the disease.

Truro Daily News, 7 January 1919, 4.

Jennie McLennan [McLellan], aged 17, died at Five Islands on 19 December [*sic*; December 10].

Truro Daily News, 24 December 1918, 2. Courtesy the
Colchester Historeum, Truro.

 MISS JENNIE MCLENNAN [MCLELLAN] DIED AT FIVE ISLANDS
Five Islands, Dec. 17, 1918. An epidemic of influenza has lately scourged our village, and widespread sympathy was aroused by the sad deth of Jennie McLennan, at the early age of 17 years [on 10 December]. Four months ago she came here from her home in Cambridge, Hants Co., to assist Mrs. MacKinley Corbett. Quiet and modest in her deman er [demeanour], she was well-liked and highly respected by all who knew her, and her deth cast a gloom over the whole village. She was one of the first to fall a victim to influenza. Pneumonia set in, and after two weeks of suffering she passed away on Tuesday morning, December 10th.

Although a stranger in a strange land, away from the tender care of loving parents and kind relatives, yet in the home of Mr. and Mrs. Corbett she was as tenderly cared for as a daughter would have been. Mr. and Mrs. Corbett, two doctors, a trained nurse and other friends, did all that human skill could do to overcome the ravages of disease, but without avail.

She was the eldest daughter of Mr. and Mrs. William McLellan, of Cambridge, Hants Co, and leaves a sorrowing father and mother, three sisters and three brothers.

The remains were taken to Cambridge for interment. The large number of sympathetic friends who attended the funeral services there on Thursday afternoon, testified to the high standing of the departed in her own community, and to the sympathy of all for the bereaved family. *Windsor Tribune*.

Truro Daily News, 24 December 1918, 2. Courtesy the
Colchester Historeum, Truro.

☞ This young woman was named McLelland, not McLennan, though each was several times used interchangeably in each newspaper entry. Note also the different death dates in these various articles. The one immediately above is the earliest, and it was published December 17, therefore Jennie couldn't have died on the nineteenth. The Death Register for Colchester County, 1918, clarifies this: "Jennie McLellan, d. December 10th, 1918." But even the registries can be confusing: there appear to be two death records for Jennie. Her return in the Colchester County Register, 1918, Book 32, Page 107, Number 405, states that she was the daughter of Mr. and Mrs. William A. McLellan, and was born in Summerville, Hants County. She was working as a "House Maid" in Five Islands, aged 17, when she died of pneumonia after influenza. A Baptist, she was buried in Cambridge, Hants County. The doctor was T. R. Johnson; Moses Leslie was the undertaker.

Her second death record appears in the Hants County Register, 1918, Book 35, Page 518, Number 480. The information is identical in almost every particular. Her father's name is given as Arthur W. McLelland, perhaps the same man as "William A.," reversed. This gives her residence as Cambridge, Hants County, aged 17, doing "Housework." Her birthplace is given as Kempt Shore. This Jennie had the same doctor during her illness, but the undertaker was one J. C. Bohner. This seems one of those occasions when a person died away from home, and thus one undertaker prepared the body for shipment, and the family used another undertaker to do the burial arrangements after receipt of the remains. Occasionally some confusion resulted, and two death records were returned—usually one from the place of death, the other from the victim's family's county of residence.

SAD DEATHS FROM INFLUENZA

Our little Village was saddened when the news came of the death of three noble young men, who died of the dread disease, 'Flu'.

Fred Chisholm, Highland, died Saturday afternoon at 1 o'clock, December 14th, at the mill camp of W.W. Giddins at Folly Mountain and was buried the same afternoon in Mahon Cemetery, Great Village. He leaves a father, Mr. Avon Chisholm, step mother; two sister, Margaret and Wilenna, and three brothers, Burnham and Judson overseas, and a younger brother, Lou, at home.

Norman Tipping was the next to join the great majority. He passed away Sunday afternoon about 3 o'clock December 15th in the same camp, and was buried Monday afternoon in the Mahom [Mahon] Cemetery.

Stewart Tipping, who was then ill, died since at the home of W. W. Giddin [Giddins], Londonderry Station, Wednesday night, Dec. 18th and was buried Thursday afternoon in the Mahon Cemetery. Miss Boomer, trained nurse, attended him through his sickness.... Great Village, Dec. 23, 1918.

Truro Daily News, 24 December 1918, 7.

NOTES FROM LONDONDERRY STATION. DEC. 21

Stewart Tipping, who was ill with Influenza at the home of W. W. Giddins, where he had been employed, died on the 18th and was buried in the Mahon Cemetery, Gt. Village on the evening of 19th.

This is the second son of Mr. Robert Tipping, Mt. Pleasant, to die of this fatal malady within a week.

Truro Daily News, 29 December 1918, 2. Courtesy the
Colchester Historeum, Truro.

ANOTHER AFFLICTION IN THE JOHN LOCKHART FAMILY

A week or two ago the well-known family of John A. Lockhart, Londonderry, was advised of the sudden deth [sometime in December] of a son, and brother, Edwin, in St. Mary's, Idaho, and on Saturday night last the doubly sad news came to Mr. and Mrs. Lockhart that a daughter, Mrs. Everett Walters of Sussex, N. B., had died of Influenza. In the immediate family Mrs. Walters leave husband and a little son, 18 months old. The deceased, formerly Miss Laura Lockhart, was well known in Truro, where she lived for six or seven years.

Truro Daily News, 23 December 1918, 4. Courtesy the
Colchester Historeum, Truro.

THE PASSING OF MISS IRENE SUTHERLAND
(Tribute by a friend)

River John Road, N.S. Dec. 23rd. A gloom was cast over the community on the 21st Inst., by the death of Miss Irene Sutherland, second daughter of Mr. Kenneth Sutherland in the sixteenth [seventeenth] year of her age. Death due to pneumonia following an attack of Spanish Influenza.

Truro Daily News, 27 December 1918, 7. Courtesy the
Colchester Historeum, Truro.

Relying on Unreliable Records

⟝⟞ The time that it took to confirm the fate of Irene Maggie Sutherland was one of the longest and most circuitous, and it shows just how even the official records that we rely on are full of inconsistencies. Irene was born in Pictou County on 25 March 1901. Her father, "William Hugh Sutherland" on the birth-record information provided by his wife, was a farmer on Mountain Road, and had died by 1944, when his wife, Hannah (née Sutherland) Sutherland, applied for her child's birth certificate. Hannah was living at the time at 251 Duncan Street in Moncton, NB, and she stated that her husband, William Hugh, was deceased. She doesn't give his death date, or whether they had moved to New Brunswick before he died. The only problem with that information, provided by the widow, is that elsewhere (newspaper death notice and death record) Irene Sutherland's father is called Kenneth, not William Hugh.

Now the only Kenneth Sutherland I found from that Pictou County area died in 1959 (Death Register, 1959, Page 2382), and I had searched a broad range of dates from all counties. The husband of Hannah, whether called William Hugh or Kenneth or both, died before October 10, 1944, the date of Hannah Sutherland's application to register the birth of her child. Perhaps the reason I can't find his death certificate is that he died in New Brunswick.

☞ Dale Swann, North Shore Heritage Society's archivist, says that in that area, people were often given nicknames or alternate names by the community, usually to differentiate them from others of that name, and there were certainly other Hugh Sutherlands alive then. Mr. Swann says that these names were even carved on their tombstones at times. Perhaps William Hugh was familiarly called Kenneth. This was confirmed by Ashley Sutherland, archivist at the Colchester Historeum.

Dale Swann to Ruth Whitehead and Janet Baker, personal communication, 11 May 2019.

☞ Let's return to the Irene Maggie who was born in Nova Scotia in 1901. It seemed odd, even considering the William Hugh and the Kenneth-named father, that there would be two Sutherland children named Irene, of approximately the same age, living in the same area as Mountain Road and the River John Road, which lie on either side of the Pictou/Colchester County line. Just in case there were, I checked the birth registers. I could only find one birth certificate for an Irene Sutherland born in Nova Scotia in 1901. I searched the records for 1890–1960: there were only two Irene Sutherlands and none of that name born previous to 1901. The only other one, Irene H. Sutherland, was born 16 years later in Halifax County, and died 16 months later of Pulmonary Tuberculosis. Her father was Roy Sutherland, a teamster born in Halifax, and her mother's name was Margaret Cossens. The family was Roman Catholic, and lived at 5 Brenton Street, Halifax. This is not our Irene. See HVS, Birth Register, Halifax County, 1917, Page 51900524, Number 51900525 and HVS, Death Register, Halifax County, 1918, Book 21, Page 460, Number 2757, father Roy Sutherland.

Here is our Irene: the child of the birth certificate filed by mother Hannah, and the young girl of the death certificate are one and the same person. That girl was named Irene Maggie Sutherland. In order to make sense of Irene Maggie's life, all we have to go on are this birth certificate, listed in the HVS search engine as filed in the 1904 register and, of course, the death record and newspaper death notice.

Let's look at the birth record first which was put in the 1904 register instead of the 1901 birth register because, back then, late applications were put in the next available blank space in the registers after the birth or death, regardless of the passage of time. Registrars sometimes left spaces blank on a six-person columned page, if they next received a packet of death returns from a different part of their district, before completing a page. They wanted a new town or village to have a page all its own. This happened rather a lot in the years before the First World War caused a paper shortage, and the Great Influenza began flooding their offices with returns.

Here's the strange part: the application is on a printed form and signed by Hannah Sutherland, who had to swear she was the mother of the child in front of a notary public. This printed form had a space for *Year of Application* that had been pre-printed as "194_," and which Hannah Sutherland herself filled in by adding a 4, making 1944. On a previous section of the form not pre-printed, she wrote the year 1944 in ink, in full. This means she applied to get her daughter a birth certificate twenty-six years after Irene had died. As a further confirmation that 1944 is correct for the year of application, the District Commissioner who later signed off on receipt of this application (name illegible, but it might be J. (or G. or F.) S. Cossens) was a commissioner under revision to an earlier law mentioned on the form title—"Chapter 5, Section 38, of the Revised Statutes, 1923." This is printed under his signature, as part of the form: HVS, Pictou County Birth Register, 1904, Page 92707443. Applied for forty-three years after Irene Sutherland's birth, on a form reading "PROVINCE OF NOVA SCOTIA / APPLICATION FOR REGISTRATION OF BIRTH / Under the Vital Statistics Act, 1923." Vital Statistics Act, RSNS 1923, c 20, pages 38-51. In handwriting, vertically, in the right the margin, he again gives his name and another title when he writes, "Filed October 25/44, J. S. Cossens, Deputy Registrar Colchester." So why apply so late? Irene would have been 43 years old in 1944 had she still been alive. We don't know any more than that.

At the time of her death, our Irene Sutherland was living on the River John Road in Colchester County, District of Waugh's River, just a few kilometers from where she had been born. Was she living with her parents then, or with relatives, perhaps working there? In any event, she died there on December 21. Her death record informant was a Lawrence Sutherland, not her mother or father. Maybe they'd gone to New Brunswick by then, or they had influenza and were unable to do it. In the end, all we really know for sure is that an Irene Sutherland, 17, of River John Road, became ill with influenza on December 10, 1918, and then died on December 21. A Doctor Gass attended, G. B. McLellan was the undertaker, and a Lawrence Sutherland sent in the death record on 9 January 1919. She was a Presbyterian and her body was buried in Waugh's River. She died the same year as baby Irene Sutherland in Halifax did.

HVS, Colchester County, Death Register, 1918, Book 32, Page 102, Number 389.

⊂⊃ Dale Swann, speaking of the local undertaker of that time, Mr. George B. McLellan, had this little story to relate about him. Mr. McLellan, he said, had a casket storage room in Tatamagouche, in a building which for the last twenty years has housed a pizza parlour. In 1918, McLellan had overseen the burials of Irene Sutherland and Gordon Millard, both flu victims.

Mr. Swann was told a story by two brothers who had been young during this period. They were talking about when their grandmother had died, and Mr. McLellan came. Their mother sent the younger children outside the house while the undertaker prepared the body. "They were told to leave the house, and not to come back in until they were called in. And Mr. Johnny McLeod was there; he ran the store in Denmark....And they were allowed back in the house eventually—one tried [to go back in], and his mother tapped on the window, 'No!' And when they came in, a truck had arrived, and Granma was in her casket. And they didn't understand."

He said that these two little brothers had gone down by the drain, when they were outside, waiting, "...and all of a sudden, some red water come out. And they didn't have a clue." One of the brothers had told Mr. Swann that years later, something triggered this memory, of the red water in the drain, and for the first time he had put it all in context.

Of course, those dying of influenza, like Irene Sutherland and Gordon Millard, couldn't be embalmed. Their bodies were required to be buried within twenty-four hours of death. Those attending to this had to keep any contact to a bare minimum.

Colchester County Deaths Continued

"FLU" IN BROOKFIELD
Suburban Brookfield is suffering from the epidemic of Influenza. It is in quite violent form. Report says a man and two children have died in a lumber camp in Upper Brookfield. They are near [New?] Brunswick people, who have been lumbering in the Brookfield woods. Little Charlie Boomer, a bright lad of some 10 years, was taken down with this disease and soon succumbed to the attack; and to add to the family affliction the father of this boy, Mr. Willard Boomer, well known in Truro, as a painter and paper-hanger, died a few days later in Hospital in Halifax from this same epidemic.

Truro Daily News, 24 December 1918, 2.

The HVS, Colchester County Death Register, 1918, Book 32, Page 118, Number 467, shows Charles Edward Boomer died on December 17, 1918, aged 9. His father, "William," was a "decorator" which is apparent because under "Occupation" of the dead person, someone mistakenly described his father's occupation. His mother's name was Grace—she sent in the return of death. The HVS, Halifax County Death Register, Book 25, Page 54, Number 323, shows Willard Boomer died on December 19, in Halifax.

Look at the entry dates (below)! This Colchester County Death Register is all over the map in Book 32, page 118:

- Number 464, Freda Wetherby, died of influenza/pneumonia on March 6, 1919.

- Number 465, Loran Harvey, died of old age on March 10, 1919.

- Number 466, Martha [Myrtle] Douthright, died 25 December 1918.

- Number 467, Charles Edward Boomer, pneumonia on December 17, 1918.

- Number 468, Emma McKenzie, died of influenza on October 30, 1918.
- Number 469, Jacob Nelson Hunt, died of pneumonia on October 19, 1918.

HVS Death Register, Colchester County, 1918, Book 32, Page 118, Number 466.

Searching Undertakers' Ledgers

👉 Undertakers' ledgers are a useful source of information for these pandemic years. An examination of Olive's ledger book shows Myrtle "Douthwright" of Upper Brookfield, dying December 21,1918, *of influenza*. She was Roman Catholic, and an E. W. Douthwright ordered the body shipped to "Riverdale, Albert County, N.B." for burial. There are seven gravestones for Douthwrights in the Roman Catholic cemetery in Riverside-Albert, NB, but she herself does not appear to have a tombstone there. E. W. Douthwright also paid for her casket and shipping.

Nova Scotia Archives, "Olive Funeral Records & Ledgers, 1899-1927," mfm # 9236. Findagrave New Brunswick, Albert County, Riverside-Albert cemetery.

👉 Could Martha/Myrtle Douthwright be one of the anonymous New Brunswick people at Brookfield, mentioned in the above newspaper article? Was it her husband and two children whose deaths are described? When I went searching for others of that surname in the death register, I found people with variants of the name. Gaps in the data for Martha/Myrtle leave her husband's first name unknown, although the death record says she was married. Her name was spelled "Douthright" in the record, but the undertaker seems to have the correct spelling—"Douthwright"—as he was paid by an in-law of that name. Myrtle, however, is definitely connected to this story, both by her date and place of death, and the fact that she was returned to "Riverdale, Albert County, New Brunswick" for burial. J. C. B. Olive records that she died of influenza, and his firm shipped the body.

Next, I found "Douchwright, Lewis Edward," according to the HVS search engine, although the surname "Douthwright" appears on the original record. Also, on the original record, the man's first name appears to me to be Laurie, not Lewis. He was 30 years old, married, a lumberman, born in Little River, NB. Little River actually has a "Douthwright Cemetery," on Highway 895 (*GPS coordinates: 45.95821N -64.96829W*), but this man does not have a gravestone there. Laurie Douthwright died in Brookfield on December 20, 1918, from influenza. The same E. W. Douthwright ordered his casket from J. C. B. Olive. His place of burial wasn't given on the death record, but undertaker Olive says his body was shipped back to New Brunswick to be buried in "Riverside, Albert County."

HVS, Colchester County Death Registry, 1918, Book 32, Page 96, Number 373. findagrave.com/cemetery-browse/Canada/New-Brunswick/Albert-County/ Little-River?id=city_542660. Nova Scotia Archives, "Olive Funeral Records & Ledgers, 1899-1927," mfm # 9236.

☞ This man's return was sent in by a "Mary Gladys Douthwright" on December 30, 1918. Now if Myrtle was his wife, she died the day after he did. Is his return being written by a relative, stepping in to take care of things after this couple became ill? Or is Mary Gladys Douthwright Laurie's wife?

☞ The *next* death record I found added more variables. This was the death record of a small boy, Vernon Duthwright, age 1 year, who died on December 17, 1918, before either Myrtle Douthright or Laurie Douthwright. Vernon's record says his father was named "Laurance Duthwright." This child had been born in Colbert, Colchester County, NS, but he has no birth record. Vernon Duthwright died of "pneumonia," and the same E. W. Duthwright sent in his return on December 18. If Myrtle and Laurie were Vernon's parents, they were probably too ill themselves to do it, as they both died shortly thereafter.
HVS, Colchester County Death Registry, 1918, Book 32, Page 96, Number 372.

☞ According to J. C. B. Olive, the undertaker, this same E. W. Douthwright, ordered the coffins for both Laurence and Myrtle Douthwright and arranged for the shipping of the bodies. He or she also provided the information for the death record of Vernon Douthwright. I think E. W. Douthwright is possibly *Lewis/Laurie/Laurance/ Laurence*'s father, and maybe Mary Gladys is the mother. They were all obviously related.

I did not find a second Douchwright/Duthwright/Douthright child. A second child did die in Brookfield during this time, but she died three days after the above newspaper article was published. Her name was Lillian Rolands. She was only 1 month old and died on December 27, 1918, from influenza, after an illness of only three days. Her death record says her father's name was G. Rolands. Her return of death was sent in by a "Nellie M. Foster" on the same day, December 27. There had been no doctor in attendance. Undertaker was Herbert Boomer. The HVS search engine gives her name as "Rowlands, Lillian U.," whereas on the original it is "Rolands, Lillian Williams."
HVS, Colchester County Death Register, 1918, Book 32, Page 115, Number 451.

More Colchester County Deaths

THE LATE MRS. JOHN E. HILL
Sad was the news at this Yuletide to the home of Mr. John E. Hill, Halifax, formerly of Onslow, when the word came that his wife on the evening of December 3 [December 30] had died at the home of her parents, Mr. and Mrs. William Cail, Economy, where she was spending the Christmas holidays. The cause of death was

pneumonia, following an attack of influenza, which she contracted at Economy. She was twenty-five years of age, and had been married but a few months.

Truro Daily News, 3 January 1919, 4. Courtesy the Colchester Historeum, Truro.

☞ The death date above seems an error and the age of Mrs. Hill is contradicted in her obituary.

OBITUARY. In early life from the world of strife there passes to the great beyond following a brief illness of Spanish Influenza and pneumonia the spirit of the late Mrs. John E. Hill, who died Monday, December 30 at the age of 27 years.

Truro Daily News, 8 January 1919, 4. Courtesy the Colchester Historeum, Truro.

☞ The HVS, Colchester County Death Register, 1918, Book 32, Page 107, Number 406, shows "Mrs. John E. Hill" (her husband's name was John Erskine Hill); they were Presbyterians. She died at Upper Economy; her father William Cail sent in the return of death. She was 25, he stated, and had died on December 30 of "Spanish Flu/Pneumonia," after an illness of two days. She had been born at Pleasant Hills, Colchester County. The body was buried in "Cemetery/Economy."

DIED OF INFLUENZA—A VERY SAD CASE

Mrs. Fred C. Manning, Falmouth, went to Sussex [New Brunswick] with her only child, Ruth, aged nearly four years, to spend Christmas with her parents, Rev. and Mrs. J. L. Tingley, formerly of Brookfield. The little girl took influenza and died [sometime in December 1918]. Mrs. Manning was so ill with influenza that her husband could not leave her to bring the remains of their child home, so the body was brought by the Rev. Mr. Tingley and interred in the Falmouth Cemetery.

Truro Daily News, 8 January 1919, 8. Courtesy the Colchester Historeum, Truro.

Word from Truro tells of the death there [on December 31, 1918] of Mrs. Vernon, who was formerly Miss Annie Dodson of New Glasgow, and daughter of the late A. Dodson. She was best known here when a little girl, and since leaving New Glasgow she had grown into beautiful womanhood, beloved and respected by a large circle of friends. She leaves a husband and family of small children, whose grief is heavy. Her death resulted from pneumonia, following an attack of influenza. [Taken from the] *Eastern Chronicle*, New Glasgow.

Truro Daily News, 6 January 1919, 1. Courtesy the Colchester Historeum, Truro.

☞ The Colchester County Death Register, 1918, Book 32, Page 92, Number 350, shows Annie T. Vernon died on December 31. The cause of death was listed merely as pneumonia. She was buried in Truro. Her husband was E. D. Vernon. The *Truro Daily News* quoted the New Glasgow newspaper *Eastern Chronicle*, which got the story, seemingly by word of mouth, and published it a week before the Truro paper said anything.

A BRAVE FIGHT—BUT DEATH WON
Mrs. Ernest D. Vernon a Victim of Pneumonia following Influenza Passes Away on Dec. 31. About five o'clock on the evening of December 31, as the last hours of the year were running out, there past away from us forever the spirit of a comparatively young life, Mrs. Ernest D. Vernon, who for some days had made a valiant fight for life against severe pneumonia, following an attack of influenza.
Truro Daily News, 2 January 1919, 4. Courtesy the Colchester Historeum, Truro.

DIED. PRATT. At Belmont, Jan. 1, 1919, of Influenza, Viola Myrtle, youngest daughter of Mr. and Mrs. John Henry Pratt, aged nine years and eight months.
Truro Daily News, 1 January 1919, 3. Courtesy the Colchester Historeum, Truro.

☞ The following is but one example of how the Great Influenza orphaned hundreds of children.

THE LATE MRS. LIZZIE FLANAGAN
Halifax, Janiary [*sic*] 8. Mrs. Lizzie Flanagan [Flannigan], wife of Thomas Flanagan, aged 35, died at the influenza hospital yesterday [January 7]. She leaves a husband and five small children. Two sisters and her mother also survive. The funeral will take place Thursday afternoon at 2 o'clock from Cruikshank's undertaking rooms. The deceased is a native of Truro, moving to Halifax a few years ago. Three weeks ago she developed influenza. This was followed by pneumonia. The entire family, seven in all—had the influenza, but the others are now improving. They were nursed by Mrs. A. Flanagan and Miss Alice Flanagan of Truro. The latter will take charge of the orphaned children at her home in Truro.
Truro Daily News, 8 January 1919, 4. Courtesy the Colchester Historeum, Truro.

☞ The HVS, Death Register, 1919, Book 25, Page 59, Number 349, shows Lizzie Flannigan had lived at 70½ Cornwallis Street. Her husband's name was Thomas Flannigan (this seems the correct spelling). She had been born in Newfoundland, was a Roman Catholic, and was buried at Mount Olivet Cemetery. Her doctor was J. F. Buckley. Undertaker: Nova Scotia Undertaking Co.

☞ Henry Copland [Kaplan?] aged 18, Indian Reserve [Millbrook, Truro District]; died 29 January 1919, Tuberculosis and Influenza, length of illness not given. Listed as "Indian" in death register, he appears as "Henry Copland," Roman Catholic. His father's name is not given. He lived and died on the Reserve, and then was buried there. The doctor's name was H. V. Kent, the undertaker was J. C. B. Olive. His return was made by persons unknown, on 29 January 1919.

This information comes from the HVS Death Register, Colchester County, 1918, Book 32, Page 111, Number 434. Copland is an odd name for a Mi'kmaw. I think someone who did not speak the language sent in this death record, and they heard the Mi'kmaw pronunciation of Kaplan as Copland. Or else he had a non-Mi'kmaw father named Copland or Copeland. This is the only example of the name, as associated with a Mi'kmaw, I have ever seen in forty-eight years of research, although Bernie Francis tells me he knows of one or more in New Brunswick.

Bernie Francis to Ruth Whitehead, personal communication, March 2020.

LONDONDERRY, COL. CO. Feb. 3. Charles Bates, a respected resident of Lornvale, passed away on the 29th [of January]. Mr. Bates contracted Influenza, which developed into pneumonia, and passed away as stated above. To the sorrowing wife, who is ill from the same malady, and daughter Myrtle, is extended the sincere sympathy of the community.

Truro Daily News, 6 February 1919, 6. Courtesy the Colchester Historeum, Truro.

MR. EDWARD WILLIAMS DIED FROM INFLUENZA

A faithful worker and a much respected colord man, Mr. Edward Williams, died early Saturday morning, the 1st [of February], from that terrible epidemic Spanish Influenza at the home of Mr. William Dulap [Dunlap], Lower Truro. Mr. Williams had been ill but a short time, had generally had good helth, but this "Flu" took a strong hold and at the comparatively early age of 45 years, he past to the great Unknown. The funeral was held at two o'clock on Monday, Feb. 3, at Zion Church the Rev. Mr. [W. R.] States of the Second Baptist Church, New Glasgow, assisted by the Rev. W. D. Perry, of Zion Church, conducted the funeral services; and interment was in the Truro Cemetery, Robie Street. An uncle of the deceased, John J. Williams, was here from New Glasgow, to attend the obsequies.

Mr. Dunlap, speaks of Edward Williams, who had been in his employ for four or five years, as a faithful honest man, esteemed by every acquaintance.

Truro Daily News, 5 February 1919, 2. Courtesy the Colchester Historeum, Truro.

☞ Mr. Williams was born at Big Tracadie, Guysborough County. He was a widower, a Baptist, and died of pneumonia on February 1, 1919, after eight weeks of illness, aged 45, at Lower Truro. The doctor was H. V. Kent, undertaker J. C. B. Olive.

Mr. Williams was buried in Truro. The return was made by his employer, William Dunlap, on February 1, who also seems to have provided information for his obituary above.

HVS, Death Register, Colchester County, 1919, Book 32, Page 117, Number 459.

A SUDDEN CALL

"Flu" that is still hovering in our midst, and about suburban Truro, carried off on Sunday [April] the 13th one of the finest young men in the Clifton district, Frank S. Crowe, the only son of Councillor and Mrs. E. E. Crowe, of Beaver Brook. This bright young man was out motoring only a few days ago and was apparently in the best of helth [sic]; but this insidious disease, with its dedly complications, seized him, and in spite of all human efforts for relief he past away on the peaceful hours of the Sabbath to his eternal rest.

Truro Daily News, 14 April 1919, 4. Courtesy the Colchester Historeum, Truro.

OBITUARY. Mrs. David Young. At her parents home, Water Street, Truro, after a brief illness, Mrs. David Young entered into rest. She developed tubercolosis [sic] from Influenza while in Waltham, and returning home six weeks ago, grew rapidly worse, passing away on Saturday, April 26th, at the early age of twenty years. Every care and attention was given her to the last. Her husband Private David Young of the 106th Batt. predeceased her a year ago.

Truro Daily News, 29 April 1919, p. 1. Courtesy the Colchester Historeum, Truro.
HVS, Colchester County, 1919, Book 32, Page 148, Number 514.

☞ This was Gertrude Young, born in Onslow, and buried there; the cause of death is listed as tuberculosis; there is no mention of influenza. Whether this was true tuberculosis, or simply compromised lungs from influenza, is a mystery.

OBITUARY. MRS. ANGUS FIELDS. At her home in Bible Hill, Thursday morning, May 1st, of pneumonia, Mrs. Angus Fields, aged 27 years passed away....A sorrowing husband and two children, Marjorie aged two years and Donald three weeks.

Truro Daily News, 2 May 1919, 4. Courtesy the Colchester Historeum, Truro.

☞ HVS Death Register, 1919, Book 32, Page 148, Number 579, gives her as Nettie Johnston Fields, age 26, born in the US, and a Baptist. Dr. C. W. McLean attended. J .C. B. Olive was the undertaker. Mrs. Fields was buried in Waterville, Kings County.

THE LATE ANTHONY BARRON

There passed away at his home in Pleasant Valley, Rawdon, May 27th, from Pneumonia, following Influenza, Anthony Barron, aged forty-four years, leaving to mourn their loss a wife and seven children, the youngest two years old....The long line of twenty-five carriages seemed to the writer to emphasize the fact that a good man had fallen, one who by his quiet, unassuming, courteous, Christian life had endeared himself to a large circle of friends and neighbors.

Mr. Barron was the son of the late Jacob and Mary Barron, and had always lived on the homestead, on the hill overlooking a wide stretch of country with the Valley Lake in the distance, and now with the trees just putting forth their leaves with low clouds over-shadowing their brightness, seeming also to reflect on the faces of his friends the thought that they too were "sorrowing most of all that they should see his face no more."

The saddest part seemed to be that there was no chance for the beautiful burial service of the Church he so loved, but the body was committed to the grave in St. Paul's Churchyard by the Rev. P. G. Corbin.

Truro Daily News, 9 June 1919, 1. Courtesy the Colchester Historeum, Truro.

ONTARIO COMMERCIAL TRAVELLER SUICIDES AT TRURO

Harvey L. Murray, son of W. R. Murray, Delatre Street, Woodstock, Ont., committed suicide in Victoria Park on Friday last. Mr. Murray was a commercial traveller. He arrived at the Stanley House Thursday evening. On Friday morning he made an appointment with Mr. B. J. Rogers of B. J. Rogers Ltd, to show samples for millinery at the Stanley Sample Rooms. He did not keep his engagement, nor did he return to the hotel that night. Mr. Stevens of the hotel became uneasy the following morning, regarding his guest, and informed Chief of Police Fraser. The Chief learned that Murray was last seen in Victoria Park, and with five men he searched the ravines, pools and reservoir unsuccessfully. At evening, a search party of 1100 men, under the Chief of the Fire Department, was sent out to sweep the woods in the Park, at eight o'clock the body was found about 100 feet off the road leading to the reservoir in a spruce thicket....

A statement found on the deceased indicated some domestic trouble and a generally [*sic*] state of depression on account of his fear that he could not earn a living. He lately had influenza and in his room in the hotel was a certificate to Murray's firm dated May 7th, that he was then on the verge of nervous prostration and not safe to send out on the road.

Truro Daily News, 9 June 1919, 1. Courtesy the Colchester Historeum, Truro.

The record in HVS, 1919, Book 32, Page 143, Number 554, doesn't have a lot of information about this sad soul: "Traveller, age not known." For residence, it just reads, "Died at Truro." The coroner, W. R. Dunbar, pronounced him dead of poisoning by carbolic acid. He was buried at Woodstock, Ontario, once his family had been contacted.

Mr. Murray was one of a number of people stricken by influenza who suffered neurological damage, with such terrible after-effects as anxiety, apathy, exhaustion, depression, paranoia, or even hallucinations, which they were unable to shake off. Such pathology caused a number of suicides.

 HAVELOCK HAMILTON. POPULAR BROOKFIELD CITIZEN DIES SUDDENLY OF PNEUMONIA

The call came suddenly to the well known Mr. Havelock H. Hamilton, blacksmith, Brookfield, Col. Co., who on the 27th ult., died from 'flu' followed by pneumonia after an illness of but three days.

Truro Daily News, 1 March 1920, page 4. Courtesy the Colchester Historeum, Truro.

Widening the Search

The following two persons, said to have been influenza victims, are not on any of Dr. Allan Marble's lists, but were found in Nova Scotia Museum records. For forty-seven years, I have thought this account was accurate. I include this story as an encouragement to researchers to dig deep and then dig deeper, evaluating sources as they find them.

4 March 1920 / Micmac Indians. Two old Indians died of influenza on last Thursday, 4th March 1920, at the new Indian reservation at Truro, N.S. They were, Delair, widow of Soolien (William) Soowa, whose age was 82 years, and Louis Jeekouse who had reached the great age of 89 years. The latter was the father of Mrs. Joe Cope, whose husband is a well-known educated Indian of Enfield, but lately of Lunenburg.

Soowa, an old Micmac word meaning 'He takes out what he brought in.'

Jeekouse, an old Micmac word meaning 'Listen!'

Nova Scotia Museum Library, Piers Papers, Ethnology: Genealogies, 24.

Because we do not know the name of the informant who gave this information to Harry Piers, we don't know what weight to put on it. Was the informant even a Mi'kmaw? If so, was Mi'kmaw their first language? For example, Jerry Lonecloud, born Germain Bartlett Alexis, was one of Piers' frequent informants, and other entries in the Piers Papers from around this time have all come from him. He, however, was born in Maine, and lived in the US with his Mi'kmaw parents until he was orphaned, after which time he was living in Nova Scotia, but he spoke English with Piers, and even his Mi'kmaw had an interesting Maine accent to it, and included sounds no longer common in the language. Piers himself spoke no Mi'kmaw, and was guessing at the spelling—of what he *thought* he heard Lonecloud give him verbally. (Other Piers records suffer from his phonetic spelling as well, which sometimes even baffles linguists who are fluent speakers themselves.)

☞ Just so you know, *Mi'kmaw* is the name of the language spoken by the Mi'kmaq of Atlantic Canada, with *Mi'kmaq* being the tribal name, and the plural form of the noun. *Mi'kmaw* is the singular form of the noun (one *Mi'kmaw*, four *Mi'kmaq*). What is then confusing to English-speakers is that *Mi'kmaw* is also the adjectival form, used whether the noun it modifies is singular *or* plural (a *Mi'kmaw* person, two *Mi'kmaw* persons).

☞ In the case of Louis Jeekouse, according to Mi'kmaw linguist Bernie Francis, this surname translation is incorrect. Jeekouse, now spelled Kji-ku's, means literally "great month," Christmas month, December. So, was this man's name Louis Noel? Perhaps. While there *were* persons living in the province named Louis Noel at this time, many of them called Lewie Newell in English spelling, no man of that name and age has been found in the Colchester Death Register, nor one with that death date. No one, man or woman, *by any name at all*, died at the Truro Reserve on March 4, 1920. So we know now that this date of death is wrong for both Louis and Delair.

Next, I tried to uncover Louis' daughter's name, the girl who was said to have married Joe C. Cope. In 1881, a Joseph Cope, aged 23, married a Rebecca "Judies," aged 14, in Dartmouth in 1881. Her last name, as written, is very odd. It is difficult to make out in the original; it could also have been Jeedus, Judees, or other recombinations. While these names are almost certainly incorrect as Piers's notes and the marriage records have it, I wonder if this might be a case of an initial mis-heard sound: not a J-sound, but a *Kji*-sound. Possibly not not *Kji-ku's* after all, but *Kji*-something-else, although *Kji-ku's* makes more sense. A simple J is unlikely, since Mi'kmaw speakers tended to replace J in a name with S, as in Jacques becoming Sack, Sark, or Sock, in English spelling, depending upon whether the bearer of the name came from Nova Scotia, PEI, or New Brunswick.

Bernie Francis to Ruth Whitehead, personal communication, March 2020.
HVS, Colchester County, Marriage Register, 1881, Book 1871, Page 102, Number 379 (Rebecca).

☞ For "Delair, wife of Soolien (William) Soowa," there is no death record under that name, but here's what little I know about her. First, she was never the *widow* of Soolian Bill—in 1920, or any other time. She and her husband had made the Truro Reserve their home, beginning in 1880, but spent time in Dartmouth during the summers. If Piers's account of her death is correct, she was living with her husband at the Truro Reserve in the winter of early 1920, when he, William, gave Jerry Lonecloud information about various kinds of whales, below. Soolian Bill appears alive in a second Piers note, dated 1920. Soolian is now written Sulia'n, from the French baptismal name Guillaume, says Bernie Francis, Mi'kmaw linguist.

📄 31 January 1920...Soolian Bill, Micmac Indian, of Truro reservation, N.S., now about 97 years of age, who formerly lived in Cape Breton, told Lonecloud (30 Jan. 1920) that in summer, about 50 years ago (say about 1870), the same season that Pigmy Sperm Whale (?) was taken off Kingsport, that a number ("numerous") animals of the same kind, which Bill also calle Ded-men-ak-pa-jet [*temnaqpajit*], came ashore in a "gut" at Whycocomagh, Bras d'Or Lake, Cape Breton Island, and Bill saw them. He agreed that they were named as above, and that they were the same as those got off Kingsport. All agree they are very rare. They had back fins. Were not Blackfish. One had a young in it when opened. Blubber made oil.

Nova Scotia Museum Library, Piers Papers, Ethnology: Zoology.

☞ In the third oral history from the Piers Papers, Lonecloud gets Prosper's age correctly, but not the date of his death. The Death Register for Colchester County, 1923, says he died on March 25. Piers quotes him as saying, "about 3rd April," so this might indicate that someone else told this to Lonecloud first. On the other hand, Lonecloud has forgotten details of what he learned when he interviewed William Prosper in 1920, and gave Piers a birthdate for him of 1822. With information, both good and bad, from Lonecloud, Piers wrote Prosper's obituary, as follows:

📄 7 April 1923. William Prosper, a very aged Micmac Indian, who was well-known as Soolian Bill, died at the Truro Indian Reservation, Nova Scotia, about 3rd April, at the very great age, it is claimed, of one hundred and one years. He was born at Bay of Islands, Newfoundland, about 1822, as it is claimed; and he had many traditions of the old Beothuk Indians of Newfoundland which became extinct between 1810 and 1825. About 1848 he came to Whycocomagh, Cape Breton Island, and about 1860 came to Halifax and attended the welcome which the Indian representatives gave the Prince of Wales in that year and received some of the bounty money which the Prince distributed among the Tribe. He was first camped on a hill near Farrell's Pond, Dartmouth Lake, and later on the side of the stream where Greenvale School now is. He was a very prominent figure in the Halifax market, always standing in front of Walsh's hardware shop. About 1880 he moved to the Indian Reservation at Truro, Colchester County, and made his headquarters there ever since, though after coming to Halifax [to sell things]....He was a big man, tall, and straight as an arrow even in his old age. He was an expert cooper in his time, but did not excel as a hunter. He had a wonderful fund of tradition, and was appealed to for information regarding the old days, and the old customs of his tribe. He contributed quite a large sum of his savings to help build the chapel on the Truro reserve. None of his children survive him. *Vide* Jerry Lone-cloud 7 April 1923.

Nova Scotia Museum Library, Piers Papers, Ethnology: Genealogies, 27.

⏷ The final piece of evidence/information found for William's wife, Delair, comes from the Nova Scotia Museum's picture collection, P113/28.192 (6382)/ N-5572. It shows William Prosper and "Madelaine" outside their wigwam, "between Tufts Cove and North Dartmouth, just north of Olands Brewery," wrote Harry Piers in the accession records. This black-and-white photograph, taken between 1909 and 1910, is the only record of Soolian Bill's wife's name. And Delain, or Madelaine, certainly resembles Delair, with the final *n* actually mistakenly written as an *r*, when Piers was copying his notes. (Madelain/Magdalen/Madeline is the English version of the French baptismal name, Madeleine. In modern Mi'kmaw orthography, it is written *Matle'n*.)

So this lady's name was Madeleine. Mi'kmaw tradition, at that time, held that women kept their father's name, using it as the new concept of surname, even after marriage. Perhaps this is why Lonecloud didn't give it. He didn't know what her father's name had been. Harry Piers, cataloguing the photograph, simply went with English tradition and referred to her as Madeline Prosper.

Alas, now comes the great disappointment: her name was Madeleine, she *was* the wife of William Prosper, but she did *not* die in 1920, according to her death record. Nor was she a victim of influenza. The Colchester County Death Register says "Madelaine [*sic*] Prosper" died on March 18, 1916, of "old age," a condition which had lasted the "length about two years." The doctor was H. V. Kent, and he seems to have had the government-appointed care of the Truro Reserve, but he lived elsewhere, his main practice was elsewhere, and his diagnoses seem a bit perfunctory to me.

Madeleine had been married to William Prosper for many years, and as she was born about 1836 in North Sydney, Cape Breton County, according to her death record, she probably met him up in Cape Breton, after he'd come over from Newfoundland in 1848. She would have been 12 years old then. He was fourteen years older than she, but outlived her by five years. Or so I originally thought.

HVS, Colchester County, Death Register, 1916, Book 31, Page 213, Number 669, where her name was spelled 'Madelaine' on the original record, and has been entered as 'Madeline' in the HVS search engine.

All this goes to show that Lonecloud made mistakes with her data, and he may have made others with "Louis Jeekouse," just as he made mistakes with William Prosper's bio. Nevertheless, I'm fairly certain that Prosper was born in Newfoundland, from corroborating detail. This brings us to the next complication: Chief Joseph Julien of the Truro Reserve was the informant for both William and Madeleine's death records. Mr. Prosper's record states he was born in Antigonish (not Newfoundland), on June 22, 1824. There are multiple errors of fact in Harry's Piers's accounts shown above. Either Lonecloud got things wrong, or Harry Piers did, unless Chief Joseph Julian, who sent in the information to the registry, was responsible for these contradictory statements.

My feeling is that perhaps each of them got some of it right, and some of it wrong, with this exception: it's hard to argue with the creation of a death record. It may spell things wrong, but it absolutely depends on there being a dead body, so one can trust that someone has died in the year the register was written, if they are in the register, and one can usually trust that their date of death is correct, at least to the year.

Madeleine died in 1916. William Prosper died in 1923, on March 25 at 6:15 P.M., of "general disability." (H. V. Kent was still the appointed doctor.) He was buried on the Reserve. J. C. B. Olive was the undertaker. The death record says that William Prosper had been living in Truro, on the reserve, "about 39 years." Perhaps he now lies next to his wife who had been laid to rest there seven years before.

HVS, Colchester County Death Register, 1916, Book 31, Page 213, Number 669 (Madeleine). HVS, Colchester County Death Register, 1923, Book 61, Page 537 (William Prosper).

More Colchester County Deaths

"Gordon Millard, 57, d. 28 March 1920, Tatamagouche, farmer," as he appears on Dr. Marble's list of Colchester County's influenza victims beginning on page 104, was the last person to die from the Great Influenza of 1918–20 in Colchester County. His doctor was Dan Murray, MD; undertaker was George McLellan, who buried him at Mattatall Cemetery—probably at Mattatall Lake, according to Dale Swann. Mr. Millard's death record lists him as from the District of Waugh's River. He had been living in Tatamagouche, where he had farmed for nine years. Previous to this, between 1892 and 1911, he had earned a living as a "Coach Man." Perhaps with the coming of the automobile, he gave it up and bought a farm, returning to Tatamagouche, where he had been born in 1863 to Peter Millard and Catherine Simpson Millard, both native Nova Scotians. He married in later life, and he and his wife, the former Mary Monk, had a son, Gordon Elmer, born in Tatamagouche in 1915. As "Mrs. Gordon Millard,"

Mary was the informant for both records—her son's birth, and her husband's death only five years later.

HVS, Colchester County Death Register, 1920, Book 61, Page 184 (Gordon).
HVS, Colchester County Birth Register, 1915, Book 469000691, Page 46900691 [odd numbering, but given by the HVS search engine] (Gordon Elmer).

COLCHESTER COUNTY, VITAL STATISTICS, DEATH REGISTER, BOOKS 32, 61

1. Bertha M. McKinnon, 38, d. 5 November 1918, Truro, housewife.

2. Catherine Paul, 11 years, d. 5 November 1918, Indian Reserve [*Millbrook, Truro District*].

3. Cecil Lingard, 71, d. 31 October 1918, Truro.

4. Sarah Glode, 5, d. 16 October 1918, Indian Reserve [*Millbrook, Truro District*].

5. Catherine Glode, 17 months, d. 16 October 1918, Indian Reserve [*Millbrook, Truro District*].

6. Adelaide Thomas, 2, d. 17 October 1918, Indian Reserve [*Millbrook, Truro District*].

7. Peter Cope, 6 weeks, d. 11 October 1918, Indian Reserve [*Millbrook, Truro District*].

8. Wilbert McDonald, 22, d. 17 November 1918, Truro, railway employee.

9. Daniel Welsh, 38, d. 4 December 1918, Truro.

10. Gertrude Lane. 35, d. 17 December 1918, Truro, housewife.

11. Joseph Works, 23, d. 26 October 1918, Truro, railway man.

12. Harry McKay, 34, d. 9 December 1918, Onslow, farmer.

13. Lewis Douchwright [*Douthwright*] 30, d. 20 December 1918, Brookfield, lumberman.

14. Irene Sutherland, 17, d. 21 December 1918, River John Road (Colchester County).

15. Hilda Esau, 14, d. 1 December 1918, Londonderry, student.

16. Barbara Patriquin, 32, d. 1 December 1918, Londonderry, housewife.

17. Viola Copp, 21, d. 22 October 1918, Great Village, housewife.

18. Percy Matthews, 2, d. 28 November 1918, DeBert [*sic*].

19. George Chisholm, 24, d. 14 December 1918, Great Village, labourer.

20. Norman Tipping, 32, d. 15 December 1918, Great Village, labourer.

21. Stewart Tipping, 30, d. 19 December 1918, Great Village, labourer. [*Norman (above) and Stewart Tipping were brothers, the sons of Robert Tipping. Both lived at "Mt. Pleasant Grt Village," and appear on the same page of the death register for Colchester County, Book 32, Page 106, Numbers 401 and 403.*]

22. Mrs. John Hill, 25, d. 30 December 1918, Upper Economy, housewife.

23. Wanda Hill, 7 months, d. 31 December 1918, Cove Road.

24. Cecil Davis, 2, d. 5 November 1918, Five Islands.

25. Mrs. David Davis, d. 5 November 1918, Five Islands.

26. Bernard Davis, 2 days, d. 5 November 1918, Five Islands.

27. Arthur Smith, 1 day, d. 18 February 1919, Truro. [*Arthur Hallet Smith died of influenza having lived only one day. Book 32, Page 109, Number 418.*]

28. Henry Copeland [*Kaplan?*], 18, d. 29 January 1919, Indian Reserve, [*Millbrook, Truro District*].

29. Viola Pratt, 9, d. 30 December 1918, Belmont.

30. Lillian Rowlands, 1 month, d. 27 December 1918, Brookfield.

31. Laurie Lansburg, 30, d. 10 January 1919, Kemptown.

32. William MacLean, 47, d. 15 January 1919, Riversdale, farmer.

33. Hazel Johnson, 18, d. 11 January 1919, Kemptown.

34. Freda Weatherby, 6 months, d. 6 March 1919, Lower Truro.

35. Emma McKenzie, d. 30 October 1918, Brookside.

36. Bertha McKay, 27, d. 9 March 1919, Riversdale, housewife.

37. Edith McKenzie, 9 months, d. 9 December 1918, Stewiacke.

38. Alonzo Ellis, 31, d. 7 January 1919, Shubenacadie, lumberman.

39. Adelaide Nelson, 16, d. 2 February 1919, Londonderry, housewife.

40. Charles Bullers, 47, d. 24 January 1919, Londonderry, labourer.

41. Irvin McNeil, 18, d. 27 March 1919, Bass River.

42. Mrs. _____ Moore, 32, d. 8 January 1919, Economy. [*HVS, Book 32, Page 137, Number 524, is difficult to read; the husband's first name, for example, appears (twice) to be Paoli, and (once) as what looks like Neale. She was born in Pembroke, Hants Count, and died aged 32.*]

43. Lillian McLellan, 35, d. 14 January 1919, Central Economy.

44. David Patterson, 8 months, d. 18 January 1919, Economy.

45. Amos McLaughlin, 54, d. 8 February 1919, Pleasant Hills, carpenter.

46. Fred D. Loomer, 24, d. 19 February 1920, Truro, D.A.R. engineer.

47. Havelock H. Hamilton, 56, d. 27 February 1920, Brookfield, blacksmith.

48. Lorinda Davison, 65, d. 8 February 1920, Portaupique [*sic*], housework.

49. Bessie M. Douglas, 6, d. 15 March 1920, North River.

50. Gordon Millard, 57, d. 28 March 1920, Tatamagouche, farmer.

Chapter VI

CUMBERLAND COUNTY

꙳ꛬꙷ꙳

IN CUMBERLAND COUNTY there were at least 153 confirmed deaths from the Great Influenza. Between October 2, 1918 and March 31, 1919—the much worse Second Wave—131 people died; between February 18 and April 15, 1920, the Third Wave took 20 souls.

INFLUENZA CLAIMS TWO PARRSBORO YOUNG PEOPLE

While there have been so far no deaths from the influenza in Parrsboro, and there are only a few cases of mild type, the bodies of two young people have been brought home for burial. On September 15, Cecil Lamb, the only remaining son of Mr. and Mrs. Augustus Lamb, died at the Marine Hospital, Chelsea, Mass., from the influenza. He was engineer on a large barge carrying coal from Virginia to Boston, and was in his 20th year. He was an excellent young man. The burial was in Parrsboro, Oct. 1. A week later, Oct. 8, Lilian L. Morrison, aged 25, died at Halifax from the same disease. She was employed [waitress] at the Green Lantern, and was a young woman of fine character. She was the only remaining daughter of Howard Morrison of Parrsboro....The interment was in Parrsboro. The sadness of the burial of these young people was increased by not being able to open the caskets or take them to the homes of their parents. The funerals were from the railway station and the Undertaker's room. The schools and churches are closed in Parrsboro, and the influenza is not making much progress.

Amherst Daily News, 21 October 1918, 3.

RECENT DEATHS

T. A. RICE [Charles Amos Rice]. Death occurred at Westchester, Cumberland Co., on Saturday, October 5th, of T. A. Rice, aged 45 years. The deceased was a son of the late Alexander Rice, formerly of Digby. The remains arrived here [Digby] on the 8th, and were taken in charge of by Mr. J. F. Rice, undertaker and the funeral was held the same day, with interment in the Baptist cemetery.

Digby Courier, 11 October 1918, 2. HVS, Cumberland County Death Register, 1918, Book 39, Page 225, Number 870.

The name on his death certificate was Charles Amos Rice; HVS database search engine only finds him if one enters "Charles Awar Rice." He had been a lumber surveyor. His death certificate lists him as an Evangelical. His doctor, R. O. Shatford, stated that he died of "Locomotor Ataxia, complicated by Influenza." He was unmarried. The undertaker in Cumberland County who prepared the body for shipment was J. C. B. Olive.

HVS, Death Register, Cumberland County, Year 1918, Book 39, Page 225, Number 870.

FOUR MORE DEATHS FROM SPANISH INFLUENZA

Wolfville is one of the few communities in Nova Scotia which has not felt the blight of the disease. There is not an accredited case, the schools and churches remain open, and the fortunate inhabitants are indulging their movie appetite to the full. The situation is very different in Parrsboro, across the Basin; there the epidemic is serious and a large number of the houses are closely quarantined, marked with a yellow flag.

Halifax Morning Chronicle, 15 October 1918, 5.

Frank Cameron, of Parrsboro, a bank clerk for a time in Middleton, died on Saturday [October 19] in Charlottetown of Influenza and pneumonia. His brother, Pte. Blair Cameron, was killed in action on Sept. 30.

Bridgetown Monitor, 23 October 1918, 3.

At least three Mi'kmaq (and possibly seven), all with the surname of Paul, died of the Great Influenza in Cumberland County in 1918:

- Joseph Paul, 39, d. 10 October 1918, Springhill Junction, labourer.
- Anthony Paul, 9, d. 14 October 1918, Springhill Junction, student.
- Joseph Paul, 27, d. 23 November 1918, Springhill Junction, labourer.

- The older Joseph Paul had been born in New Brunswick, was married, and worked as a labourer in Springhill Junction—possibly having gotten a job there because of the war, with its shortage of able-bodied men. He died on October 10, 1918, after an illness of seven days, of "Influenza and Pneumonia." He was the father of Anthony Paul (see next page). Dr. A. E. Forbes attended him. Alexander Paul sent in the return of death.

HVS, Cumberland County Death Register, 1918, Book 39, Page 303, Number 1199.

- Anthony Paul, son of Joseph, was 9 years old. He died four days after his father, on October 14; cause of death: Influenza and Pneumonia. He had been ill for only five days. Anthony had been born in New Brunswick, and was living in the family home in Springhill Junction. His doctor was the same A. E. Forbes. Alexander Paul sent in the return of death form to the registrar.

     HVS, Cumberland County Death Register, 1918, Book 39, Page 303, Number 1200.

- Joseph Paul the younger, aged 27, was also a married labourer living in Springhill Junction. He died on November 23, 1918, of "Influenza/Pneumonia," following an illness of twelve days. A later entry to his record, done in pencil in a different hand, stated that he had been born in Pictou County. No doctor or undertaker was listed, but he was buried in the Catholic cemetery in Springhill. Noel Tobin sent in the return on November 25.

     HVS, Cumberland County Death Register, 1918, Book 39, Page 304, Number 1206.

☞ Now we come to the suspected—the plausible—victims of influenza, all Mi'kmaq, and all with the surname Paul, all from the same general area, all dying within five weeks of one another. Influenza had already taken the lives of two Pauls when the others fell ill and died; influenza would take another, in week five.

- Daniel Paul, Jr., son of Daniel Paul, Sr., was 7 months old when he died on 11 October 1918. He lived in Springhill Junction, with his father—and presumably his mother. A. E. Forbes is listed as the doctor. The cause of death was originally entered as "Cholera," but this was later changed (in pencil) to "Marasmus / Inanition." Alexander Paul sent in the death record on 15 October. Daniel was buried in the Catholic cemetery in Springhill.

     HVS, Cumberland County Death Register, 1918, Book 39, Page 303, Number 1202.

☞ Marasmus is malnutrition; inanition is starvation. This child was unable to absorb nutrients—but why? Two of the symptoms of the Great Influenza were severe diarrhea and vomiting.

- Noel Paul, aged 75, a widower, lived at the Indian Reserve, Halfway River, which is just off Route 2, leading into Springhill. Mr. Paul fell sick on about October 19, and then sometime during the week he was ill, he was taken to Amherst to the hospital, dying there on October 26, 1918. Cause of death was listed as "Pneumonia, ill about one week"—another reason for assuming that all this information came via the Amherst Hospital, which only saw him in extremis from his pneumonia.

Furthermore, because this "about one week" is an estimate, the doctor attending, R. Jeffers [sp?], MD, was in all likelihood on the hospital staff at Amherst, and not the federally appointed doctor who (in theory, anyway) would have attended any ill Mi'kmaw people at Halfway River—Dr. A. E. Forbes. An undertaker named John Pickard prepared the body for burial, as well as for transport to the Roman Catholic cemetery in Parrsboro. The priest, Rev. Houlihan Kennal [sp?] O R S Fran., sent in the return of death to the district registrar.

HVS, Death Register, Cumberland County, Year 1918, Book 39, Page 308, Number 1221. Noel Paul was brought to our attention by researcher Linda Littlejohn, Parrsborough Historical Society, Parrsboro.

- On October 20, 1918, at the Indian Reserve of Halfway River, a child named Martin Laurence Paul died. No doctor attended, no length of illness was given, nor cause of death. His father's name was not given. The Catholic priest, Rev. Houlihan Kennal [sp?], O R S Fran., sent in the return of death to the District Registrar. It was entered into the register and later, a different hand provided, in pencil, as cause of death "Cholera Infantum." As no doctor attended, and the initial return left this category blank, one wonders who made this later diagnosis? I mention this to show that medical care was sketchy on the Halfway River Reserve.

HVS, Cumberland County Death Register, 1918, Book 39, Page 308, Number 1219.

☞ As discussed in the first chapter, the Great Influenza pandemic was sometimes diagnosed as cholera (among other things), due to the unusual ways it could present. This child, for all we know, could have died of the Great Influenza. There is no way to verify this, or the cause of the other deaths mentioned here, and so this remains in the realm of speculation. But there is, here, a suggestive cluster of Paul family deaths, either in Springhill Junction or in Halfway River, located just off Route 2, south of Springhill.

- The last one of this group is Lennith Nichols Paul, a Mi'kmaw child aged 2 years, who died April 15, 1918, in Amherst. He had been born in Big Cove, New Brunswick, to the family of Eddie Paul. As this family was residing in Springhill Junction when the child took sick, he presumably was taken to the Amherst hospital, where he died after an illness of one week. The home doctor was, again, A. E. Forbes. The cause of death was given as "Heavy Cold," written in ink; in pencil was added later, "pneumonia." This child may have had influenza with pneumonia, and if that were indeed his cause of death, he would have been one of the victims we know about who died in the First Wave of the Great Influenza, which took the lives of a number of Nova Scotians, beginning about March or April 1918. The child was buried in the Roman Catholic cemetery in Amherst on April 16.

HVS, Cumberland County Death Register, 1918, Book 39, Page 207, Number 800.

- Agnes McAloney, aged 19 years 5 months, single, was residing at Springhill when she was taken sick. Born in Cumberland County, her parents were Thomas and Eleanor Stevenson McAloney. She died at Amherst on November 8, 1918, of influenza and pneumonia, and was buried at Maccan, Cumberland County.

  Information found by Linda Littlejohn. HVS, Death Register, Cumberland County, Year 1918, Book 39, Page 303, Number 1183.

- Howard Angus Brown died at the age of 5 years 6 months. He was born in Springhill, and lived at East Mapleton. Matthew Brown was his father. He died in Amherst on November 15, 1918, of influenza, after an illness of two days, and was buried in Mapleton. The family was Methodist.

  Information found by Linda Littlejohn. HVS, Death Register, Cumberland County, Year 1918, Book 39, Page 303, Number 1204.

- Eliza Adelaide Mills Brown, formerly of East Mapleton, aged 38, married to Aaron Gilroy Brown of East Maitland, Hants, died at Amherst of influenza and pneumonia on November 19, 1918, after an illness of one week. She was buried at Mapleton Cemetery, Cumberland County.

  HVS, Death Register, Cumberland County, Year 1918, Book 39, Page 304, Number 1205.

- Philomen [Philomène] Landry (female), 20, died on November 20, 1918, in Amherst. Dr. Allan Marble added this gender clarification to his list here; the original death record, however, clearly records her as "male." (Acadian-born contributor Angela Buckles assures me that she has never seen this name carried by any but females.) She must have been a woman, however, judging by the rest of the death record: a husband is listed. His name seems to be "Dos. D. Landry," and her occupation is "housework." The couple lived at 13 Princess Street in Amherst. Her doctor was F. E. Boudreau; no place of burial is recorded.

  HVS, Death Register, Cumberland County, Year 1918, Book 39, Page 258, Number 985. Angela Buckles to Ruth Whitehead, personal communication, September 2019

- Leonard Johnson Brown, aged 28, single, born in Cumberland County, but more recently of South Maitland, East Hants, died in Amherst on 25 November 1918. A soldier, he spent eight months in the trenches, had been gassed, and contracted influenza upon returning home to Nova Scotia. The combination of the two killed him. He was the son of A. H. Brown, and was buried at South Maitland.

> HVS, Death Register, Cumberland County, Year 1918, Book 39, Page 268, Number 1042.

 SCOTT. At River Hebert, N.S., Dec. 18th, of pneumonia, Abbie B., daughter of Mr. J. O. Scott, aged 19 years.

> *Truro Daily News*, 30 December 1918, 2. Courtesy the Colchester Historeum, Truro.

Her death record (1918, Book 39, Page 282, Number 1115), says that she died December 13, after one week of influenza and pneumonia. A Methodist, she was buried in River Hebert at the New Cemetery.

THE LATE MARION ELIZABETH PURDY
The death occurred at 1 Milford Street, Amherst, N.S., of Marion Elizabeth Purdy, at the early age of 26 years. Deceased had been sick only a short time with influenza and pneumonia, and despite the best medical attention and loving care of her Mother and Sister, she sank rapidly, passing away in the early hours of Christmas morning....She was the third daughter of Mr. and Mrs. Thomas W. Purdy, Millvale, N.S.

> *Truro Daily News*, 7 January 1919, 6. Courtesy the Colchester Historeum, Truro.

SMITH. At Amherst on Feb. 20th of pneumonia, Mrs. Matthias L. Smith, leaving her husband and eight sons to mourn the loss of a kind and efficient mother. She was the daughter of Mr. Joseph Shipley of Leicester.

> *Truro Daily News*, 10 March 1919, 2. Courtesy the Colchester Historeum, Truro.

Parrsborough Shore Deaths from the Great Influenza

This chapter is fortunate in having for inclusion a number of articles, book extracts, memoirs, and unpublished documents by a variety of Cumberland County residents, or modern researchers and journalists. First is a compilation of information on victims within the "Parrsborough Shore" area. This is the old District name for the communities of Cumberland County you will see featured in the following section.

Using Dr. Allan Marble's list of victims by county, Harriet McCready of the Parrsborough Shore Historical Society has arranged the Parrsborough Shore victims' names by communities within her part of the county. Her document now includes some victims native to, or residents of, the county, whether or not they died therein. This list has been conflated with Linda Littlejohn's research, providing more data on victims' families. Linda Littlejohn has also uncovered names missing from Allan Marble's list for this county. These have been edited for consistency, with some supplemental HVS research. What follows here are the listings submitted by Harriet McCready to this book, organized according to the communities along the Parrsborough Shore. She says to remember that Black Rock, West Bay, and Parrsboro Roads are all just different names for the same place, adjoining Parrsboro.

Apple River

Smith, Elizabeth O., 19, East Apple River. Her parents were George W. and Sarah G. Smith. She died on 22 November 1918, after five days' illness, of influenza and pneumonia. A Methodist, she was buried at Advocate Cemetery, Advocate Harbour.

> HVS, Death Register, Cumberland County, Year 1918, Book 39, Page 309, Number 1229. See also, *Amherst Daily News*, 26 November 1918, 3 (described as "Miss").

Taylor, Lee, 29, of Apple River, died in Massachusetts before 7 January 1919.

> See *Amherst Daily News*, 7 January 1919, 3

Shulie

Mills, William, aged 32. A native of Shulie; he died in Halifax on 31 October 1918, ill 18 days with Influenza and broncho pneumonia. A soldier, he was buried at Fort Massey, the military cemetery on Queen Street, Halifax. He was the brother of Charles Mills, below. Their parents were Enos and Prudence Ripley Mills. His religion is given as Christian.

> HVS, Death Register, Halifax County, Year 1918, Book 21, Page 587, Number 3519.

Mills, Charles E., aged 30. A native of Shulie, single, and a lumberman, he died at River Hebert on December 1, 1918. Dr. William Rockwell attended. A Presbyterian, his burial was in the Baptist Cemetery, River Hebert. Brother to William Mills, above.

> HVS, Death Register, Cumberland County, Year 1918, Book 39, Page 281, Number 1111. See also, *Amherst Daily News*, 7 January 1919, 3.

Advocate

Bennet, Clarence, aged 33, married to Kathleen Morris Bennet; his parents were Alexander and Mary Bennet, and he was born somewhere along the Parrsborough Shore, in one of the communities stretching to the west of Parrsboro, around Cape Chignecto, and north as far as Apple River. He died at Amherst on November 14, 1918 of pneumonia, having been ill for two weeks. He was buried at Advocate Harbour, which may have been where he was born and had family.

HVS, Death Register, Cumberland County, Year 1918, Book 39, Page 309, Number 1228.

Morris, Dimmock, aged 33, born in Advocate, married to Gladys Vernon Lunn Morris. He was a carpenter who lived in Advocate Harbour. He died on 25 October 1918 of pneumonia, after being sick eight days. The doctor was M. J. Tillimore; undertaker S. R. Canning. Buried in Advocate Harbour.

HVS, Death Register, Cumberland County, Year 1918, Book 39, Page 309, Number 1225. A notice of the death of Dimmock Morris appears in the *Amherst Daily News*, 30 October 1918, 4, as "Dimock Morris, Advocate."

Fox River

Maud Grant, 32, was the wife of James Leonard Grant of Fox River. She died of influenza and pneumonia, after an illness of 11 days, and was buried at the Methodist cemetery, Port Greville.

See Mrs. Leonard Grant, Fox River, *Amherst Daily News*, 27 December 1918, 3.

No record found on HVS Database.

Hughes, Mabel, aged 44, wife of Robert Hughes of Fox River. She died November 16, 1918, after two days of illness, and was buried in the Methodist Cemetery, Fox River/Port Greville.

See Mrs. Robert Hughes, *Amherst Daily News*, 21 November 1918, 3. HVS, Death Register, Cumberland County, Year 1918, Book 39, Page 309, Number 1214.

Graham Hughes, aged 17, single, of Fox River, died in Amherst on November 18, 1918 of Spanish Influenza and pneumonia. His parents were Robert and Bessie "Mabel" Hughes. His mother had died two days earlier, of the same disease. He is buried in the Methodist Cemetery, Fox River/Port Greville.

HVS, Death Register, Cumberland County, Year 1918, Book 39, Page 309, Number 1215.

Port Greville

 Ells, Harley Edward, aged 3, of Port Greville, Cumberland County, died there on November 21, 1918. His parents were Blanchard and Emma Ells.

Amherst Daily News, 21 November 1918, 3; with supplemental family information by Linda Littlejohn. No death record found in HVS database under Ells.

Parrsboro

 Lamb, Cecil F., aged 19, a native of Parrsboro, died in Boston, Massachusetts, on September 15, 1918.

See above, from the *Amherst Daily News*, 4 October 1918, 3, for the full story.

 Morrison, Lillian L., aged 25, a native of Parrsboro, d. Halifax, Nova Scotia, on October 8, 1918.

See above, from the *Amherst Daily News*, 4 October 1918, 3, for the full story.

Desmond, Beatrice, aged 13, of Parrsboro; died at Amherst on October 23, of influenza and pneumonia, having been sick for four days. Her parents were John and Emma Phinney Desmond. The family was Roman Catholic, and she was buried in the Roman Catholic cemetery in Parrsboro.

HVS, Death Register, Cumberland County, Year 1918, Book 39, Page 308, Number 1220.

Hunter, Edna May, aged 23, Parrsboro Roads, died in Amherst on November 27, 1918, of Spanish Influenza and pneumonia. She had been ill only two days. Her parents' names were Norman and Hannah Hunter.

HVS, Death Register, Cumberland County, Year 1918, Book 39, Page 305, Number 1210. See also, *Amherst Daily News*, 29 November 1918, 3.

Brown, Tressa Diana, aged 41, married to Leslie Brown of Parrsboro. She died at Amherst on February 14, 1919, having been ill for twelve days. She is buried in the Anglican cemetery, Parrsboro. The HVS search engine calls her "Brown, Tressa Dianna," but the actual record reads "Diana."

HVS, Death Register, Cumberland County, Year 1918, Book 39, Page 349, Number 1383.

Smith [Smythe], James V., aged 10 months, of Cross Roads, Parrsboro. He died on February 26, 1919, ill for ten days. His surname was really Smythe, according to his relative, Harriet McCready. His parents were James V. and Bessie Rector Smythe, and he was buried at the Methodist cemetery, Parrsboro. His actual death record shows "Smythe, James U." [*sic*], but the HVS search engine only shows him if one types in "Smith, James D." His tombstone says his name was "Vincent J."

HVS, Death Register, Cumberland County, Year 1918, Book 39, Page 353, Number 1393.

Seaman, Elizabeth Ruth, aged 3 years, of Parrsboro, died February 26, 1919, after an illness of ten days. Her parents were Alonzo and Lillian M. McArthur Seaman. Elizabeth Ruth died of pneumonia, and was buried at Union, in Halfway River.

HVS, Death Register, Cumberland County, Year 1918, Book 39, Page 350, Number 1385.

Bennett, Almadine, aged only 3 weeks, of Parrsboro, died at Amherst on February 27, 1919. As she was ill with influenza almost immediately after her birth, it was probably caught from her mother or a close family member. She was ill for the entire three weeks of her short life. Isaac Bennet was her father's name. This baby was buried at the New Methodist Cemetery, Parrsboro.

HVS, Death Register, Cumberland County, Year 1918, Book 39, Page 350, Number 1386.

Anderson, Florence Susan, aged 6 weeks, born in Parrsboro, died at Amherst on May 4, 1919, having been ill one week from influenza. Her parents were James and Sadie M. (Parsons?) Anderson. Burial was in the Anglican cemetery, Parrsboro.

Family information from Linda Littlejohn. No record found in HVS, Death Register, for her, in the period 1918–1920, or for any Anderson infants at all.

Lakelands

Fulton, Elsie Ray, aged 14, was the child of Arthur and Alida (Brown) Fulton of Lakelands. She died at Amherst on 01 November 1918, after being ill five days with influenza and pneumonia. She was buried at the Methodist Cemetery, Lakelands, on November 2.

HVS, Death Register, Cumberland County, Year 1918, Book 39, Page 307, Number 1212. See also, *Amherst Daily News*, 15 November 1918, 4.

Henwood, Hesley [Wesley] aged 3 weeks, of Lakelands. His name was really Wesley, according to Harriet McCready. He was the son of Silas and Annie Dowe Henwood. He died at Amherst on April 7, 1919, after having been sick only three days, from Influenza. He was buried at Union, Halfway River.

No record of him in the HVS Death Register.

Black Rock

Henwood, Blanch, aged 15, of Black Rock, Cumberland County, died in Amherst of Spanish Influenza on October 16, 1918, after being ill ten days. She and her sister Lilla, below, were the children of Harvey D. and Mary Harrington Henwood. They were both buried in the Baptist Cemetery, Black Rock.

HVS, Death Register, Cumberland County, Year 1918, Book 39, Page 308, Number 1222.

Henwood, Lilla, aged 13, of Black Rock, Cumberland County, died in Amherst of Spanish Influenza on October 20, 1918. Length of illness is not given. She and her sister Blanch, above, were the children of Harvey D. and Mary Harrington Henwood. They were both buried in the Baptist Cemetery, Black Rock.

HVS, Death Register, Cumberland County, Year 1918, Book 39, Page 308, Number 1223.

Places searched with no deaths: Fraserville, Ward's Brook, Ratchford River, Diligent River, Wharton, Two Islands, Green Hill, West Bay (found only the one in Cape Breton), Parrsboro Roads, Prospect, Moose River, West Brook…. Remember that Black Rock, West Bay, and Parrsboro Roads are all just different names for the same place on the outskirts of Parrsboro.

Harriet McCready, from information provided by Dr. Allan Marble and Linda Littlejohn. Supplemental research by the editor.

Chignecto Mines

INFLUENZA IN CUMBERLAND
The Mines at Chignecto have been temporarily shut down owing to the epidemic at that place. There is hardly an occupied house in that village, but has one or more persons suffering from influenza. There is also a serious outbreak in River Hebert, but so far the Joggins Mines is free from the disease.

Amherst Daily News, 22 October 1918, 3.

All the mines mentioned above, as well as the mines at Maccan, upriver from Chignecto, were established to work the same coal seam, which ran from Springhill down to Joggins, in Cumberland County. One by one, the mineworkers and their families began to come down with influenza. The crowded working conditions made it easy for the contagion to pass on, and poor air quality (low in oxygen and high in coal dust) affected the lungs, even before the horrific pneumonia which accompanied the influenza struck the miners.

A local woman, years later, wrote a small self-published book about the Chignecto mines. One chapter covered the effect the Great Influenza had on these mines, miners, and their families.

Extract from Myrtle Chappell's Memoir

THE SPANISH FLU. The Spanish Influenza raced through Chignecto at about the end of World War I and some recall there were about 10 deaths. Mrs. James McCarthy recalls her mother, Mrs. James McMaster, who was pregnant at the time and who never took the flu, going from house to house to help out, and she, as a little girl, carrying hot soup and hot tea to houses and setting them on the doorsteps of home where all were sick, and someone would reach out as she was leaving, to pick it up.

She recalls Dr. Forbes, from Maccan, Dr. Boudreau, and Dr. Goodwin, from Amherst, who brought nurses out with them, coming to care for the sick. She says her mother wore a scarf around her face that was soaked with disinfectant, and kept brandy in her mouth. She says one of the nurses died before midnight after being in there with the doctors during the day.

When someone died, their family had to put the body outside to be picked up, and Mrs. Percy Field [née Ripley] says that Robie Furlong told her when her father, John Ripley, died, that Mr. Ripley was the man who make [sic] the pick-ups, and he [Furlong] felt that he [Ripley] may have spared the life of his father, Tom Furlong, who [otherwise] would have had to go to Chignecto for the bodies, and might have taken the disease. Also Brad Bowlsby took bodies out. Some residents, who were children or young people, who did not survive were Winnie McDonald, Fronie O'Brien, Ada Everill, Alex Drousbeck, Rosie Schlosser, Mrs. Bill Seaman, two McPhee children, Ezra Ripley, Jim Henderson, and other names have not been recalled, and they say families were nearly wiped out.

Myrtle Chappell. *The Chignecto: St. George and Fenwick Mines*. Self-published, 1977. Courtesy the generosity of Frank Allen, who had an extra copy which he gave to Harriet McCready, who lent it to Ruth Whitehead.
Myrtle Chappell died at the age of 97.

Myrtle Chapell's informants had remarkably accurate memories. Here are the flu victims remembered in the memoir:

- Winnifred McDonald, aged 6, was born in Chignecto Mines; her father was Rupert McDonald. She died on October 28, 1918 in Amherst; of pneumonia, and had been ill only for one day. She was buried in Fenwick, NS.

HVS, Death Register, Cumberland County, Year 1918, Book 39, Page 267, Number 1035.

☞ Jim Henderson's name does not appear in Allan Marble's lists, although a *Harry* Henderson on the Marble lists appears a likely candidate: "Henderson, Harry, 28, Chignecto Mines, 18 October 1918, ill 7 days." Dr. Marble also found him in the *Amherst Daily News*, 19 October 1918, 4.

• Harry Clinton Henderson was born in Wallace, NS. He was 28 at the time of his death, and was a Baptist, married, working as a stoker, and living in Chignecto Mines. He died of influenza, having been ill only one week. His doctor was A. E. Forbes; and the return was sent in to the registrar by Mrs. Robert McPhee.
HVS, Death Register, Cumberland County, Year 1918, Book 39, Page 265, Number 1027. See below for further information.

VICTIMS OF INFLUENZA AT AMHERST. October 19
Influenza is claiming a number of victims in this county and, rather remarkable to say, the rugged and robust are the first to succumb. Word was received here this afternoon that Harry Henderson, formerly of the Amherst police force, had died last evening at Chignecto from influenza. The deceased was about 28 years old, and a native of Middleboro. He returned east about two years ago and accepted a position on the Amherst police force. He resigned from the force some months [past].
Halifax Evening Mail, 21 October 1918, 2.

☞ Alex Drousbeck appears on Dr. Allan Marble's lists as Droesbeck: "Droesbeck, Alex, 25, Chignecto Mines, 22 October 1918, [days ill] 09."
See also, *Amherst Daily News*, 29 October 1918, 4.

• Alex Droesbeck, aged 25, was born in Belgium and resided at the time of his death in Chignecto Mines, where he was a coal miner. He died of influenza after nine days illness, on October 22, 1918. A Catholic, he was taken upriver to Maccan for burial. His doctor was F. E. Boudreau, his undertakers Christie Brothers.
HVS, Death Register, Cumberland County, Year 1918, Book 39, Page 266, Number 1029.

☞ Rosie Schlosser appears on Dr. Allan Marble's list: "Schlosser, Rosie, 17, Maccan, 24 October 1918, days ill not given."

• Rosie Schlosser, aged 17, was single and lived in Maccan. Her father's name was Frank Schlosser. Death came on October 24, 1918, caused by influenza. A lot of this record was then left blank, down to place of burial. She was interred at Maccan. Someone unnamed returned her particulars to the registrar on October 31.
HVS, Death Register, Cumberland County, Year 1918, Book 39, Page 266, Number 1033.

☞ Ada Everill appears on Dr. Allan Marble's lists as "Everill, Ada." She appears on Linda Littlejohn's list as "Ada Lena Everill, 16 months, father William Everill, Chignecto Mines, N.S. Burial—Nappan." Ada died on October 28, 1918, of influenza, ill with it only one week.

- Ada Lena Everill was born in Chignecto Mines and lived to the age of 16 months there; she died, still at home in Chignecto Mines, on October 28, 1918. Her father's name was William Everill. Cause of death was influenza, after a week's illness. The doctor was F. E. Boudreau. She was buried at Nappan. Her mother, "Mrs. William Everill," sent in her daughter's return on November 11.

  HVS, Death Register, Cumberland County, Year 1918, Book 39, Page 267, Number 1036.

☞ Mrs. Bill Seaman appears on Dr. Allan Marble's lists as "Lida Seaman."

- Lida May Seaman, 22, living at Chignecto Mines, was married to William Seaman, who was born in St. George, Maine. [*She appears in the Myrtle Chappell memoir as Mrs. Bill Seaman.*] She died October 30, 1918, at Amherst, from heart failure and influenza, after an illness of twenty-four hours. She was buried at Maccan, Cumberland County, just upriver from Chignecto Mines.

  HVS, Death Register, Cumberland County, Year 1918, Book 39, Page 267, Number 1037.

- Fronie O'Brien: It appears her name was Sophia Isabell; 'Fronie' was apparently a nickname. Fronie appears on Dr. Allan Marble's lists as "O'Brien, Sophine, 05, Chignecto Mines, 30 October 1918, [days ill] 07." She appears in Linda Littlejohn's list as "Sophia Isabell O'Brine of Chignecto Mines. Died in Amherst age 5 years 8 months, Influenza x 1 week. D/O Ernest O'Brine. Burial, Nappan." She appears in the Death Register for 1918, and even in the HVS search engine, as Sophia Isabell O'Brien, 5 years, 8 months, Chignecto Mines, father, Ernest O'Brine [*sic*]. She died of influenza, after an illness of one week, attended by Dr. F. E. Boudreau. Her death return was sent in by Vance Stiles, J. P., on November 9, 1918.

  HVS, Death Register, Cumberland County, Year 1918, Book 39, Page 267, Number 1038.

- Ezra Ripley appears on Dr. Allan Marble's lists as Ezra Richard Ripley: "Ripley, Ezra Richard, d. Fenwick, aged 22. *Amherst Daily News*, 5 November 1918, 3." He appears on Linda Littlejohn's list as aged 21, single, died Amherst, November 14, 1918. "Res. Fenwick. Pneumonia x 2 weeks. S/O George W. Ripley. Burial Fenwick." Ezra's name appears on his death certificate as "Ripley, Ezra T., aged

21, single, Methodist; father George W. Ripley. He lived at "Fenwick Road," and was buried in "Fenwick," but he died in Amherst on November 4, 1918, after a two-week illness ending in pneumonia. No doctor or undertaker's name appears on the entry for him.

HVS, Death Register, Cumberland County, Year 1918, Book 39, Page 267, Number 1040.

The Two McPhee Children

☞ Racheal [Rachael?] McPhee, 13 months, died at Chignecto Mines, on April 15, 1919, of Influenza and Bronchial Pneumonia, after an illness of 3 days. Her parents' names are not given, nor is her place of burial, only her doctor's name, A. E. Forbes, who obviously didn't know the family well, or at all. (He was just helping out from Maccan.) He did report that the family was Methodist. Rachael was perhaps just buried by a family member or family friend. She is the only McPhee child during this epidemic who has a death certificate, unless the second victim is entered under a wildly different variant (a number of which were tried).

HVS, Death Register, Cumberland County, Year 1918, Book 39, Page 365, Number 1452.

☞ The 1911 Census for Cumberland County, Nova Scotia, Chignecto Mines, shows a George McPhee, born 1881, and wife, Anna, born 1882, with three girls and two boys. They may have been Rosie's parents. As to the memoir's other child, either they or any of the boys enumerated in this or other McPhee families at Chignecto Mines could have gotten married and had children, one of whom died. We may never know anything more than this about Rachael McPhee or the other McPhee child who fell victim to the flu.

There were other deaths, up and down that coal seam, at many different mines. Here are the flu victims who died at the locations closest to the Chignecto Mines. The final column of numbers represents the length of the illness for each victim:

Smith, Jennie	20	Fenwick	01 November 1918	06 [days ill]
Ripley, Ezra Richard	22	Fenwick	04 November 1918	2 weeks
Webb, Hazel	16 m.	Fenwick Mines	26 November 1918	05
Harrison, Freeda	35	Fenwick Mines	27 November 1918	not given
St. Peter, Olive June	12	Maccan	04 November 1918	04
Rector, Christy	10	Maccan	27 November 1918	07
Rector, Harry	08	Maccan	26 November 1918	04
Rector, Wesley	09	Maccan	01 December 1918	07
Wood, Mrs. W.W.	40	Maccan	04 March 1919	07
Bridge, John	40	Maccan	04 March 1919	07

Hall, James	55	River Hebert	10 October 1918	07
LeBlanc, Zelda	34	River Hebert	14 October 1918	07
Burke, Annie	27	River Hebert	21 October 1918	03
Hoeg, Florence	49	River Hebert	10 November 1918	not given
Mills, Charles	30	River Hebert	01 December 1918	05
Wood, Stella	26	River Hebert	10 December 1918	07
Scott, Abbie	19	River Hebert	13 December 1918	07
Morris, Giles	49	Joggins Mines	14 November 1918	10
Morris, William	40	Joggins Mines	16 November 1918	04
McGovern, William	28	Joggins Mines	17 November 1918	10
McGovern, Chester	24	Joggins Mines	21 November 1918	08
Belliveau, Evelyn	24	Joggins Mines	08 December 1918	08
Como, Amos	38	Joggins Mines	16 March 1919	3m
Legere, Malinda	36	Joggins Mines	30 March 1919	10
Smith, Christina	63	Joggins Mines	31 March 1919	11
White, Robert	4m	Joggins Mines	22 November 1918	05

Compiled from Dr. Allan Marble's list, Cumberland County Vital Statistics,
at the end of the chapter.

 James Hall, whose father was the late William Hall, formerly manager of the Springhill mines, and the first mayor of that town, was buried at Springhill on Friday. He contracted influenza followed by pneumonia while working at River Hebert and died after a few days' illness.

Halifax Evening Mail, 21 October 1918, 12.

THE LATE ELISHA R. MILLS, DIED NOV. 10.

A Hero of Many Fights Gone to His Rest

The sad news reached Truro, on the 11th, of the deth at Pugwash, of Elisha R. Mills, son of Mr. and Mrs. McLeod Mills, Victoria Street, Truro, the deth [*sic*] having occurred on Sunday, Nov. 10th.

The deceased at the outbreak of the war enlisted with the 40th Battalion, trained at Valcartier and was wounded twenty-eight times during the second battle of Ypres and Hooge. He returned to Canada something over a year ago with the loss of one eye. He recovered sufficiently to take the position of Collector of Customs at the Port of Pugwash, was late married and has been living their [*sic*] performing the duties since.

A few weeks ago he was stricken with Spanish Influenza and was seriously low and recovered and was up around when he took a relapse and passed away, quickly, as stated. He is survived by his wife, formerly Miss Clark, of Pugwash.

Truro Daily News, 12 November 1918, 5. Courtesy the
Colchester Historeum, Truro.

✑ A week after I'd finished this book manuscript, an email came from Dale Mills, who had made contact after a reading an interview featuring Dr. Allan Marble and myself. He wrote:

✉ I just read an interesting and appropriate article by Moira Donovan and in it there was a story about a Pugwash man that you had presented to her. I am the grandson of Elisha Raymond Mills, the man who was referenced in the article. Actually, he wasn't shot 28 times. He had 28 wounds with 3 gunshot wounds (maybe) and the rest (perhaps all) were from shrapnel. He spent about 5 months in three different hospitals recuperating. I have his medical records. He married my grandmother Susan (Clarke) and they both had the Spanish flu in the fall of 1918, with Susan surviving. Unfortunately, my grandfather died from the Spanish flu before my father was born.

✑ I gratefully replied to him, and a day later, he sent a huge packet of his sources on his grandfather, as well as photographs (see page 124), and some of the research he and his nephew Eric Mills had put together earlier. He said his grandfather, Elisha Raymond Mills, was born March 15, 1897, in Benton, NB. His parents, McLeod and Nora Mills, moved to Truro, NS. In August 1915, their son enlisted in the 40th Battalion, "basically a replenishment unit for other units in France, thus the transfer to the 5th Battalion Canadian Mounted Rifles (5CMR) in the fall of 1915."

Dale Mills to Ruth Whitehead, 21 December 2019, email.

Dale and Eric Mills' Research

✉ Elisha Raymond Mills—Brief History
Born March 15, 1897 Benton, New Brunswick
Parents: Nora and McLeod Mills and family moved to Truro, N.S....

- Feb 16 1916 in Belgium.
- Payroll records show he was paid $1.00 per day and received an extra $.10 a day for being in the trenches (field).
- June 1916 reported Killed In Action.
- He was 19 years old weighing 140 pounds when wounded on June 2, 1916 at the Battle of Mount Sorrel, the 5CMR's first battle honour.
- June 12 telegram to his mother Nora Mills reported he was dangerously ill with gunshot wounds to the arm, chest and head.

In Ypres France [Belgium] on June 2nd he received 28 wounds with 3 gunshot wounds (maybe) and the rest (perhaps all) were from shrapnel. While on a stretcher, a bomb exploded nearby burying him with some dirt likely causing blindness in his left eye. We are skeptical about gunshot wounds (GSW) even though it was on several of the reports. We think it was all shrapnel. None of the detailed medical reports or disability reports mentioned GSW's. Unless we missed something... there was a lot of paperwork! Regardless he sustained several very serious injuries including a punctured lung.

Patient was at several hospitals for 5 months—Boulogne Hospital, Bagthorpe Hospital, Eye & Ear Hospital (Folkestone), Ramsgate Hospital.

- Dec 1916 Returned to Canada, convalescent home in St. John, NB May 31, 1917.

- Discharged at the rank of lance-corporal.

- Collector of Customs at Pugwash June 1917.

- Member of Canadian Order of Forresters.

- Married Susan Catherine Clarke, June 28, 1918.

- Both Elisha and Susan came down with the Spanish flu in October 1918. Susan recovered. Elisha was well on his way to recovering when suddenly he ended up with cerebral meningitis, the cause of which the doctor attributed likely to shrapnel being embedded in his skull. Date of Death Nov. 10, 1918 the day before the Armistice.

- Son Elisha Raymond Clarke Mills Born Jan. 24, 1919.

- Susan raised Raymond on Pugwash Point on her family's homestead. She never remarried, became a nurse, delivered many babies as a midwife and she took care of her elderly parents. She corresponded with a cabinet minister to get war widow pension. Their son Ray served in RCAF in WWII. Susan lived until 1992, aged 97, outliving her son Raymond who passed in 1990. She used to reminisce about her husband 'Millsy'.

- An interesting piece of information was that her son said that he had very bad teeth and had to have dentures at a very early age, saying that when his mother had the Spanish flu, it was at a time when teeth buds in the fetus were forming.
  Dale and Eric Mills to Ruth Whitehead, email, 31 December 2019.

Elisha R. Mills. Pugwash, Nov. 18, 1918. The death of E. R. Mills, Collector of Customs here, which occurred on Sunday Evening, 10th inst., cast a deep gloom over this community. The deceased was among the first in town to be stricken with Spanish Influenza. He seemed to be recovering, however, and on Friday sat up for a few hours. On Saturday alarming symptoms appeared and his father was sent for. Meningitis developed and after intense suffering, he passed away on Saturday ⌈Sunday⌋ evening as stated above.

Unattributed newspaper clipping (Amherst Daily News?) provided by
Dale and Eric Mills, 31 December 2019.

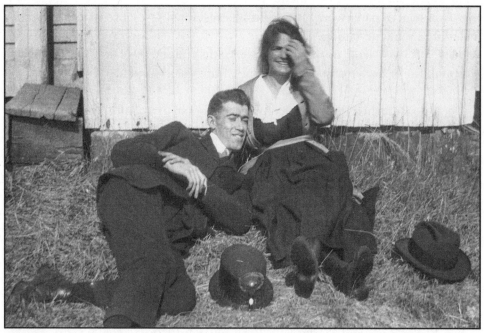

Elisha and Sue Mills, Pugwash, ca.1918. Both caught influenza in October 1918. Susan and their unborn son survived. Elisha died on November 10. *(Courtesy Dale Mills (grandson), Eric Mills (great-grandson); photographer unknown)*

HUGHES. At Port Greville, N. S., Nov. 15th, 1918, of Spanish Influenza, in her 45th year, Mrs. Robert S. Hughes, for many years a faithful and loyal member of the Methodism ⌈*sic*⌋ Church.

Truro Daily News, 4 December 1918.

Writers Describe 1919 Deaths

In 1968, Canadian author Will R. Bird, who was born in East Mapleton, Cumberland County, wrote a memoir of his time in the First World War. He had served two years in Europe with the 42nd Battalion. This book, with the evocative title, *Ghosts Have Warm Hands*, contains an experience with "Spanish Influenza." He and his friend Tommy were back in London in 1919, waiting to be sent home. Just as they began to realize they had survived some of the worst fighting of any war, Tommy took sick. The following is an extract from this memoir:

Tommy roused me at noon and said he was feeling feverish. He dressed, and the attendant at the place where we stayed mixed him a concoction of some nature but it was no help. At four in the afternoon, I began trying to locate a doctor. There was no luck on the telephone. Always a female answered and assured me the doctor had more than he could handle, since a 'flu epidemic was raging'. So out I went, and after an hour of searching, helped wonderfully by a huge bobby, I contacted a doctor and told him the circumstances. He looked a tired man but he went with me, and in half an hour Tommy was on his way to a hospital. I followed by taxi to make sure there were no difficulties....

That night I did not go out and the next morning tried in vain to get in touch with the doctor. After two in the afternoon, the suspense became too much, and away I went in search of the hospital. It took me until four o'clock in the afternoon to find it, and then I had quite a battle to gain admittance. When another doctor came to my rescue, I went with him. I had to put on a mask before we went into a long ward. Tommy looked wretched but managed a grin at my appearance, then urged me to get out before I caught influenza too.

It was dark by the time I got back and I had no heart to go out for any entertainment. The next forenoon seemed an eternity and then I followed the route again, but in a shorter time since I had learned to watch for various landmarks. Again there was the refusal of admittance and again I stayed in the waiting room. Eventually a doctor appeared. Although he was obviously annoyed by my persistence, he went to see if I could visit the ward. He was back quickly and his message stunned me. Tommy had died that morning!

The world crashed around me. It was dark when I found myself back at the quarters we had shared, and midnight before I stopped pacing the room. But there was simply nothing I could do.

William R. Bird. *Ghosts Have Warm Hands: A Memoir of the Great War, 1916–1919.*
First edition, 1968. Paperback edition, 1997, 176–7.

"Story from River Herbert" by Charles Thompson: The following is a memoir about influenza deaths in the author's family.

My great grandparents died from the Spanish Flu in 1919 in River Hebert, leaving my grandmother and her siblings orphans. Up until now I only really knew the basics of it, but wanted to learn more about it as it certainly changed the direction of my family's history. The six children were sent to live with various relatives. They lived in River Hebert at the time of their death.

My great grandfather was Gordon Argyle Rector who died on April 1, 1919. The Rector family was originally from Parrsboro, more specifically at Lakelands. My great grandmother, Mamie Beatrice (Nuttall) Rector died three days later on April 4, 1919, just four days after giving birth to their sixth child. Mamie was born in New Salem and was a teacher in Brookville on the Parrsboro Shore for a couple of years before getting married. So growing up I had always heard of the story of them dying young and my grandmother and her twin sister being sent to live with the Nuttall grandparents in New Salem, and how the other siblings were sent to various Rector aunts and uncles.

I just live in Truro so not far away and would love to keep in touch and learn more about this and would be willing to help where I can. I know River Hebert is not on the Parrsboro Shore but if my great grandparents' information is useful to any work, I would gladly supply what I can. Sadly, I did not get interested in this all until after my grandmother and all her siblings passed so was what I know is what I remember from stories as a kid. Although do have a write up from the Amherst paper and a photo of them and five of their six children a year or two before they passed....Yes, feel free to share it. It was a very sad story as I am sure so many were in that time between the war and the flu taking so many young and otherwise healthy people and leaving behind widows, single parents or orphans....If there is anything else I can do please let me know.

Charles Thompson, Truro, to Harriet McCready, Parrsboro, via Facebook Messenger, 13–14 November 2018. Slightly condensed and edited for clarity.

☞ See page 127 for a photograph sent by Charles Thompson, with the following note: "Photo of the whole family; we are guessing it was from late 1917 or early 1918, as Dorothy the baby was born June 1917. So left to right it is Marion 'Aileen' Rector (1914–2007), Gordon Argyle Rector (1886–1919), Georgina Berle Rector (1912–2008), Margaret Merle Rector (1912–2004), Mamie Beatrice (Nuttall) Rector (1887–1919)—she is holding Dorothy Nema Rector (1917–2001); Beatrice Evangeline Rector (1915–2003). We are not sure which twin is which in the middle, I think my grandmother Margaret is sitting and Aunt Georgie is standing, but it is just a guess based on subtle differences."

Cumberland Roots. River Hebert. This community was greatly saddened on Tuesday morning the 1st inst., when the death of Gordon Rector was reported, the whole family including Mr. Rector and his wife and six children was stricken down with influenza almost at the same time, when Mr. Rector in doing all he could to alleviate the condition of the family developed pneumonia with the fatal result. A few hours previous to his death a baby boy was born and the nurse on

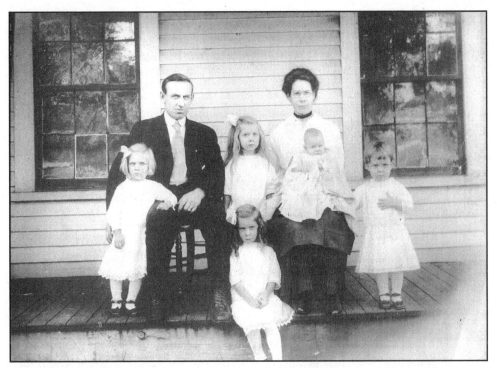

The Gordon Rector family, from left: Marion "Aileen" Rector (1914–2007), Gordon Argyle Rector (1886–1919), Georgina Berle Rector (1912–2008) [possibly the twin standing at centre], Margaret Merle Rector (1912–2004) [possibly the twin seated in front], Mamie Beatrice (Nuttall) Rector (1887–1919) holding Dorothy Nema Rector (1917–2001); Beatrice Evangeline Rector (1915–2003). Parents Gordon and Mamie died of influenza less than a year after the photo, just after Mamie had given birth to a son. *(Courtesy of Rector descendent Charles Thompson, Truro, who provided photo and identifications. Photographer unknown)*

showing him the new born baby, the first boy in the family, he replied that it was too late; and on Friday, Mrs. Rector passed away, leaving six orphan children, the eldest, twin girls, being only six years old. Mr. Rector was in his thirty-first year, and his wife who was a Miss Mamie B. Nuttall before marriage, in her 32nd year. The late Mr. Rector in May of last year purchased a house and five acres of land at a cost of $1200 and on the Saturday previous to his illness he paid the last cent of the purchase money, getting his release of mortgage, showing how industrious and careful he was getting along. Both he [and his wife are] buried in River View Cemetery at River Hebert.

Amherst Daily News, 15 April 1919, 7. Courtesy of Charles Thompson, Truro.

The Amherst Internment Camp for Prisoners of War

"Amherst Internment Camp. Between 1914 and 1920 thousands of Ukrainians and other Europeans were needlessly imprisoned as 'enemy aliens' during Canada's first national internment operations, as were prisoners of war. This plaque commemorates those held on this site, in the Malleable Iron Works, between April 17, 1915 and September 27, 1919."

> Commemorative plaque at the site of the former Malleable Iron Works, Park Street, Amherst, NS. The inscription has a border of barbed wire around it, and is in English, French and Ukrainian. The building itself no longer exists, but there is a local museum on the property. The plaque is affixed to its outside wall.

☞ One of this camp's most famous prisoners was Leon Trotsky. After leaving New York in 1917 to return to Russia, he and his wife, Natalia Sedova, and their children were taken off a Norwegian ship which had called at Halifax Harbour. He was eventually sent to Amherst; his family was put up in a local hotel in Halifax. He described conditions at the camp, as follows:

The Amherst Concentration camp was housed in an old and very dilapidated iron foundry that had been confiscated from its German owner. The bunks were arranged in three tiers, two deep on each side of the hall. About 800 of us lived in these conditions. The air in this dormitory at night can be imagined. Men hopelessly clogged the passages, elbowed their way through....in spite of the heroic efforts of the prisoners to keep themselves physically and morally fit, five of them had gone insane. We had to eat and sleep in the same room with these madmen.

> *My Life*, by Leon Trotsky. New York: Charles Scribner's Sons, 1930.

☞ Influenza flourished in crowded situations such as this camp. At its worst, it held 834 prisoners. They were crammed into a building a quarter of a mile long, but only one hundred feet wide. In addition, there were, at peak, 256 guards, most of them Amherst men.

INFLUENZA OUTBREAK

There has been a serious outbreak among the interned prisoners. There are over one hundred and twenty cases in the Military hospital in the Drill Hall, and there are a number of prisoners in the hospital in connection with the camp which will be transferred to the Drill Hall as soon as possible. The News understands that Lt. Dr. Goodwin has asked the military authorities in Halifax for an Assistant Doctor and other additional Red Cross [*sic*; the typesetter left out all the rest of this sentence except the final letters 'inen' – probably the word 'linen']. The influenza was evidently brought into camp by working parties of prisoners that had been out in effected [*sic*] districts. At the opeulug [opening] of last week, there was [had been] practically no patients in the Military hospital here.

Amherst Daily News, 12 February 1919, 3.

☞ Lt. Dr. B. E. Goodwin must have worked miracles with his patients, because only one—possibly two or three—of them died of influenza during this time. The only recorded "Spanish Influenza" death was that of Heinrich Harms, who died on January 14, 1919. Two pneumonia deaths could also have resulted from influenza, but as it is not certain, we cannot count these two: William Wegner, who died on February 15, 1919, and Joachim Tiedemann, who died on November 18, 1918. Wegner and Tiedemann, of course, do not appear on Dr. Allan Marble's list.

- Heinrich Harms, aged 45, married, sea pilot, warrant officer [German navy or merchant marine], was held at the Amherst Internment Camp, where he died on January 14, 1919, three months after the war ended. According to his death certificate, he had been born in "Amt Jeve, Oldenburg." This is Jever, a city in northwest Germany, situated near the Baltic Sea coast around Oldenburg in Holstein. Oldenburg is the "Amt" of Jever, and lies to the southeast; an Amt is a "collective municipality," according to its Wikipedia entry. "Seat of the Amt" implies "a county, a shire, or a township, but not part of it."

  Harm's wife, Johanna Harms, is actually listed in the death certificate—the only time during this period that a wife's name was given on a death record. The spousal space reads, "If married, give name of husband." A wife's name was considered non-essential.

  HVS, Death Register, Cumberland County, Book 39, Page 312, Number 1241.

- Joachim Tiedemann, aged 23, was born in Hamburg, Germany, father's name unknown, single. He was held in the Internment Camp, Amherst, as a German prisoner of war. He died of pneumonia on November 18, 1918. His doctor was Lt. B. E. Goodwin. Christie Brothers Co. buried him at Amherst.

  HVS, Death Register, Cumberland County, Year 1918, Book 39, Page 258,
Number 983. He is a possible Influenza/Pneumonia victim.

- "William Wegner #519," as the name is written on his death certificate, is listed as having been born in Germany, aged 26, single; a German soldier being held at the internment camp in Amherst. He died February 15, 1919 of pneumonia. The doctor treating him was "Dr. B. E. Goodwin, Lieut." Undertaker was F. M. Brown, who also sent in the death return; burial was at Highland Cemetery. No one seems to have known much about him.

  HVS, Death Register, Cumberland County, Year 1919, Book 39, Page 315,
Number 125. He is a possible Influenza/Pneumonia victim.

- Harms and Tiedemann are among those commemorated on a stone—paid for by the prisoners themselves—headed "DEN VERSTORBENEN KRIEGS-GEFANGENEN DEUTSCHEN" ["To the late German prisoners of war"], in Amherst Cemetery. Thanks to the Brigitte Neumann for the German translation.

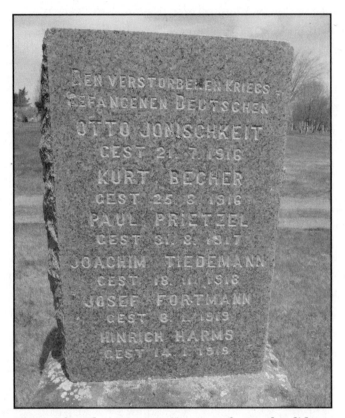

Memorial to the German prisoners-of-war who did not survive the First World War Internment Camp, Amherst. Three of these died from the Great Influenza. The stone was paid for by fellow prisoners. (*Courtesy of Harriet McCready*)

1920 Deaths

⟐ Maude Bourgeois's death on February 18, 1920, was the first one recorded for influenza's Third Wave in Cumberland County. Perhaps the doctor was exhausted, because somehow her death records states that she was born in Amherst on February 25, 1920, which was eight days after the date of her death. In fact, Bourgeois lived all her 34 years, 11 months and 18 days at the same address, 16 Mill Street. Her father, Ferdinand Bourgeois, was born in Newfoundland, and her mother, Mary Gaudet Bourgeois, was born in New Brunswick. F. E. Boudreau was the doctor's name; he states he saw her last on February 17, and that she died at 2:00 A.M. the following morning. She was buried at St. Charles cemetery, Amherst, on the same day, February 18.

HVS, Cumberland County Death Register, 1920, Book 63, Page 179.

⟐ **CHARLES A. NELSON DIED MARCH 18 AT LOWER WENTWORTH**
There past [*sic*] away on Thursday March 18 at his home in Lower Wentworth, Cumb. Co., Charles A. Nelson...after an illness of but two weeks. Death was due to Influenza, followed by pneumonia....The deceased was forty years of age. He leaves a widow and two small children.

Truro Daily News, 24 March, 1920. Courtesy the Colchester Historeum.

⟐ Euphemia Hope [Hape] was the final victim of this Third Wave of influenza in the county. She was 29 years, 2 months and 14 days old when she died on April 15, 1920. She had been born in 1891, in Denmark, Colchester County, to John (a farmer) and Mary Langille Cole. On April 30, 1919, at the time of her marriage to Percy E. Hape, or Elias Percy Hape, as his name appears on her death record, she was living in Wallace Highlands, as were her parents and at least one brother. Before her marriage, she had been working for nine years as a servant. Her husband, Elias Percy Hape, was of Dutch extraction, the son of Henry and Adeline Pye (or Pyle) Hape, both born in Nova Scotia. Percy and Euphemia Cole Hape were married in Wallace. He was Anglican, and she was a Baptist. Euphemia and her husband Percy witnessed the marriage that same year of an older brother, John Mitchell Cole, in Tatamagouche on November 3, to Mabel Murphy McNeil, a widow.

Euphemia Hape died fifteen days short of her first wedding anniversary. She had been ill from influenza for ten days, then pneumonia developed and she fought it off for seven more days, but died at noon on April 15. She was buried in "Bay Head," i.e., Bayhead, near Tatamagouche, Colchester County. The undertaker was R. C. McLellan of Tatamagouche. Her parents were also buried there: John in August 1919, Mary in May 1948. Elias Percy Hape, her husband, died on an Acadian Lines bus somewhere in or close to Amherst, on 14 April 1952. An inquest showed that the cause of death was coronary thrombosis. He had remarried and was resident in Malagash Mines, but was buried in Bayhead, as his first wife, Euphemia, had been.

HVS, Cumberland County Death Register, 1920, Book 63, Page 325 (Euphemia).
HVS, Cumberland County Marriage Register, 1919, Book 38, Page 896, (Percy Hape, Euphemia Cole). The HVS search engine has the bridegroom's name as "Hope," but he signed the register as "Hape."
HVS, Cumberland County Death Register, 1919, Book 39, Page 417, Number 1630 (John Cole Sr.)
HVS, Colchester County Marriage Register, 1919, Book 44, Page 767 (John Mitchell Cole, Mabel McNeil).
HVS, Colchester County Death Register, 1948, Page 3042 (Mary Langille Cole).
HVS, Cumberland County Death Register, 1952, Page 2864 (Percy Hape). His name is written "Hope" here, but corrected in parentheses to "Hape."
HVS, Cumberland County Death Register, 1963, Page 5202 (John Mitchell Cole, "retired carpenter," resident in Wallace Highlands).

CUMBERLAND COUNTY, VITAL STATISTICS, DEATH REGISTER, BOOKS 39, 63

1918

1. Charles Rice, 45, d. 2 October 1918, Westchester, surveyor of lumber.

2. Robert Jobe, 18, d. 4 October 1918, Westchester Station, farmer. N.P. [*No one by this name found in HVS database. Dr. Marble's list has "N.P. (called Weldon Job)," but that's not in there either. Dr. Marble used "N.P.," he says, to mean "not present" in the original register. He may have gotten this death listing, and subsequent N.P. names, out of newspaper references.*]

3. Harold Scott, 17, d. 14 October 1918, Westchester, labourer.

4. Elizabeth Patriquin, 35, d. 22 October 1918, Greenville Station, housewife.

5. Abraham Cormier, 76, d. 17 October 1918, Amherst. N.P.

6. Carl Pipes, 28, d. 21 October 1918, Amherst, mail carrier. N.P.

7. Dora Kent, 14 months, d. 22 October 1918, Amherst.

8. Bernice Cormier, 7 months, d. 24 October 1918, Amherst.

9. Blair Cormier, 35, d. 30 October 1918, Amherst, blacksmith.

10. Vera Dunphy, 28, d. 31 October 1918, Amherst, housewife.

11. Noel Russell Fraser, 27, d. 31 October 1918, Amherst, skipper. N.P.

12. Alphonse Papineau, 23, d. 3 November 1918, Amherst, [soldier and] toolmaker. [*Alphonse's residence was in Ontario (name of town illegible); he had been born in "St. Joseph" and was buried in "St. Joseph's." Cumberland County Death Register, 1918, Book 39, Page 255, Number 969.*]

13. Mrs. Blair Cormier, 35, d. 4 November 1918, Amherst.

14. Clodia Bourque, 1, d. 6 November 1918, Amherst.

15. Margaret Butler, 34, d. 11 November 1918, Amherst.

16. Cassie Manslip, 20, d. 13 November 1918, Amherst.

17. Philomen [*Philomène*] Landry, female, 20, d. 20 November 1918, Amherst, housework.

18. Norman Ells, 30, d. 24 November 1918, Amherst, trunk factory.

19. Carl Bishop, 16, d. 25 November 1918, Amherst.

20. Maggie Melanson, 18, d. 26 November 1918, Amherst.

21. Cyril Doncaster, 2, d. 11 December 1918, Amherst.

22. Eloise LeBlanc, 31, d. 12 December 1918, Amherst.

23. Elizabeth Gardiner, 22, d. 21 December 1918, Amherst.

24. Grace Mills, 7, d. 23 December 1918, Amherst.

25. Harry Henderson, 28, d. 18 October 1918, Chignecto Mines, stoker.

26. Alex Droesbeck, 25, d. 22 October 1918, Chignecto Mines, coal miner.

27. Rosie Schlosser, 17, d. 24 October 1918, Maccan.

28. Ada Everill, 16 months, d. 28 October 1918, Chignecto Mines.

29. Lida Seaman, 22, d. 30 October 1918, Chignecto Mines, housework.

30. Sophina [*Sophia Isabell*] O'Brien, 5, d. 30 October 1918, Chignecto Mines. [*See essay for Cumberland County for discussion of her first name, which appears as "Sophia" on the original record.*]

31. Jennie Smith, 20, d. 1 November 1918, Fenwick.

32. William Morris, 40, d. 16 November 1918, Joggins Mines, miner.

33. Leonard Brown, 28, d. 25 November 1918, South Maitland, soldier, "influenza and gassed during war."

34. Hazel Webb, 16 months, d. 26 November, Fenwick Mines.

35. Harry Rector, 8, d. 26 November 1918, Maccan.

36. Christy Rector, 10, d. 27 November 1918, Maccan.

37. Freida Harrison, 35, d. 27 November 1918, Fenwick Mines.

38. Wesley Rector, 9, d. 1 December 1918, Maccan.

39. W. B. Gould, 33, d. 11 January 1919, Nappan, meat dealer.

40. Mrs. Minnie Thomas, 26, d. 19 November 1918, Thompson, housewife.

41. Mrs. Olive Rushton, 57, d. 22 November 1918, Westchester Station, housewife.

42. Ruliph [Ralph Alexander] Adams, 14 months, d. 24 November 1918, Westchester. [Book 39, Page 273, Number 1068.]

43. Orland [Orland Levi] Adams, 8 days, d. 4 December 1918, Westchester.

44. Charles Moore, 22, d. 3 November 1918, Oxford.

45. Wentworth Callow, 14 months, d. 4 November 1918, Oxford. [Buried in Advocate, NS, per Harriet McCready.]

46. Alberta Embrie, 11, d. 29 November 1918, Oxford.

47. Frank Dotton, 28, d. 16 October 1918, Oxford Junction, main dispatcher.

48. Sarah Gordon, 28, d. 15 December 1918, Oxford Junction.

49. Florence Hoeg, 49, d. 10 November 1918, River Hebert, housewife.

50. James Hall, 55, d. 10 October 1918, River Hebert, bookkeeper.

51. Zelda Le Blanc, 34, d. 14 October 1918, River Hebert, housewife.

52. Annie Burke, 22, d. 21 October 1918, River Hebert, housekeeper.

53. Giles Morris, 49, d. 14 November 1918, Joggins Mines, miner.

54. William McGovern, 28, d. 17 November 1918, Joggins Mines, miner.

55. Chester McGovern, 24, d. 21 November 1918, Joggins Mines, miner.

56. Robert White, 4 months, d. 22 November 1918, Joggins Mines.

57. Charles Mills, 30, d. 1 December 1918, Shulie.

58. Evelyn Belliveau, 24, d. 8 December 1918, Joggins Mines. [She was the daughter of Amos Belliveau, single, Catholic, and died of Influenza and Pneumonia. Her doctor was William Rockwell. Book 39, Page 282, Number 1113.]

59. Stella Wood, 26, d. 10 December 1918, River Hebert, postmistress. [She was single, the daughter of Charles R. Wood, died of Influenza and Pneumonia, and is buried in the Baptist Cemetery, River Hebert. Book 39, Page 282, Number 1117.]

60. Abbie Scott, 19, d. 13 December 1918, River Hebert.

61. Frank Demings, 21, d. 6 October 1918, Pugwash, soldier.

62. William King, 18, d. 29 October 1918, Pugwash, farmer.

63. Willard Woodward, 26, d. 9 November 1918, Middleboro, farmer.

64. Elisha Mills, 21, d. 10 November 1918, Pugwash, customs officer.

65. *Infant* Hudson, 5 months, d. 27 November 1918, Hertford ["Hansford?"; note by Dr. Marble. Book 39, Page 287, Number 1132 says his residence was "Hartford," his father was James Hudson].

66. Truman Carter, 20, d. 3 December 1918, Pugwash, farmer.

67. Lewis Teed, 21, d. 26 December 1918, Pugwash, labourer.

68. Ernest Teed, 15, d. 26 December 1918, Pugwash, labourer.

69. _____ McLeod, 21, d. 29 December 1918, Pugwash, farmer. [*Book 39, Page 288, Number 1142, gives no first name; name of his father was "Hirman McLeod."*]

70. Annie Card, 3 months, d. 28 October 1918, Springhill.

71. Gertrude Swanwick, 35, d. 28 October 1918, Springhill, housewife.

72. Effie Colwell, 1, d. 31 October 1918, Springhill.

73. Bedford Miller, 39, d. 31 October 1918, Springhill, labourer.

74. Katherine Wilson, 54, d. 2 November 1918, Springhill, housewife.

75. Eldora McKay, 3, d. 31 October 1918, Springhill.

76. Alexander Crowe, 8, d. 2 November 1918, Springhill, student.

77. Peter Legere, 1, d. 3 November 1918, Springhill.

78. John Pettigrew, 17, d. 6 February 1919 [*sic*], Springhill, miner.

79. May Jewkes, 30, d. 4 November 1918, Springhill, housewife.

80. Samuel Bennett, 42, d. 6 November 1918, Springhill, labourer.

81. Thomas Caulder, 5 months, d. 6 November 1918, Springhill.

82. Alden Spence, 14, d. 28 December 1918, Springhill.

83. Ida Chandler, 28, d. 28 December 1918, Springhill, schoolteacher.

84. Elizabeth Van Buskirk, 28, d. 31 December 1918, Springhill, housewife.

85. James Matthews, 33, d. 31 December 1918, Springhill, coal weigh clerk.

86. Belle Anderson, 22, d. 7 November 1918, Springhill, housewife.

87. Murray McPherson, 35, d. 8 November 1918, Springhill, miner.

88. Agnes McAloney, 19, d. 3 November 1918, Springhill.

89. Annie Colburne, 33, d. 11 November 1918, Springhill, housewife.

90. John Casey, 15, d. 13 November 1918, Springhill, labourer.

91. Mary Havelock, 49, d. 13 November 1918, Springhill, housewife.

92. Gladys Brown, 1, d. 19 November 1918, Springhill.

93. Torlyer Ripley, 3, d. 21 November 1918, Springhill.

94. Hugh Wilson, 3, d. 29 November 1918, Springhill.

95. Charles Cudhea, 2, d. 22 December 1918, Springhill.

96. Joseph Paul, 39, d. 10 October 1918, Springhill Junction, labourer.

97. Anthony Paul, 9, d. 14 October 1918, Springhill Junction, student.

98. Olive St. Peter, 12, d. 4 November 1918, Maccan.

99. Ada Melanson, 8, d. 28 October 1918, Springhill Junction.

100. Howard Brown, 5, d. 15 November 1918, East Mapleton.

101. Eliza Brown, 38, d. 19 November 1918, housewife.

102. Joseph Paul, 27, d. 23 November 1918, Springhill Junction, labourer.

103. Edna Hunter, 23, d. 27 November 1918, Parrsboro.

104. Elsie Fulton, 14, d. 1 November 1918, Lakelands.

105. Mable Hughes, 44, d. 16 November, Fox River.

106. Graham Hughes, 17, d. 18 November 1918, Fox River.

107. Beatrice Desmond, 13, d. 23 October, Parrsboro.

108. Blanch Henwood, 15, d. 26 October 1918, Black Rock.

109. Lilla Henwood, 13, d. 20 October 1918, Black Rock.

110. Elizabeth Smith, 19, d. 22 November 1918, East Apple River, student.

111. Elizabeth Gardner, 22, d. 21 December 1918, Amherst.

1919

112. Frederick Bumpstead, 10, d. 11 January 1919, Amherst, student.

113. Heinrick Harms, 45, d. 14 January 1919, [*prisoner*] Amherst Internment Camp; [*formerly a German*] warrant officer.

114. Margaret Melanson, 77, d. 15 February 1919, Amherst.

115. Rella Smith, 29, d. 18 February 1919, Amherst, housewife.

116. Ella Stewart, 52, d. 19 March 1919, Amherst, housewife.

117. Leah Smith, 15, d. 4 January 1919, Pugwash.

118. Harold Fanning, 1, d. 16 January 1919, Port Howe.

119. Benjamin Chapman, 63, d. 28 January 1919, Fort Lawrence, farmer.

120. John Bridge, 40, d. 4 March 1919, Maccan, farmer.

121. Allen Boulter, 47, d. 12 January 1919, Westchester Station, lumberman.

122. Mrs. W. W. Wood, 40, d. 4 March 1919, Maccan, housewife.

123. Thomas Brown, 84, d. 6 March 1919, Little River, farmer.

124. Amos Como, 38, d. 16 March 1919, Joggins Mines, miner.

125. Malinda Legere, 36, d. 30 March 1919, Joggins Mines, housewife.

126. Christine Smith, 63, d. 31 March 1919, Joggins Mines, housewife.

[*Number 127, following in Dr. Marble's list of actual entries in the original register, is a repeat of Leah Smith, 117. This has been corrected here so that the number of the dead is accurate.*]

127. Wesley Piers, 62, d. 26 February 1919, Wallace, merchant.

128. Bernice Budd, 33, d. 15 February 1919, Springhill, housewife.

129. Robert Newman, 21, d. 1 January 1919, Springhill, miner.

130. Oliver Wade, 67, d. 1 January 1919, Springhill, labourer.

131. Sophia Johnson, 34, d. 2 February 1919, Springhill, housewife.

132. Tressa Brown, 41, d. 14 February 1919, Parrsboro, housewife.

133. Almadine Bennett, 3 weeks, d. 27 February 1919, Parrsboro.

Register searched to the end of March 1919.

1920

134. Maud Bourgeois, 34, d. 18 February 1920, Amherst.

135. Minnie Steeves, 18, d. 20 February 1920, Amherst.

136. Katherine Read, 26, d. 21 February 1920, Stanley.

137. Elizabeth McLellan, 17, d. 27 February 1920, Chignecto, housewife.

138. Priscilla Tattrie, 88, d. 24 February 1920, Lower Wentworth, housewife, [died in:] County Asylum, Pugwash.

139. Jane Russel [Russle], 20, d. 29 February 1920, Spring Hill, [died in:] County Asylum, Pugwash.

140. Sarah Layton, 61, d. 14 February 1920, Parrsboro, housewife.

141. Lawrie Aberley, 43, d. 14 March 1920, Amherst Emergency Hospital, farmer.

142. Annie Dow, 14, d. 3 March 1920, Athol.

143. James Smith, 55, d. 6 March 1920, Nappan, farmer.

144. Georgie Colburn, 42, d. 30 March 1920, Oxford, housekeeper.

145. Karl C. Black, 41, d. 6 March 1920, Salem, farmer.

146. Charles A. Nelson, 40, d. 18 March 1920, Wentworth, farmer.

147. Frank Wilson, 2, d. 23 March 1920, Wallace.

148. Tamalia McIvor, 35, d. 25 March 1920, Fox Harbour.

149. Jessie Rutledge, 26, d. 9 April 1920, Amherst.

150. Amos B. Colborne, 81, d. 1 April 1920, Oxford, carpenter.

151. Susie Stone, 23, d. 8 April 1920, Oxford Junction, housekeeper.

152. Duncan McInnis, 70, d. 4 April 1920, Wallace Ridge, farmer.

153. Euphemia Hope [*Hape*], 29, d. 15 April 1920, Wallace Grant, housewife.

Chapter VII

DIGBY COUNTY

IN DIGBY COUNTY, there were at least ninety-five confirmed deaths from the Great Influenza of 1918–20. The record of these deaths in Digby starts in the county's death register for 1918, with Book 33. The first page in this ledger is numbered 509 (not 001). The first *deaths* entered in this ledger, on this page, date from December, and are of persons from the town of Digby itself.

We know, however, that Digby County people were dying earlier, in October, even in September. For example, Mrs. Stillman Yorke became ill on September 26 and died on October 2. This, perhaps, was a month when everyone was so ill they weren't able

Death records for St. Bernard Parish, Digby County. (*Nova Scotia Archives*)

to do more than the bare minimum. Medical reports were not sent in and the registrar did not receive returns. Whatever the reason, October deaths begin to appear in Book 33 only by page 524, this time from smaller venues like Riverdale or Weymouth Falls or Danvers. It's somewhat confusing. Anyone now opening Ledger 33 might think influenza didn't strike in Digby County until December. Deaths were recorded not by date of death, but just when they were sent in from any one location to the registrar. People were often behind with these and one can understand why.

See an exact copy of the Digby Death Register's 1918–20 influenza-death records at the end of this chapter, followed by a table showing the date of onset of illness for the victims.

October was a time of death after death in Digby, during the Second Wave of influenza. The neighbouring District of Clare reached epidemic status by early October. It is not surprising that there are almost no Digby newspaper accounts for that period, and not surprising that doctors were late sending in returns for the dead. The Nova Scotia Archives, for example, contains almost no *Digby Courier* newspapers at all for October; it may be that few were printed. November and December were not much better. Into 1919, the influenza continued to kill through to July 3. In early 1920, a Third Wave of influenza manifested, and took its first victim on January 15, but thereafter ten more, with the final death occurring April 16.

RECENT DEATHS

T. A. RICE [*Charles Amos Rice*]. Death occurred at Westchester, Cumberland Co., on Saturday, October 5th, of T.A. Rice, aged 45 years. The deceased was a son of the late Alexander Rice, formerly of Digby. The remains arrived here [*Digby*] on the 8th, and were taken in charge of by Mr. J.F. Rice, undertaker and the funeral was held the same day, with interment in the Baptist cemetery.

Digby Courier, 11 October 1918, 2. HVS, Cumberland County Death Register, 1918, Book 39, Page 225, Number 870.

The name on the death certificate was Charles Amos Rice; HVS database search engine only finds him if one enters "Charles Awar Rice." This may be the only *Digby Courier* publication I have found. Charles Amos Rice had been a lumber surveyor. His death certificate lists him as an Evangelical. His doctor, R. O. Shatford, stated that he died of Locomotor Ataxia, complicated by influenza. He was unmarried. The undertaker in Cumberland County who prepared the body for shipment was a Mr. Olive, possibly J. C. B. Olive.

HVS, Death Register, Cumberland County, Year 1918, Book 39, Page 225, Number 870.

1916 Recruitment Poster, for CEF No. 2 Construction Battalion of Nova Scotia. An example of the overt or subtle racism that can also be seen in death records for Black persons during this period. *(1900.237-WWI/31 NO.2 CONSTRUCTION BATTALION FOR COLORED MEN OF CANADA, World War One Poster Collection, Esther Clark Wright Archives, Acadia University)*

THE INFLUENZA AT METEGHAN

METEGHAN, October 21—At the time of writing there does not appear to be any diminution of the ravages of this terrible scourge and at least four fatalities have occurred entirely attributable to its attacks. Three funerals took place at Meteghan on Sunday and a fourth today. The authorities have sent Dr. George Deveau from Halifax, and his work in the midst of so much sickness will be very highly welcomed. Lack of proper nurses is very keenly felt, and there are instances where sufferers have had no personal attention at all. There is a general feeling of depression and even strong men express in bated breath the fear that is uppermost in their thoughts should they fall victims. Few houses are free from the unwelcome visitor, and medical aid is nothing like adequate to cope with the sufferers.

Halifax Evening Mail, 22 October 1918, 16.

☞ The progress of influenza must be ascertained through outside newspaper accounts, which are sparse.

DEATHS AT HILLSDALE
Sent in by a correspondent. The community of Hillsdale has been made sad by the sudden and early death on Oct. 11, of Ellsworth Mullen. He was sick only a few days with Spanish influenza followed by the dread disease, bronchial pneumonia. He was 25 years of age. The deceased was the fifth son of Mrs. Stephen Mullen of that place.

The community was again doubly saddened on Oct. 18th, when death visited the home of Judson Mullen and took Lennie, his beloved wife, in the 27th year of her age. She was sick only a few days with Spanish influenza followed by bronchical [*sic*] pneumonia. [She was the daughter of] Mr. and Mrs. Henry Lewis of Danvers.

Digby Courier, 8 November 1918, 4. These October deaths were not published until November.

FIFTY NEW CASES OF SPANISH INFLUENZA
The Epidemic Is Spreading Throughout The Province—The Department Of Public Health Issues Important Circular Regarding The Disease.

...During the forty-eight hours ending at noon October 14th, the cases of epidemic influenza reported from Nova Scotia to the Provincial Health Officer numbered 731. Several of these, however, are from belated returns. Recent deaths reported from this disease numbered 15.

☞ The provincial health officer, Dr. W. H. Hattie, also provided the newspaper with the status in Nova Scotia of the last twenty-four hours, ending at noon, October 15. This is the number of cases and deaths by community for just one day; Digby locations are bolded.

LOCATION	CASES		DEATHS
Welmouth [*Weymouth*] Mills	01		—
Halifax	46		—
Springhill Junction	four families		02
Digby	06		—
Pictou	06		—
Pictou [County?]	46	*[This entry may be a typographical error.]*	—

Clare Municipality	epidemic	—
Port Bickerton	08	—
Goldenville	01	—
Sherbrooke	02	—
Yarmouth	02	—
Newport	03	—
Scotch Village	01	—
Ellershouse	01	01
Martin's Point	01	—
Glace Bay	18	02
Bayview	04	—
Weymouth Falls	**19**	—
New Tusket	04	01
Lunenburg	08	01
Trenton	05	—
Lockeport	epidemic	03
Truro	04	—

Halifax Morning Chronicle, 16 October, 1918, 2.

👉 This is the first published information that influenza in any Nova Scotia community had reached epidemic status. Digby County locations are highlighted. Richmond County had not yet reported. They had reached epidemic status as well, but the doctors were either too ill, dead, or run off their feet to send in the paperwork, which had to be sent to Halifax by telegraph or telephone, where available. Cases everywhere in the province were massively under-reported.

📰 MRS. INNOCENT COMEAU. A very sad death took place at Concession, Digby Co., yesterday when Mrs. Innocent Comeau passed away after an illness of only a few days of influenza and pneumonia....She leaves a family of fourteen children, the youngest of whom is an infant of two days.

Yarmouth Telegram, 1 November 1918, 1.

📰 MRS. W. S. WINCHESTER. The death of Georgie, the loving wife of Councillor William S. Winchester, took place last Friday morning, Nov. 1st, at her house on Warwick Street [in Digby....She left] four children, five stepchildren, an aged mother, Mrs. Seraph Daley, Culloden.

Digby Courier, 8 November 1918, 2.

DEATHS AT BELLIVEAU'S COVE

The Parish of St. Bernard's was the scene of four deaths within a few days, three of whom were victims of the dreaded Spanish Influenza:

Mr. Joseph Buckly [Buckley], son of Mr. James Buckly, aged about 25 years. [Joseph Buckley was a ship carpenter.]

Elisee [Elisé] and Fred Gaudet, aged 23 and 18 years respectively, sons of Oyesiphore [Telesphore] Gaudet, all of Whites Cove. [Elisé was a ship caulker; Fred was a ship carpenter.]

Mrs. Pat [Polycarp] Gaudet (nee Elizebeth [Elizabeth] Melanson), aged 30 years, leaving to mourn their loss a husband and two children, one daughter aged 5 years, and an infant son...."

Digby Courier, 8 November 1918, 2.
HVS, Digby, 1918, Book 33, Page 531, Number 1386.
(Elisé Gaudet. Died of influenza; ill 5 days.)
HVS, Digby, 1918, Book 33, Page 531, Number 1387.
(Joseph Buckley. Died of influenza; ill 8 days.)
HVS, Digby, 1918, Book 33, Page 531, Number 1388, 1386.
(Fred Gaudet. Died of influenza; ill 12 days.)
HVS, Digby, 1918, Book 33, Page 531, Number 1389.
(Elizabeth Melanson Gaudet). She died of convulsions after childbirth, possibly from influenza.

SMITH'S COVE....Mrs. Spurgeon Weir has about recovered from a severe case of la grippe.

Digby Courier, 8 November 1918, 2.

INFLUENZA IN DIGBY

Many Cases and Several Deaths Within the Past Few Days.

Digby's second attack of influenza is far worse than the first. In fact, it is the worst epidemic disease that has ever visited the town. It is said that there are in the vicinity of one hundred cases, and there have been four deaths within the past few days. Perhaps the saddest of all is that of Private C.W. Muise, who returned from overseas just a week before his death. He was aged 54 years and was for many years one of Digby's best known merchant tailors. He died Friday [December 6] and was buried Saturday. Monday afternoon his wife also passed away and was buried yesterday. [His wife was Sarah Muise, 54; she also died of influenza, on 9 December; Book 33, Page 512, Number 1330.]

Mr. Kenneth Skinner, a very popular salesman in H.T. Warne's grocery, passed away Saturday night, aged 24 years, after a week's illness....The remains were taken to Berwick via Monday's express, where interment took place the same afternoon.

On Sunday, Norman van Tassel, aged 15, died at his home on the Corner of Prince William street and Maiden Lane....

On the same day, Mrs. Charles Wilson died at her home in Bear River, aged 51 years.

Bridgetown Monitor, 11 December 1918, 8.

VAN TASSEL. At Culloden, Digby Co., N.S., Dec. 13th, Mrs. Augustus VanTassel, aged 26 years. Just two days after the remains of Mr. VanTassel's wife was laid to rest, his two children, Wm. Benedict VanTassel, aged 3 years, and Augustus Charles VanTassel, aged 1 year, succumbed to Influenza.

Truro Daily News, 30 December 1918, 2. Courtesy the
Colchester Historeum, Truro.

The news has been received in Little Brook, Digby Co., of the death of Dr. Winifred [*sic*] McDonnell, which occurred in England on Nov. 19, after a short illness of influenza and pneumonia. The deceased was a native of Sydney, C.B., and graduated in medicine at Dalhousie in 1910. He married Miss Celeste Lombard, of Little Brook [Digby County], who was a graduate nurse on the staff of the Victoria General Hospital, Halifax. When the St. Francis Xavier Hospital Unit was organized for work overseas, Dr. and Mrs. McDonnell offered their services, were accepted and crossed to England and later to France, where for many months both saw much active service and underwent many thrilling experiences during the Hun air raids on hospitals and casualty dressing stations. He was about 35 years of age and leaves, besides his widow, one child, which was born in England. Mrs. McDonnell, writing to friends in Little Brook, states that she, with her infant, will return to her home at the earliest opportunity.

Yarmouth Telegram, 13 December 1918, 1.

The people of Digby and vicinity are still suffering with the influenza. There have been eleven deaths, since Thursday, some of which were from other causes.

Mrs. Augustus VanTassell and two little sons have passed away.

Rev. Father Grace conducted three funerals in the Catholic cemetery yesterday morning.

The list of the dead since Thursday are as follows:

Dec. 12th At Culloden. Mrs. Augustus VanTassell, aged 25 years. Funeral 13th.

Dec. 14th At Hill Grove, Mr. Amero, aged 80 years. Funeral 15th.

Dec. 15th Wallace Stark, son of Mr. and Mrs. Wallace Stark, aged 4 years. Funeral 16th·

[Dec. 15th] Gladys Melanson. Aged 8 years. Funeral 16th.

Dec. 16th At Culloden, Fred Hersey, aged 25 years. Funeral 17th.

Dec. 16th At Digby, Michael Rogers, aged 62 years. Funeral 17th.

[Dec 16th] Wm. Benedict VanTassell, aged 3 years, and brother Augustus Charles VanTassell, aged 1 year. Funeral 17th.

[Dec 16th] Mrs. Agnes Pyne, aged 32 years. Funeral 17th.

[Dec 16th] Wm. McKinnon, aged 70 years. Funeral 17th.

There are a number who are not expected to live. Undertaker J. F. Rice is working almost day and night and the doctors are also having very busy times. Everything possible is being done to prevent further spread of the epidemic.

Bridgetown Monitor, 18 December 1918, 8.

HVS, Digby County, 1918, shows that these people did not die of Influenza: Henry Amero (Book 33, Page 516, Number 1345), died of Bronchial Asthma and Heart Failure; Agnes Pyne (Page 514, Number 1333) either had pneumonia, which caused a miscarriage, or contracted it after a miscarriage, or she may have had that fatal combination of influenza/pneumonia, causing miscarriage, but there is no way to know. Michael Rogers (Book 33, Page 514, Number 1332) died of Bright's Disease; HVS search engine gives his name as Micheal Rogers; the original record shows Michael.

ALICE HANDSPIKER. Miss Alice Handspiker, daughter of David J. and the late Rebecca Handspiker, passed away at the home of her sister, Mrs. Chas. R. VanTassel, Mt. Pleasant, yesterday at the age of 52. She had been an invalid practically all her life, but died from influenza. She leaves, besides the sister with whom she resided, two brothers, Freeman Handspiker, Mt. Pleasant, and Jeremiah, of Oguincuite [Ogunquit], Maine.

Digby Courier, 3 January 1919, 5.

DELTA MAUDE THURBER. It is with great sorrow we are called on to report the passing away of one of Freeport's young girls, in the person of Delta Maude, daughter of Mr. and Mrs. Albert W. Thurber, aged 20 years. Delta had been sick since Christmas, having contracted the dread disease Influenza, through her kindly ministrations to a sick girl friend. Her mother was called to her bedside, doctors and nurses gave help to the utmost of their ability, but all in vain. Though she seemed better from her first disease, and all were hopeful for her recovery, suddenly her lungs were overflowed with a fluid, which proved fatal....She had made many friends also in St. John, where she and her sister Lillian worked with the New Brunswick Telephone Co., and attended the Central Baptist Church and Sunday School.

Digby Courier, 24 January 1919, 5.

MRS. EDDIE MALLETT. A sudden death took place at Mavilette on Tuesday of last week, when Mary Esther, beloved wife of Eddie Mallett, passed away after only a brief illness of influenza and pneumonia. The deceased was the only daughter of the late Anselm D'Eon, of West Pubnico, and was by her kindly manner dearly beloved by all who knew her, not only in Mavilette but also by many in and about the Pubnicos. Mrs. Mallett was 38 years of age and leaves, besides her husband, five young sons and one daughter; also six brothers, Anthony and Eloi, of West Pubnico; George, Alphee and Raymond, in Massachusetts; and J.E. of Metegan River. The funeral took place at Salmon River on Wednesday.

Digby Courier, 24 January 1919, 5.

ALBERT SAULNIER. Albert, son of Mr. and Mrs. Monde Saulnier, died at their home at Saulnierville, Digby Co., on Saturday after only four days' illness of pneumonia, which developed from a severe attack of influenza. He was a ship carpenter of considerable ability and as such was well known all along the St. Mary's Bay shore. Mr. Saulnier was 30 years of age.

Digby Courier, 26 March 1919, 5.

DIED OF "FLU" IN A LUMBER CAMP

A gloom was cast over North Range, Digby Co., when it became known that Oscar Andrews had been called away in his 29th year, by death, to his home beyond. Mr. Andrews was cook in Dickie's Lumber Camp in South Range. On Friday the 11th, he was smitten with that dread disease influenza, was brought to his home [in North Range] in the Dr.'s car, but medical aid and tender nursing could not save him, for he passed away just one week later, April 18th.

Truro Daily News, 9 May 1919, 4. Courtesy the Colchester Historeum, Truro.

Oscar Andrews (above) was the son of William and Levile (Lucile?) Andrews of North Range. William was a farmer. When Oscar married Miss Grace Adelaide Bent on 30 October 1918, in Bridgetown, Annapolis County, he stated he was a bachelor, a farmer, and aged 29. She was a spinster, Church of England, and had been born in Young's Cove, Annapolis County, to William D. and Mary Roland (?) Bent. Her father was also a farmer. When Oscar died in April of 1919, he and Grace had been married less than a year.

Oscar Andrews appears twice in the Digby County Death Register, Book 33. The two records are largely identical except for the dates of death: Mr. Andrews thus apparently died, aged 29 and 10 months, on April 17, 1919. He apparently died again (I'm not serious) at age 30, on July 3, 1919. The first return of death was sent in on May 14, 1919, by his wife who, as a bride of less than six months, signed her name firmly as "Mrs. Oscar Andrews." Cause of death was "Spanish Influenza and Lobar Pneumonia," after an illness of seven days. Dr. W. R. Dickie attended; Fred Rice was the undertaker, and burial was in North Range. Oscar had been a Baptist, and spent his whole life in North Range, where he was born, lived and died. This report was sent in on July 15, 1919 by District Registrar Hanford Van Blascom, for the period ending June 30, 1919.

Oscar Andrews's second death record was sent in on October 8, 1919 by John Daly or Daley, a different District Registrar, for the period ending September 30, 1919. Mr. Andrews' occupation was given as "chef"; the date of death is July 3, 1919; his length of illness was written either as a 4 or as an 11 (it looks like a capital H); cause of death was merely "Flu," and the return was made by "Dr. Dickie" (who usually signed as W. R. Dickie, MD).

Possibly the second registrar overlooked the first record, and in scrambling to get another one together, got several things wrong. This wasn't the only mistake John Daly made. There is also on the same page a death record for D'Arcy James Spencer, a "Protestant Irish" fisherman born in Trout Cove, who died of "Flue" after an illness of six days. An addendum to it reads, "Died in Halifax," which means it shouldn't have been in there at all.

HVS, Annapolis County Marriage Register, 1918, Book 1, Page 603.
HVS, Digby County Death Register, 1919, Book 33, Page 583, Number 1550.
It is the first and only entry on an otherwise blank page.
The second entry is as follows: HVS, Digby County Death Register, 1919,
Book 33, Page 607, Number 1611.

IN BELLIVEAU'S COVE
The Parish of St. Bernard's has had many deaths within the last two weeks of pneumonia.

On the 15th instant [March], Ulysses L. Doucette, aged 23 years; on the 21st, Emile D. LeBlanc, aged 14 years; and Françoise C. Doucette aged 79 years, widow of the late Charles B. Doucett.

On the 22nd Charles Jos. Comeau, aged 42 years, leaving a wife and five young children to mourn.

On the 29th inst. Celeste aged 14 years, only daughter of Mr. and Mrs. Siffroi L. Comeau, leaving six brothers besides her father and mother to mourn.

Digby Courier, 2 April 1920, 5.

This article has errors; see below for corrections.

- Ulysse Doucet, aged 25, 15 March 15, at 8:00 A.M. His parents were Leslie Doucet and Eva Comeau Doucet. He had worked at home all his life as a labourer, according to his death record, and died of "Influenza complicated by Broncho pneumonia." Dr. E. J. Elderkin was his doctor, and J. Thibodeau was the undertaker.

HVS, Digby County Death Register, 1920, Book 66, Page 119.

- Charles Comeau was born on January 15, 1875. His parents were Joseph and Maryann LeBlanc Comeau. When he was twenty, he went to sea and worked as a sailor for fifteen years. By 1910, he was on shore again, making a living as a farmer, and marrying wife Alma. They produced five children. He died aged 45 on March 21, 1920; his doctor was E. J. Elderkin. The cause of death was pneumonia. Alma Comeau sent in his return of death.

HVS, Digby County Death Register, 1920, Book 66, Page 121.

- Emile LeBlanc was born January 15, 1907, and aged 13 years, 2 months, and 6 days when he died on March 20 at 9.00 A.M. Under "Occupation," someone has scrawled diagonally across the page, "This boy was born a simpleton." The cause of death was pneumonia. His parents were Dreme and Alma LeBlanc. Mr. LeBlanc had been born in St. Bernard; his wife Alma was born in "New Edingburg."

HVS, Digby County Death Register, 1920, Book 66, Page 122.

- Françoise Doucet, a widow living in Belliveau's Cove, died March 22, 1920. The cause of death was "Influenza; contributary Pneumonia." She was 76 years, 2 months, and 12 days old. Her parents were Joseph and Mary Amero Doucet. Her death record lists her life's occupations as "Service girl, about 10 years/ Household duties, 30 years." Her son-in-law, surname also Doucet, sent in the death return. Her father, husband and son-in-law were all Doucets. Dr. E. J. Elderkin of Weymouth was her doctor.

HVS, Digby County Death Register, 1920, Book 66, Page 123.

- Celeste Comeau was born to Siffroi and Edesse Belliveau Comeau, on November 20, 1908. Edesse had been born in Grosses Cocques, and Siffroi in Belliveau's Cove, where the family lived. Daughter Celeste contacted influenza March 24, 1920, and died five days later, on March 29. Cause of death is listed as "Influenza," with "contributary pneumonia."

HVS, Digby County Death Register, 1920, Book 66, Page 124.

☞ Influenza in Digby County quickly reached epidemic status, but Digby had less newspaper coverage than any county outside of Cape Breton, relative to its high death rates. Although at least ninety-five people died of the Great Influenza in this county between the fall of 1918 and the spring of 1920, we were only able to find a handful of newspaper death notices or obituaries.

Because there is such a paucity of information for this county, and because portions of it reached epidemic status, at the end of this chapter I have included—in addition to the usual deaths by county list—a table of onset dates for the county dead, showing when and where the Great Influenza first infected, and then killed, its victims.

DIGBY COUNTY, VITAL STATISTICS, DEATH REGISTER, BOOK 33, 66

1918

1. Percy Pyne, 35, d. 22 December 1918, Digby, labourer.

2. Villa Handspiker, female, 7 months, d. 22 December 1918. [*Villa Parker Handspiker was 7½ months old when she died; perhaps in Digby, as her name appears in a lengthy bunch of Digby town death returns. There is no birth record, but her death record states she was born in Culloden, to Mr. and Mrs. Wallace Handspiker. The family was Methodist. They didn't have a doctor attending. There is no place of burial given, but they did have an undertaker (J. F. Rice), who sent in the return of death to the registrar. Book 33, Page 516, Number 1342.*]

3. Dustin Vantassell [*Van Tassell*], 6 months, d. 23 December 1918, Digby.

4. Mrs. Stillman York, 21, d. 2 October 1918, Digby.

5. Ethel York, 4, d. 24 October 1918, Digby.

6. Georgie Winchester, female, 41, d. 1 November 1918, Digby.

7. Cyrial Muise, 54, d. 6 December 1918, Digby.

8. Kenneth Skinner, 24, d. 7 December 1918, Digby, grocery clerk.

9. Norman Van Tassell, 18, d. 8 December 1918, Digby.

10. Sarah Muise, 55, d. 9 December 1918, Digby, housewife. [*Widow of Cyrial Muise, above.*]

11. Fred Hersey, 18, d. 14 December 1918, Culloden, fisherman.

12. Mrs. Augustus Van Tassell, 23, d. 14 December 1918, Mt. Pleasant, housewife.

13. William McKinnon, 78, d. 15 December 1918, Alms House, Maybelltown.

14. Gladys Melanson, 8, d. December 1918, Alms House [*Maybelltown?*].

15. Wallace Stark, 4, d. 18 December 1918, Digby.

16. Agnes M. Pyne, 32, d. 16 December 1918, Digby.

17. William Van Tassell, 3, d. 16 December 1918, Mt. Pleasant.

18. Augustus Van Tassell, 1, d. 16 December 1918, Mt. Pleasant.

19. Wallace Stark, 33, d. 19 December 1918, Digby, fisherman.

[*The succeeding number (20) on Dr. Marble's list shows there was a repeat of the death record for Mrs. Augustus Van Tassel in the register, so the list has been amended here to reflect accurately the number of deaths in the county during this epidemic.*]

20. Mary Amero, 40, d. 13 December 1918, Doucetteville.

21. Viney Melanson, 31, d. 24 December 1918, Plympton Station.

22. Ernest O'Neill, 19, d. 28 December 1918, Plympton, labourer.

23. Edmund Hogan, 57, d. 7 November 1918, Weymouth, clerk.

24. Annie Hainey, 33, d. 17 November 1918, Weymouth, companion.

25. Ernest Rodney, 3, d. 27 November 1918, Weymouth.

26. Edith Fowler, 6, d. 8 December 1918, Weymouth.

27. Nancy Bell, 22, d. 15 October 1918, Riverdale, housewife.

28. Donald Langford, 17, d. 16 October 1918, Danvers, labourer.

29. Blanche Jarvis, 5, d. 25 October 1918, Weymouth Falls.

30. Vaughan Young, 7, d. 26 October 1918, Weymouth.

31. Myrtle Gidney, 27, d. 23 November 1918, Mink Cove, housewife.

32. Elisé Gaudet, 23, d. 31 October 1918, St. Bernard, ship caulker.

33. Joseph Buckley, 30, d. 3 November 1918, St. Bernard, ship carpenter.

34. Fred Gaudet, 21, d. 3 November 1918, St. Bernard, ship carpenter.

35. Nina Gaud [Gaudet?], 6 weeks, d. 29 October 1918, _____ville. [This child does not appear in the HVS Database, even under any reasonable variation of her name. Her residence may have been in Saulnierville. Dr. Marble's list reflects his search in the original death registers, so she must have a record there.]

[The succeeding number (36) in the Marble list shows "Donald Langford, 16, d. 17 October 1918, Danvers ...." (Book 33, Page 532, Number 1395). This is a repeat of the death record for a "Donald Langford, 17, d. 16 October 1918, Danvers" (Book 33, Page 524, Number 1366). This second entry bears a note from the registrar, saying "By mistake, I had entered this once in _____ {illegible; 'the form'?} H.H." This list has been amended to reflect the actual number of deaths in the county.]

36. Rosie Gaudet, 43, d. 31 October 1918, Concession, housekeeper.

1919

37. Ambroise Comeau, 30, d. 3 January 1919, Grosses Coques, carpenter.

38. Marie Boudreau, 76, d. 12 February 1919, Church Point, housekeeper.

39. Ellsworth Mullen, 25, d. 12 October 1918, Havelock, farmer.

40. Elizabeth Mullen, 6, d. 14 October 1918, Easton.

41. Lennie Mullen, female, 30, d. 18 October 1918, Havelock, housewife.

42. Marie Saulnier, 5, d. 8 November 1918, Meteghan.

43. Edmund Dugas, 24, d. 19 October 1918, Meteghan, farmer.

44. Louise Saulnier, 3, d. 19 October 1918, Meteghan.

45. Robert Robichaud, 15 months, d. 24 October 1918, Meteghan.

46. Joseph B. Comeau, 25, d. 27 October 1918, Meteghan River, labourer.

47. Harvey Trahan, 20, d. 30 October 1918, Meteghan, farmer.

48. John Ford, 33, d. 20 October 1918, Meteghan, mariner.

49. Mary Rombolt, 40, d. 30 October 1918, Meteghan, housemaid.

50. Philippe Doucet, 26, d. 7 November 1918, Meteghan.

51. Jéréme [Jérémie] Deveau, 30, d. 28 October 1918, Lake Doucette, ship carpenter.

52. Abroise [Ambroise] Doucette, 25, d. 25 November 1918, Mavillette, fisherman. [The HVS search engine names him Ambroise Doucet (sic), Book 33, Page 546, Number 1444; this 1444 is a renumbering from the original number, 82. His father's name was Benjamin Doucette, they were Roman Catholic, and Ambroise was buried in Salmon River.]

53. Elise Leblanc (female), 40, d. 13 November 1918, Meteghan River, housewife.

54. Evangeline Eimothe [Timothé], (female), 53, d. 14 November 1918, Saulnierville, housewife. [Book 22, Page 547, Number 1447.]

55. Leonce Smith, 18, d. 21 October 1918, Saulnierville Station, farmer.

56. Grace Thibault, 25, d. 27 October 1918, Saulnierville Station, housewife.

57. Rose Gaudet, 8, d. 1 November 1918, Saulnierville Station.

58. Marguerite Deveau, 17, d. 6 November 1918, Meteghan Station.

59. Aleise [*Alice*] Handspiker, 52, d. 2 January 1919, Mt. Pleasant.

60. Mary Pictou, 17 months, d. 8 February 1919, Bear River.

61. Oliver Pictou, 15, d. 8 February 1919, Bear River, pupil.

62. Fred Nickerson, 44, d. 22 February 1919, Weymouth, labourer.

63. Genéve [*Marie Geneviève*] Dugas, 59, d. 14 March 1919, Belliveau's [*sic*] Cove, housewife. [*Book 33, Page 567, Number 1507, shows her first name was entered as "Genive," which was later crossed out with a pencil, and written in as "Mary Genevieve."*]

64. Florence Melanson, 32, d. 30 January 1919, Corberrie, housework.

65. Marie Deveau, 96, d. 23 March 1919, Meteghan, inmate in Poor House.

66. Louis Saulnier, 3 months, d. 31 March 1919, Meteghan.

67. Mrs. Esther Maillet, 37, d. 14 January 1919, Mavillette, housewife, "epidemic influenza."

68. Joseph Thibault, 30, d. 10 April 1919, Acaciaville, farmer.

69. _____ [*Elmira*] Bacon, female, 76, d. 11 April 1919, Hill Grove. [*Book 33, Page 579, Number 1535 shows a name several times written over, but which appears to be "Elmira"; the search engine for the database has it as Elmira Bacon. She was a widow, formerly married to Edward Bacon, 76. The record describes her as a "Baptist/Anglo-Saxon." Hill Grove is in the Municipality of Digby, Digby County.*]

70. Isabell Marshall, 39, d. 20 April 1919, South Range.

71. William Ross, 53, d. 2 April 1919, Roxville, farmer.

72. Oscar Andrews, 29, d. 17 April 1919, North Range.

73. Florence Hooper, 27, d. 5 May 1919, Sandy Cove, music teacher.

74. Seymour Gidney, 2, d. 3 May 1919, Sandy Cove.

75. Joseph Doucet, 7, d. 24 May, Little Brook Station.

76. Arsène Bonafant, 79, d. 30 June 1919, Grosses Coques, housekeeper, widow. [*This woman does not appear on the HVS data base, even searching for 'B' surnames for 1919, all counties. Dr. Marble's list must have found the original record in the register, but it isn't in the HVS database.*]

77. John Blinn, 64, d. 29 June 1919, Corberrie, farmer.

78. Benoît Deveau, 13 months, d. 9 June 1919, Meteghan.

79. Marc Saulnier, 80, d. 3 June 1919, Meteghan Center, farmer.

80. Charles Thibodieu, 54, d. 5 April 1919, Meteghan Center, farmer.

81. Marie Comeau, 3 months, d. 27 April 1919, Meteghan.

82. Blanche Comeau, 3 months, d. 29 April 1919, Meteghan River.

83. Celestin Trahan, 71, d. May 1919, Meteghan, shoemaker.

84. Emile Deveau, 16, d. 26 May 1919, Mavillette.

[*Number 85 on Dr. Marble's list shows "_____ Andrews." The death record gives his first name as Oscar. This is a copy of Entry 72, and has thus been removed to give an accurate total of the county deaths.*]

[*Number 86 on Dr. Marble's list shows D'Arcy Spencer, aged 68, who died in Halifax on 11 May 1920. This entry has been moved to Halifax County, since he died there.*]

1920

85. Joseph Le Blanc, 63, d. 15 January 1920, Lower Saulnierville, farmer.

86. Madelaine Boudreau, 98, d. 24 February 1920, Meteghan.

87. Joseph Saulnier, 35, d. 29 February 1920, Meteghan, carpenter.

88. Sarah Riley, 73, d. 27 March 1920, Digby.

89. Charles White, 39, d. 18 March 1920, Ashmore, farmer.

90. Ulysse Doucet, 25, d. 15 March 1920, St. Bernard, labourer.

91. Françoise Doucet, 76, d. 22 March 1920, Belliveau's [*sic*] Cove, housework.

92. Celeste Comeau, 100, d. 29 March 1920, Belliveau's [*sic*] Cove.

93. Marie Baudrian [*Boudreau*], 66, 30 March 1920, Church Point, housework. [*HVS, Digby County Death Register, Book 66, Page 128, gives her name as Marie Boudreau, daughter of Augustin and Catherine Comeau Boudreau. She was single. Her death return was sent in by Adeline Thibodeau of Church Point.*]

94. Alonzo Grant, 79, d. 1 April 1920, Weymouth, carpenter.

95. John A. Morrisey, 81, d. 16 April 1920, Gilbert Cove, farmer.

DIGBY COUNTY, VITAL STATISTICS, BOOKS 33, 66

Onset on:	Death on:	Name, Age, Location, Occupation, Length of illness
1918		
1918 09 26	1918 10 02	Mrs. Stillman York, 21, d. 2 October 1918, Digby; ill 1 week.
1918 10 03	1918 10 12	Ellsworth Mullen, 25, d. 12 October 1918, Havelock, farmer; ill 9 days.
1918 10 05 (or 10 09)	1918 10 16 (or 10 17)	Donald Langford, 17, d. 16 October 1918, Danvers, labourer; ill 10 days. Second record states "d. 17 October, ill 8 days."
1918 10 05	1918 10 15	Nancy Bell, 22, d. 15 October 1918, Riverdale, housewife; ill 10 days.
1918 10 07	1918 10 19	Edmund Dugas, 24, d. 19 October 1918, Meteghan, farmer; ill 12 days.
1918 10 07	1918 10 14	Elizabeth Mullen, 6, d. 14 October 1918, Easton; ill 7 days.
1918 10 08	1918 10 18	Lennie Mullen, female, 30, d. 18 October 1918, Havelock, housewife; ill 10 days.
1918 10 11	1918 10 20	John Ford, 33, d. 20 October 1918, Meteghan, mariner; ill 9 days.
1918 10 11	1918 10 21	Leonce Smith, 18, d. 21 October 1918, Saulnierville Station, farmer; ill 10 days.
1918 10 15	1918 10 25	Blanche Jarvis, 5, d. 25 October 1918, Weymouth Falls; ill 10 days.
1918 10 15	1918 10 27	Grace Thibault, 25, d. 27 October 1918, Saulnierville Station, housewife; ill 12 days.
1918 10 16	1918 10 19	Louise Saulnier, 3, d. 19 October 1918, Meteghan; ill 3 days.
1918 10 16	1918 10 30	Mary Rombolt, 40, d. 30 October 1918, Meteghan, housemaid; ill 2 weeks.
1918 10 17	1918 11 01	Rose Gaudet, 8, d. 1 November 1918, Saulnierville Station; ill 15 days.
1918 10 17	1918 10 24	Ethel York, 4, d. 24 October 1918, Digby, ill 1 week.
1918 10 17	1918 10 27	Joseph B. Comeau, 25, d. 27 October 1918, Meteghan River, labourer; ill 10 days.
1918 10 17	1918 10 30	Harvey Trahan, 20, d. 30 October 1918, Meteghan, farmer; ill 13 days.
1918 10 19	1918 10 24	Robert Robichaud, 15 months, d. 24 October 1918, Meteghan; ill 5 days.
1918 10 20	1918 10 28	Jérémie Deveau, 30, d. 28 October 1918, Lake Doucette, ship carpenter; ill 8 days.
1918 10 22	1918 10 29	Nina Gaud [*Gaudet?*], 6 wks, d. 29 October 1918, ____ville [*Saulnierville?*]; ill 7 days.
1918 10 23	1918 10 24	Vaughan Young, 7, d. 26 October 1918, Weymouth; ill 3 days.
1918 10 25	1918 10 31	Marie Saulnier, 5, d. 8 November 1918, Meteghan; ill 15 days.
1918 10 25	1918 11 01	Georgie Winchester, female, 41, d. 1 November 1918, Digby; ill 1 week.
1918 10 26	1918 10 31	Elisé Gaudet, 23, d. 31 October 1918, St. Bernard, ship caulker; ill 5 days.
1918 10 26	1918 11 03	Fred Gaudet, 21, d. 3 November 1918, St. Bernard, ship carpenter; ill 12 days.
1918 10 26	1918 10 31	Rosie Gaudet, 43, d. 31 October 1918, Concession, housekeeper; ill 6 days.
1918 10 27	1918 11 03	Joseph Buckley, 30, d. 3 November 1918, St. Bernard, ship carpenter; ill 8 days.
1918 10 28	1918 11 06	Marguerite Deveau, 17, d. 6 November 1918, Meteghan Station; ill 10 days.

1918 10 31	1918 11 07	Philippe Doucet, 26, d. 7 November 1918, Meteghan; ill 8 days.
1918 10 31	1918 11 14	Evangeline Eimothe [*Timothé*], 53, d. 14 November 1918, Saulnierville, housewife; ill 15 days.
1918 11 01	1918 12 08	Edith Fowler, 6, d. 8 December 1918, Weymouth; ill 5 weeks.
1918 11 01	1918 11 07	Edmund Hogan, 57, d. 7 November 1918, Weymouth, clerk; ill 6 days.
1918 11 03	1918 11 13	Elise Leblanc (female), 40, d. 13 November 1918, Meteghan River, housewife; ill 10 days.
1918 11 09	1918 11 17	Annie Hainey, 33, d. 17 November 1918, Weymouth, companion; ill 8 days.
1918 11 13	1918 11 23	Myrtle Gidney, 27, d. 23 November 1918, Mink Cove, housewife; ill 10 days.
1918 11 14	1918 11 25	Abroise [*Ambroise*] Doucette, 25, d. 25 November 1918, Mavillette, fisherman; ill 11 days.
1918 11 20	1918 11 27	Ernest Rodney, 3, d. 27 November 1918, Weymouth; ill 1 week.
1918 11 24	1918 12 08	Norman Van Tassell, 18, d. 8 December 1918, Digby; ill 2 weeks.
1918 11 30	1818 12 06	Cyrial Muise, 54, d. 6 December 1918, Digby; ill 1 week.
1918 11 30	1918 12 08	Kenneth Skinner, 24, d. 7 December 1918, Digby, grocery clerk; ill 1 week.
1918 11 30	1918 12 14	Fred Hersey, 18, d. 14 December 1918, Culloden, fisherman; ill 2 weeks.
1918 12 02	1918 12 09	Sarah Muise, 55, d. 9 December 1918, Digby, housewife, widow; ill 1 week.
1918 12 02	1918 12 16	Augustus Van Tassell, 1, d. 16 December 1918, Mt. Pleasant; ill 2 weeks.
1918 12 03	1918 12 13	Mary Amero, 40, d. 13 December 1918, Doucetteville; ill 10 days.
1918 12 07	1918 12 28	Ernest O'Neill, 19, d. 28 December 1918, Plympton, labourer; ill 3 weeks.
1918 12 07	1918 12 14	Mrs. Augustus Van Tassell, 23, d. 14 December 1918, Mt. Pleasant, housewife; ill 1 week.
1918 12 10	1918 12 15	William McKinnon, 78, d. 15 December 1918, Alms House, Maybelltown; ill 5 days.
1918 12 10	1918 12 16	Agnes M. Pyne, 32, d. 16 December 1918, Digby; ill 6 days.
1918 12 11	1918 12 15	Gladys Melanson, 8, d. 15 December 1918, Alms House [*Maybelltown?*]; ill 4 days.
1918 12 12	1918 12 22	Percy Pyne, 35, d. 22 December 1918, Digby, labourer; ill 10 days.
1918 12 12	1918 12 18	Wallace Stark, 4, d. 18 December 1918, Digby; ill 4 days.
1918 12 12	1918 12 19	Wallace Stark, 33, d. 19 December 1918, Digby, fisherman; ill 1 week.
1918 12 14	1918 12 13	Viney Melanson, 31, d. 24 December 1918, Plympton Station; ill 10 days.
1918 12 15	1918 12 22	Villa Handspiker, female, 7 months, d. 22 December 1918, [*in Digby?*]; ill 1 week.
1918 12 18	1918 12 23	Dustin Vantassell [*Van Tassell*], 6 months, d. 23 December 1918, Digby; ill 5 days.
1918 12 22	1919 01 03	Ambroise Comeau, 30, d. 3 January 1919, Grosses Coques, carpenter; ill 12 days.
1918 12 26	1919 01 02	Aleise [*Alice*] Handspiker, 52, d. 2 January 1919, Mt. Pleasant; ill 1 week.

1919

1919 01 06	1919 01 14	Mrs. Esther Maillet, 37, d. 14 January 1919, Mavillette; ill 8 days, "epidemic influenza."
1919 01 25	1919 01 30	Florence Melanson, 32, d. 30 January 1919, Corberrie, housework; ill 5 days.
1919 01 30	1919 02 08	Mary Pictou, 17 months, d. 8 February 1919, Bear River; ill 10 days.
1919 01 30	1919 02 08	Oliver Pictou, 15, d. 8 February 1919, Bear River, pupil; ill 10 days.
1919 02 01	1919 02 22	Fred Nickerson, 44, d. 22 February 1919, Weymouth, labourer; ill 3 weeks.
1919 02 04	1919 02 12	Marie Boudreau, 76, d. 12 February 1919, Church Point, housekeeper; ill 8 days.
1919 02 27	1919 03 14	*Genevieve* Dugas, 59, d. 14 March 1919, Belliveau's [*sic*] Cove, housewife; ill 16 days.
1919 03 16	1919 03 22	Marie Deveau, 96, d. 23 March 1919, Meteghan, inmate in Poor House; ill 1 week.
1919 03 23	1919 03 31	Louis Saulnier, 3 months, d. 31 March 1919, Meteghan; ill 8 days.
1919 03 28	1919 04 10	Joseph Thibault, 30, d. 10 April 1919, Acaciaville, farmer; ill 10 days.
1919 03 30	1919 04 11	*Elmira* Bacon, female, 76, d. 11 April 1919, Hillgrove; ill 12 days.
1919 04 06	1919 04 27	Marie Comeau, 3 months, d. 27 April 1919, Meteghan; ill 3 weeks.
1919 04 10	1919 04 17	Oscar Andrews, 29, d. 17 April 1919, North Range; ill 1 week.
1919 04 12	1919 05 03	Seymour Gidney, 2, d. 3 May 1919, Sandy Cove; ill 3 weeks.
1919 04 13	1919 04 20	Isabell Marshall, 39, d. 20 April 1919, South Range; ill 1 week.
1919 04 14	1919 05 05	Florence Hooper, 27, d. 5 May 1919, Sandy Cove, music teacher; ill 3 weeks.
1919 04 22	1919 04 29	Blanche Comeau, 3 months, d. 29 April 1919, Meteghan River; ill 1 week.
1919 04 28	1919 05 26	Emile Deveau, 16, d. 26 May 1919, Mavillette; ill 4 weeks.
NO DATA	1919 04 02	William Ross, 53, d. 2 April 1919, Roxville, farmer; "Influenza & Bright's Disease," ill 2 years. No onset date for the Influenza.
NO DATA	1919 04 05	Charles Thibodieu, 54, d. 5 April 1919, Meteghan Center, farmer; "La Grippe & T.B.," ill 4 years. No onset date for the Influenza.
1919 05 02	1919 05 09	Celestin Trahan, 71, d. May 1919, Meteghan, shoemaker; ill 7 days.
1919 05 19	1919 05 24	Joseph Doucet, 7, d. 24 May, Little Brook Station; ill 5 days.
1919 05 26	1919 06 09	Benoît Deveau, 13 months, d. 9 June 1919, Meteghan; ill 2 weeks.
1919 05 31	1919 06 03	Marc Saulnier, 80, d. 3 June 1919, Meteghan Center, farmer; ill 4 days.
1919 06 17	1919 06 29	John Blinn, 64, d. 29 June 1919, Corberrie, farmer; ill 12 days.
1919 06 28	1919 06 30	Arsène Bonafant, 79, d. 30 June 1919, Grosses Coques, housekeeper, widow; influenza, ill 2 days.

1920

1920 01 08	1920 01 15	Joseph Le Blanc, 63, d. 15 January 1920, Lower Saulnierville, farmer; ill 7 days.
1920 02 18	1920 02 29	Joseph Saulnier, 35, d. 29 February 1920, Meteghan, carpenter; ill 11 days.
1920 02 20	1920 02 24	Madelaine Boudreau, 98, d. 24 February 1920, Meteghan; ill 4 days.
1920 03 08	1920 03 15	Ulysse Doucet, 25, d. 15 March 1920, St. Bernard, labourer; ill 7 days.
1920 03 10	1920 03 18	Charles White, 39, d. 18 March 1920, Ashmore, farmer; ill 8 days.
1920 03 14	1920 03 22	Françoise Doucet, 76, d. 22 March 1920, Belliveau's [*sic*] Cove, housework; ill 8 days.
1920 03 15	1920 03 30	Marie Baudrian, 66, 30 March 1920, Church Point, housework; ill 15 days.

1920 03 23	1920 03 27	Sarah Riley, 73, d. 27 March 1920, Digby; ill 4 days.
1920 03 24	1920 03 29	Celeste Comeau, 100, d. 29 March 1920, Belliveau's [*sic*] Cove.
1920 04 09	1920 04 16	John A. Morrisey, 81, d. 16 April 1920, Gilbert Cove, farmer; ill 7 days.
NO DATA	1920 04 01	Alonzo Grant, 79, d. 1 April 1920, Weymouth, carpenter.

Chapter VIII

GUYSBOROUGH COUNTY

❦

PARTS OF THIS county got off relatively lightly in the Great Influenza. There were forty-seven confirmed deaths of Guysborough County natives. Fewer than ten people, however, died in western Guysborough, in St. Mary's District. Deaths seem clustered more around fishing ports such as Canso

Up to the present time of writing Canso is one of the places, possibly in Nova Scotia, which has practically escaped Spanish Influenza. Several cases of a suspicious nature were treated for Spanish Influenza, wisely as we believe; as a result, there has been so far no spread of the disease. No results have been reported and it is confidently hoped that the town will escape the scourge, which has attacked so many towns all over the continent.

Some weeks ago, the trawler 'Ran' arrived in Canso, reporting some of her crew ill, and while the disease could not at that time be recognized as Spanish Influenza, precautions were taken to isolate the steamer and other means were taken to guard against contagion. Two or three other cases in the town apparently developed but with the exception of one case, these were very mild, and we are glad to report that all have recovered.

On the advice of the Health Officer, on the first indication of the disease, the Moving Picture theatre, Pool Room and Post Office corridor were closed to the public and remained closed for about a week, when they were re-opened. It was thought that these were the most likely places to be visited by strangers, who might possibly carry the disease. All will commend the efforts of the Health Officer and Board in taking every precaution to guard against a spread of this dread disease.

Canso News, 26 October 1918, 1.

Sadly, this escape from influenza in Canso did not last. Hundreds became ill; twelve died. A number of the victims were fishers or their relatives.

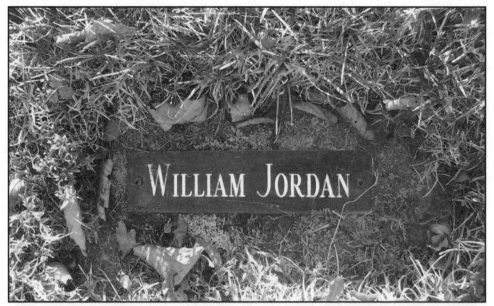

A modern grave marker in Argyle Sunset Cemetery, Guysborough County. William Jordan, of Eight Island Lake, lies in the older part of the cemetery, next to his parents, and close to various Feltmates and Masons—Eight Island Lake neighbours who also lost members to the flu. (*Ruth Legge*)

Eight Island Lake, Guysborough County

Sometimes all it takes is one person to infect a whole community, but often there is no record of who that person was, or how it all happened. The story of the Eight Island Lakes victims is therefore of interest because the way it had been transmitted to the community has been identified.

Three people died at Eight Island Lake, Guysborough County, in late 1918. This is a very isolated community, and all three became ill at around the same time. How death came to this tiny little community, off the main road between Sherbrooke Village and Antigonish, is an astonishing story. A number of people contributed in this effort, especially Ruth Legge, a researcher and historian in Guysborough County. See section beginning on page 162 for a selection of her emails to me.

A search for anything on Eight Island Lake's victims, in the HVS death registration database, revealed that all three victims were listed as Baptists, buried at Goshen, a few miles away. This was confirmed by researcher Ruth Legge. Later, thanks to Dr. Allan Marble's newspaper references list, I found this newspaper report:

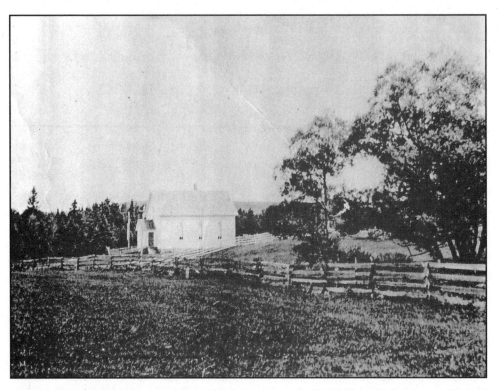

Goshen Baptist Church, Guysborough County, was destroyed by a lightning strike and fire, August 1918; afterwards, services were held for a while in the Eight Island Lake School. *(Courtesy of Lewis MacIntosh, who writes, "It was located just up the road from where I live." Photographer unknown)*

[F]rom Goshen, Guysboro County, comes a story that indicates how alarmingly contagious an infection influenza really is. A Baptist clergyman visited the Mission to hold Divine Service on a recent Sunday. He had the disease in its incipient state. Apparently all who attended the service became sick, also all the members of the household at which he was a guest. Altogether there were some fifty cases of influenza at Goshen. At least one death has occurred there from influenza.

Pictou Advocate, 6 December 1918, 4.

☞ The last sentence refers either to the death of Mrs. Henry Mason of Eight Island Lake, on November 30, or that of William Jordan, on December 4. Those three Baptists who died at Eight Island Lake are all on the same page in the death register, Book 32, Page 313, Numbers 233–5. If indeed they were infected by a visiting minister, one of the contributing factors was that the Goshen Baptist church had burned down in August 1918, and the congregation was holding services crammed into a small schoolhouse. In addition, because pastoral visits were infrequent, surely everyone in the congregation strove to attend. Note the date of the newspaper story, December 6, 1918, which was a Friday. The minister probably visited Goshen on or before Sunday, November 24, in order for Mrs. Henry Mason to fall ill by November 26–28 (see below). Two subsequent deaths occurred shortly thereafter.

- Mason, Mrs. Henry. This young woman was aged 23 years, married to Henry Mason of Eight Island Lake. She died on November 30, 1918, and her illness has to have manifested somewhere between November 26 and November 28—a range of two to four days previous to her death—for a note on the death record to say that she had only been ill "a few days." The family were Baptist, so she was buried at Goshen. No doctor attended, but the name of a "Trained Nurse, Miss Stewart" is written in the space for "Doctor in Attendance." Undertaker was J. J. McIntosh. The return was sent in by "Nichols George" [*George Nichols?*] on December 22, 1918.
  HVS Death Register, Year 1918, Book 32, page 313, No 233.

☞ Ruth Legge reports plenty of Nichols's still living in the area, but no George surnames. The District Registrar must have been a Nichols.

- Jordan, William. Aged 25, single, he was a farmer in Eight Island Lake. He first manifested symptoms of influenza on November 28, and died on December 4, 1918. The family being Baptist, he too was buried at Goshen, in the Argyle Cemetery. Dr. McDougall attended. Undertaker was J. J. McIntosh. The return was sent in by his mother, Mrs. Orman Jordan, on December 6, 1918.
  HVS Death Register, Year 1918, Book 32, page 313, No 235.

- Feltmate, _____ (infant, female). Aged 1 year, 3 months, this unnamed child's father was Elijah Feltmate of Eight Island Lake. She was ill for a week and died December 21, 1918, so her onset of illness was around December 14. Again, the family was Baptist, and she was almost certainly buried at Goshen's Argyle cemetery, as her father's headstone is there. No doctor attended, and again the name of "Trained Nurse, Miss Stewart" is in the space "Doctor in Attendance." Undertaker was J. J. McIntosh. The return was sent in by "Nichols George." [George Nichols] on December 22, 1918.
  HVS Death Register, Year 1918, Book 32, page 313, No 234.

✐ At the bottom of the death registration page where all these names were written, the district registrar stated, "I forwarded the cards belonging to these deaths at once. There are no other deaths in this District [St. Marys, Guysborough] this Quarter ending December 31. Given under my hand this 3rd January 1919, A.F. McNaughton, District Registrar."

There is no way of knowing who else in Eight Island Lake, Goshen, or elsewhere in the district contracted the disease at Goshen church, apart from the newspaper account (above), which states that fifty people were infected. We only know the names of the dead.

Eight Island Lake Deaths, Correspondence with Ruth Legge

✐ Beginning in April 2018, Ruth Legge began a correspondence with me that reveals a year's work to bring some clarification to the deaths at Eight Island Lake. The following are her emails, in chronological order:

✉ Last evening someone mentioned a mutual friend that I could ask about Mrs. Henry Mason of Eight Island Lake. I looked up Mrs. Mason's obituary [death record] and noticed that the other two on the same page were also from Eight Island Lake and all three had died within about a month in late 1918. I missed those when I initially went through Dr. Marble's listing, so perhaps I've missed some others. I will go back over his list. But it seems there WAS a little outbreak there in that community. [I had asked her about the hamlet.] All three are buried in Goshen and were Baptists. I will do a bit of digging on that. I also talked to the woman that was suggested to me and she will see if she can find anything out. So stay tuned on that!

✉ This morning I trolled around in the Excel sheet that I copied and pasted from the Open Site. I found the next quarterly return for the Goshen area finally by spot checking records based on local names. Here is the only death [Alexander Cumings] that was recorded for the January to March 1919 quarter: novascotiagenealogy.com/ItemView.aspx?ImageFile=32-351&Event= death&ID=113778.

✉ Since Alexander Cummings died on January 4, 1919, of old age and there were no other deaths in that quarterly return, I think the three deaths we have are the only three from that epidemic. I also found and checked the April to June 1919 return and there were no flu deaths in that return either.

✉ I went back to the Goshen Community Centre website with the history of the area and reread about the United Baptist Church. There was never actually a church built at the cemetery site. The church that burned was close but not there. If you look at the map I sent, stay on the road that runs along the top, going east out of Goshen, and just past the little road that runs down to the cemetery heading east along that road on the top of the map, the church was on the right near the road. Lloyd Sinclair says there is a bit of a depression on the side of the hill where the old church sat. He is not aware of there being a cemetery there by the old church site (maybe some graves of children near the old church according to rumor) and the Argyle Sunset Cemetery, that I sent photos of, was the only cemetery for that congregation as far as he knows. The congregation was without a church building until the 1940s when Goshen Gospel Church was built. Same congregation of people. As it says on the website, the congregation had gotten materials from an old building that was taken apart and had planned to build a new church where the cemetery is, but it was never built.

✉ Lloyd confirmed that William Jordan did have a twin brother, Charles, who is buried beside him, BUT did NOT think that Charles died of Spanish Influenza. I don't either since I've not found his death registration.

✉ You already have this, from the cemetery listing webpage, but here it is anyway. His parents are to his left and on his right is a Charles Jordan, then two markers that say Baby Jordan.

This is what local people refer to as the old part of the cemetery. Elijah Feltmate, father of the unnamed Feltmate girl, is buried nearby. There is also a broken marker that says Mason and a death date, but in the 1930s, therefore not Mrs. Henry Mason but perhaps him? It is very close to the Jordans.

All of this is just to give you some background in your head as we pursue this.

☞ She included photographs. Ruth Legge to Ruth Whitehead, 16 May 2018:

✉ I think I've come to an end of what I can dig up on the Eight Island Lake epidemic. Here is a photo of the Baptist Church of which the three victims were members. HOWEVER, it had apparently burned down by the time the Spanish Influenza made its way to Eight Island Lake/Goshen area. The photo comes to us courtesy of Lewis MacIntosh. He states: "On the back of one of the pictures it said the church was hit by lightening [*sic*] in August 1918."

✉ It was a bad year for that Baptist congregation! I've determined that the Argyle Sunset Cemetery was already in use by this Baptist congregation by the time the church burned down. There are a number of graves from before 1900 in the cemetery. I have a deed that I believe is for that land, dated 1877, and the cemetery is shown on Ambrose F. Church's Guysborough County map ca 1876, and so is the church, just a very short ways from the cemetery. The people I've talked to are in agreement that services were held in the Eight Island Lake School after the church burned, so I think we are safe in saying that is where the visiting clergyman preached his sermon and spread the influenza. According to the deed I found (St. Mary's Deeds, Book F, pages 416-7), the church was known as Goshen Baptist Church (not Argyle Baptist as Lewis MacIntosh labelled the photo).

As I mentioned the other day, I am pretty confident that only three people died in the Eight Island Lake/Goshen area, due to the next two quarterly returns not showing any influenza deaths.

➡ Ruth Legge on Calvin Breen:

✉ Calvin Breen: Dr. Marble's list indicates that he died in Marie Joseph, Guysborough County, but my reading of his death record is that he was BURIED at Marie Joseph; his place of residence is listed as Halifax. He was 17 years old and no occupation is listed. I am not sure why he was in Halifax, perhaps living with relatives and going to school? He was enumerated with his family in Marie Joseph in 1911 (age 10) and his parents' family was also enumerated in Marie Joseph in 1921, so I don't think the whole family moved to Halifax, but that is just a guess on my part. His parents were James and Mary Breen. The 1911 Census shows elder siblings Gertie M (19) and Roy C (17). In 1921, Roy is enumerated with James and Mary, the parents.

Calvin's death record link: novascotiagenealogy.com/ItemView aspx? ImageFile=25-56&Event=death&ID=102032.

I would question his actually dying in Guysborough County. [Yes, I've already got that.] He was the son of James and Mary (Noye) Breen. Born in Marie Joseph, Guys. Co, in 1900 or 1901 and died 4 January 1919, aged 17 [Halifax County Deaths, 1919, Book 25, Page 56, # 334]. His residence at the time of his death is listed as Halifax on the death record. I have no idea why he was in Halifax. He was enumerated with his parents on the 1911 Census in Marie Joseph, Guysborough County, at the age of 10 (birth given as August 1900), and his parents were enumerated there again in 1921. In the 1911 Census, his name was given as Calvan G. but on his tombstone it is George C.

George Calvin was not enumerated with his family in 1901, although the 1911 Census says he was born in August of 1900. I cannot find him elsewhere in that

Census. I think perhaps the birth year of 1900 on the 1911 Census was in error and he was born in August 1901 instead, and that was probably AFTER the enumeration took place. His tombstone says 1901 and that would jive with his age being 17 at death.

1901 Census: data2.collectionscanada.ca/1901/z/z001/jpg/z000039039.jpg
1911 Census: data2.collectionscanada.gc.ca/1911/jpg/e001969780.jpg

✉ He seems to be the youngest of the family. His siblings: Arthur Henry Breen; James Stowel Breen (died at 18 and buried with Calvin and their parents—see tombstone); Martha Gertrude "Gertie" Breen; Roy Charles Breen (the only one enumerated with the parents in 1921). They are buried in the old Anglican cemetery at Fancy's Point, Marie Joseph, where the first Anglican church was built. It was later replaced with a new church and cemetery, St. Matthew's Anglican, Marie Joseph.

✎ And further from Ruth Legge:

✉ This [photo of family headstone] is for Calvin Breen—apparently his name was George Calvin Breen. He is buried in Fancy's Point cemetery, the old Anglican cemetery in Marie Joseph. I did not have to drive out...found a photo on the internet (guyscogene.net/cem/fancyspt.html and the listing and photo are by Maureen Brown.)

✎ Ruth Legge later went to the cemetery herself, in December 2019, but she and her husband were unable to find this stone. Ruth Legge on Edwin Lawson:

✉ The only names I have identified as actually dying IN the Municipality of St. Mary's (western section of Guysborough County) from Dr. Marble's list are: Edwin R. Lawson and Mrs. Henry Mason [for Mrs. Henry Mason, see Eight Island Lake, above, and Ruth Legge's correction as she found two more names of flu victims]. Lawson, Edwin, 54, St. Mary's (River), [died] 29 Oct. 1918, [days ill] 09. (Allan Marble List.)

St. Mary's River is a tiny settlement just downriver from Sherbrooke. Keith Gallant recalls being shown "Lawson's field" in that area. As for Edwin Lawson: He is supposed to be buried in Riverside Cemetery in Sherbrooke, but thus far I have not been able to locate his gravestone. I do have info on his wife and children, which I will compile and send. He was listed as "cook on steamer" at the time of his death, and I would suggest this explains his contracting the Spanish Influenza when no one else in his family or community seems to have done so. I have found reference to Edwin's middle name as being Ruthvin and Ruthrum. Not sure which might be correct. In 1911, Edwin Lawson was enumerated as "Edward" and he was married with a large family. He is listed as a cook, with place of employment as "cook house." At the time of his death, however, he was listed as a cook on a steamer...my best guess as to how he contracted the illness.

1911 Census: data2.collectionscanada.gc.ca/1911/jpg/e001969871.jpg

✉ When he married Eva McConnell on 4 April 1894, he was a "steward" and aged 29, born and resident in Sherbrook (sic), the son of William Lawson, a farmer. His wife, Eva, was born and resident in Port Hilford, Guyborough County, aged 22, the daughter of James McConnell, sea captain, and Sarah A. McConnell. They were married in the Port Hilford Baptist Church: novascotiagenealogy.com/ItemView.aspx?ImageFile=1814179&Event=marriage&ID=42759. Their children: Edwin Lester, b ca 1896; Minnie Elizabeth, b ca 1898; William Vincent, b 1899; James McConnell, b 1902 in Sherbrooke; Estella Mary, b 1904 at St. Mary's River; Edison, b ca 1906: Sarah Marion, b ca 1912. Edwin Lawson's age at death looks like 54 and that is what is on his tombstone. When he was married in 1894, his age was given as 29, which would basically agree, so he was born ca 1865. Link to death record: novascotiagenealogy.com/ItemView.aspx?ImageFile=32-348&Event=death&ID=113776.

✉ In 1921, Eva, his widow, was enumerated with several of their children. The first one, Mrs. Geo. Fader, was crossed out and then she is listed farther down in the enumeration. This would be Minnie Elizabeth who married George Fader. Minnie was listed as a teacher, public school. Her place of residence was written as Halifax but then crossed out. The next two are sons: Wm. and J McC (William Vincent and James McConnell). Unfortunately, their professions have been written over, but they were working in sawmills. My guess would be millhand and custodial?? Stella, Edison, and Marion were all listed as students. The next household enumerated is that of Edwin and Eva's son, Lester, and wife Jennie, so it would seem that Eva's family were there for her after Edwin passed away. In the margin on that page of the Census is written "St. Mary's River." Edwin is buried in Riverside Cemetery in Sherbrooke, as are his parents, William G Lawson and Eliza McDaniel, and his sister Ada S. Lawson. He is not buried in the same plot with them, but a distance away.

1921 Census: central.bac-lac.gc.ca/.
item/?app=Census1921&op=img&id=e002902774

Marriage Bond for Edwin's parents (1862):

novascotiagenealogy.com/ItemView.
aspx?ImageFile=180010592&Event=marriage&ID=201184

This research by Ruth Legge demonstrates the very many ways one has to use local resources, and in particular, the importance of the rural cemeteries along the backroads of Nova Scotia. This was the extent of our exchange about Eight Island Lake and other deaths.

Guysborough County Deaths Continued

FRANK SUTHERLAND. Not only on the battlefields of Europe are Canso's young men giving up their lives, but on this side of the water, far removed from the danger of cannon balls and bullets, many of Canso's young men are being taken off. The death of Frank Sutherland, son of Mr. and Mrs. Roderick Sutherland of Canso, took place in Gloucester [Massachusetts] recently, caused by Spanish Influenza. Frank Sutherland was a capable, straightforward, manly young fisherman, whose prospects of success in life were very bright, but like so many men in like circumstances he contracted the dread disease and his young life was quickly snuffed out.

Canso News, 26 October 1918, 4.

MRS JOSEPH BOND. The circumstances in connection with the death [on 19 November 1918] of Mrs. Joseph Bond were sad indeed....Mr. and Mrs. Bond with a family of seven children were taken with the influenza all about the same time. The mother, with an infant six months old, labored beyond her strength to care for the sick ones and succumbed to the disease. Mrs. Bond was a native of Port Felix. The funeral took place from the Star of the Sea Church.

Canso News, 30 November 1918, 2.

The HVS record for Guysborough County Death Register, 1918, Book 32, Page 383, Number 348, shows that Mrs. Bond died after an illness of two days, namely of influenza and pneumonia. She was 48, a Catholic, and was buried in Canso. Her first name isn't given, only that of her husband.

VIGNAULT. At Mulgrave, after a brief illness with Spanish influenza, Captain Samuel Vignault, in his 40th year. Funeral will take place [in Halifax] from Snow and Co.'s undertaking rooms today, November 25, at 3 p.m. to Mount Olivet cemetery.

Halifax Evening Mail, 25 November 1918, 1.

DEATH AT MULGRAVE

Samuel Vignault, captain of the steamer Kinburn, plying between Pictou and P. E. Island for the last twenty-four years, died at Mulgrave on Sunday after a brief illness with Spanish influenza. He was in the 40th year of his age, and is survived by his wife and two children.

Sydney Daily Post, 28 November 1918, 3.

George H. Smith, aged 19, single, of Canso/Port Greville, Guysborough County, and son of George H. Smith of Canso, died 30 November 1918, after an illness of seven days' Influenza and pneumonia. He was buried in the Protestant Cemetery in Canso.

Information provided by Linda Littlejohn and Harriet McCready, Parrsborough Shore Historical Society, who were just making extra sure that this "Port Greville" was in Guysborough County, and not in Cumberland County.

AUGUSTUS HANLON. Among the sad events in connection with the visit of influenza in Canso was the carrying off of several young men, among whom was Augustus Hanlon, who died on November 28th. Mr. Hanlon was a successful young fisherman and leaves and wife and one child.

Canso News, 28 December 1918, 2.

GEORGE RHYNOLD. Following a severe attack of influenza, George Rhynold passed away on November 28th at a comparatively young age. He was a fisherman and at the time of his death resided with his sister Mrs. Stephen Barss.

Canso News, 28 December 1918, 2.

INFLUENZA

Contrary to hope Canso and district did not escape Spanish Influenza which has been epidemic in so many countries and throughout Nova Scotia. Fortunately, up to the present few fatal cases have occurred. Perhaps Canso learned a good deal from other towns which were visited by the disease before it arrived at the Seaport Town. The most effective means of combatting the onset of the 'Flu' seems to be in taking care, on the first symptoms to consult the Doctor, and then rigidly carrying out his instructions. Many people have lost their lives by trying to keep around when they should be in bed under the Doctor's care.

For the past four weeks the Churches, Schools, Theatres, and places of public gatherings have been closed. Notwithstanding this precaution the disease has practically gone through the community....

Some will be inclined to criticize the action of the Health Officer and the Board of Health, but this officer and the Board have come to expect such things. All will agree, however, that no measures have been taken in any arbitrary spirit but with the good and safety of the community uppermost.

Canso News, 30 November 1918, 1.

 MISS EMMA HURST. The death of Miss Emma Hurst took place at the home of her brother, Seymore Hurst, on Monday the 18th last. Miss Hurst had recovered from an attack of influenza, but not being of a robust constitution, heart failure followed, and she quietly passed away. The deceased was a daughter of the late William Hurst.

Canso News, 30 November 1918, 2.

 MRS. DAVID SHRIDER [Shrader]. All that medical skill could do did not prevent the death of Mrs. David Shrider, which took place on Wednesday morning twentieth from influenza. Double pneumonia and other complications developed and for days the doctor had small hopes of her recovery. Mrs. Shrider had a family of grown up children. Her husband predeceased her some years.

Canso News, 30 November 1918, 2. HVS, Guysborough County Death Register, 1918, Book 32, Page 301, Number 204.

The original record has her name as Mrs. David Shrader. The HVS search engine has her as Schrader. She was a widow, aged 64, and had been born in Half Island Cove. Her doctor was Hugh Ross; the undertaker Jarvis Charles Knight. She was buried in Canso.

 GEORGE SMITH. Another bright Canso boy passed away on November 30 in the person of George Smith, son of Mr. and Mrs. George R. Smith.

Canso News, 28 December 1918, 2. HVS, Death Register, Guysborough County, Year 1918, Book 32, Page 302, Number 209.

George Smith was a fisherman. He died of influenza and pneumonia.

 FRED SCELES. The death of Fred Sceles took place at Canso on December 1st. Never of a robust constitution, he succumbed to an attack of influenza. He leaves a wife who is a resident of Canso. Burial took place at Half Island Cove.

Canso News, 28 December 1918, 2.

 MRS. SYLVESTER FANNING. The death of Mrs. Sylvester Fanning took place on December 2nd, following an attack of influenza. Mrs. Fanning was a comparatively young woman and leaves three small children with her husband to mourn their loss. The funeral took place from the Star of the Sea church.

Canso News, 28 December 1918, 3.

Sergeant Major J. A. Chisholm has just returned to his military duties at Halifax, after a ten days furlough spent with his wife at Guysboro. He has about recovered from a serious attack of influenza and pneumonia.

Antigonish Casket, 12 December 1918. Courtesy the Antigonish Heritage Museum.

Mulgrave had a severe influenza epidemic, occasioned, it is said, by contact with the crew of a schooner who were suffering. The Captain of the schooner died. Altogether Mulgrave had fully a hundred cases. Business at Mulgrave felt the disease to some extent. The local Bank had to close its doors for several days because of the flu gripping the staff.

Antigonish Casket, 19 December 1918. Courtesy the Antigonish Heritage Museum.

Mrs. Laura Skinner, aged 32, married, kept house for her husband, John G. Skinner. They lived at "Guysboro." Listed as "mulatto" in the death register, she had been born in Tracadie, Antigonish County. Mrs. Skinner died December 27, 1918, of "Influenza and Pneumonia," ill seven days. Her death was further complicated by premature labour. The attending doctor was G. E. Buckley; he made the return on December 28. Mrs. Skinner was a Baptist, so was buried in the Baptist Cemetery, Guysborough.

HVS, Death Register, Guysborough County, 1918, Book 32, Page 294, Number 187.

BREEN. On January 4th, at Marie Joseph, of influenza, Calvin G. Breen, son of Mr. and Mrs. James Breen, age 17 years.

Halifax Evening Mail, 23 January 1919, 1.

This newspaper account is incorrect. Calvin G. Breen, or George C. Breen, depending on whether one reads his tombstone or the newspaper, was buried in Marie Joseph, Guysborough County, but he died in Halifax, and his death certificate, in the registration book for Halifax County, so states: he died in Halifax. See the earlier section in this chapter for further Breen information collected by Ruth Legge.

JOHN De RABBIE. Another Canso boy passed away at Halifax recently, in the person of John DeRabbie, who was attached to the Military there. He contracted Influenza and passed away very quickly. He was the son of Mr. and Mrs. George DeRabbie of Hazel Hill. Interment took place at Halifax.

Canso News, 25 January 1919, 1.

LEANDER PYCHE. The death of Leander Pyche in young manhood took place on February 6th, leaving a wife and five small children. Some months ago, Mr. Pyche contracted Influenza from which he never totally recovered, but continued to fail in health until death overtook him on the date mentioned. He was a son of Mr. George Pyche of the Public Building staff.

Canso News, 28 February 1919, 1.

Mary McFhee [MacPhee], aged 54, married, housework, lived at Upper Big Tracadie. She died 15 March 1919, of Influenza and Pneumonia, after an illness of sixteen days.

Listed as "African" in the death register, her name is given as McFhee on Allan Marble's rough draft list above, but the original death record shows, both for her and her husband, the surname McPhee. Mrs. McPhee was born in Tracadie, resided in Upper Big Tracadie, and was married to Mr. Archie McPhee. "Dr. Cameron, MD" was her doctor; the undertaker was P. Floyd. A Baptist, she was buried at the Baptist Cemetery, Big Tracadie. John J. Williams sent in the return on March 15th.

HVS, Death Register, Guysborough County, 1918, Book 32, Page 357, Number 303.

Upper Big Tracadie was then in Guysborough County, Guysborough District; it is now in Antigonish County.

Influenza has paid a second visit to Tracadie, Antigonish. Two weeks ago, all the workmen at a lumber camp were taken sick. Thirty men comprised the camp, which was operated by Mr. Haggerty of Mulgrave, and was in [the] charge of Mr. George Cameron of Melrose, Guysborough Co. The workmen were also from Guysborough County districts—East River, St. Mary's, Melrose and vicinity. Herbert Maclachlan, one of the workmen, developed pneumonia. He was conveyed to Antigonish for treatment. Owing to the hospital being overcrowded, other accommodation was found, a vacant office. Two nurses attended him, and every attention was given him, still he passed away on Wednesday evening [March 19], a few minutes before his wife reached his bedside. Besides his wife, he leaves five children. As the men recovered strength, they returned to their several homes, so the camp is now practically deserted.

Antigonish Casket, 27 March 1919. Courtesy of the Antigonish Heritage Museum.

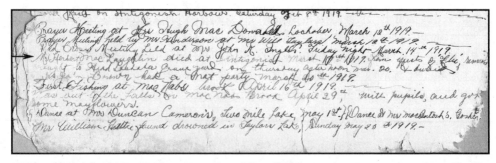

Note on burial of Mr. Herbert MacLaughlan. "This entry was a note written in the school register by teacher Mary A. Cameron, from the West Lochaber Schoolhouse, Section #44, for the school year ending July 1919. She made notes on a variety of events, natural occurrences, etc." *(Antigonish Heritage Museum)*

✏️ This man's name was actually Herbert McLaughlan. Aged 35, he was born in West Lochaber, Antigonish County. Married and a farmer, he resided in Glenelg, Guysborough County. He must have been trying to bring in some winter cash by working in a lumbering camp. He died on March 19, 1919, of influenza and pneumonia. Dr. MacDonald attended. A Presbyterian, Herbert was buried at the Head of Lochaber; P. S. Floyd was his undertaker. A Mrs. Lauchlan Thomas sent in the return to the registrar on March 27, 1919. A note in a school register, by teacher Mary A. Cameron, West Lochaber Schoolhouse, Section #44, reads, "Mr. Herb't MacLaughlin died at Antigonish, March 19, 1919, from effects of 'Flu', remains brought to Head Lochaber grave yard on Thursday after noon, & buried."

> HVS, Death Register, Antigonish County, Year 1919, Book 26, Page 527, Number 1114. Antigonish Heritage Museum, Antigonish. See photograph of schoolteacher's note, courtesy of Jocelyn Gillis, the curator.

✏️ Strangely, there are two records for a Herbert McLaughlan. Their particulars are identical in every way *except* that the residence of the second Herbert is shown as Lochaber, not Glenelg. Both were married farmers, aged 35, both had a Dr. MacDonald/McDonald attending, and P. S. Floyd as undertaker. However, this second (earlier entered) record does not name his place of birth, or place of burial. This undated return was sent in by a different person, a Billy McLaughlan. Billy was obviously a relative, but seems to have left spaces on the return blank. A "Mac Lauchlan, Thomas" made the return of death on the second entry. If these records are not for one and the same person, these Herbert McLaughlans must have been related somehow. What is more likely, however, is that there were two returns for the same man, the man who farmed in Glenelg. Number 1114 has better information, but only Number 1083 appears on Dr. Allan Marble's List by Counties.

> HVS, Death Register, Antigonish County, Year 1919, Book 26, Page 517, Number 1083.

RICHARD MCDONALD. The death of Richard McDonald took place at the home of his sister, Mrs. D. Wilson, on Sunday 16th inst. Mr. McDonald contracted influenza some months ago which left him in a weakened condition from which he never fully recovered. He was sixty-two years of age and unmarried.

Canso News, 29 March 1919, 1.

James W. Taylor, aged 72, of Crossroads Country Harbour, Guysborough County, died 29 April 1919 in Guysborough (town) after six weeks ill with Spanish Influenza, according to Dr. Allan Marble's lists. His wife was Caroline E. Holly.

Supplemental information provided by Linda Littlejohn of the Parrsborough Shore Historical Society.

JAMES KAVANAGH. The death of James Kavanagh took place on February 29th, following a severe attack of influenza. Mr. Kavanagh was one of Canso's energetic fishermen and leaves a widow and one child.

Canso News, 25 March 1920, 1.

MRS. JOHN JARVIS. The circumstances of the death of Mrs. John Jarvis are sad indeed. Having recovered from an attack of Influenza and able to be about her house again, she suddenly became ill and passed away quite quickly. She leaves a family of young children....Mrs. Jarvis was a daughter of James Rhynold of Fox Island and a sister of Mrs. John Dort, Canso.

Canso News, 25 March 1920, 1.

ROBERT WILLIAMS. The community was shocked on the 14th instant at the news of the death of Robert Williams who was cut down in the midst of life. Only a few days before the serious illness overtook him, he was about as usual. He was of a strong robust constitution but quietly wilted before the onslaught of Influenza.

Canso News, 25 March 1920, 1.

Sophie Jordan, aged 1 year, 4 months and 10 days, lived and died on the "Guysboro Road" at Upper Big Tracadie; died March 26, 1920 of Influenza and Pneumonia, after an illness of seven days. Her mother's name is given as "Miss Victoria Jordan," born in Nova Scotia; her uncle, "Charless Reddish" [Charles Reddick] of Upper Big Tracadie is listed as the informant returning the information. Listed as "African" in the death register.

Guysborough County, Year 1920, Book 68, Page 112. Upper Big Tracadie was then in Guysborough County, Guysborough District; it is now in Antigonish County.

- Mrs. Mary Clyke, aged 18, lived in Guysborough, and did housework. She died April 30, 1920, of complications of pregnancy and Influenza, ill two months. She was listed as "coloured" in the death register. Her husband, Mr. Archie Clyke, returned the information on March 2, 1920, saying her father's name was unknown to him, her mother's maiden name had been Annie Laurenson, and that Mary had lived at her place of death for seven months before passing on. The death record also says that in addition to pregnancy and influenza, she died of uremia, followed by coma. Her doctor, G. S. Buckley, certified that he had attended her first on February 7, and last saw her on the day of her death, April 30.

Guysborough County, Year 1920, Book 68, Page 121

Death record for Margaret Cohoon, who died October 5, 1920—the last person in the county to die of the Great Influenza. (*Nova Scotia Archives*)

Last known death in Nova Scotia.

Influenza could wreck the health and linger on for months in some cases. A prime example is that of Margaret Cohoon, widow of Moses Cohoon. She had been born July 2, 1842, a daughter of Patrick Curry, a native of Ireland, and his wife, who had been a McGuire. The parents emigrated to Canada before their daughter was born, as her death record states she had lived in the province for her "Lifetime," and had resided in Guysborough for forty-five years before her death. She became ill with influenza late in 1919, or early in the year of 1920. On March 25, the *Canso News* printed a message of support for her children: "Much sympathy is expressed for the family of Mrs. Moses Cohoon in their anxiety in regard to the serious illness of their mother who for many weeks has been lingering between life and death. Only a few weeks ago the husband and father passed away."

Canso News, 25 March 1920, 1.

☞ There does not appear to be a death record in the HVS database for Margaret's husband Moses. Unless he is in the death register but has not made it into the database, he must have gone unreported, or he died outside Nova Scotia. All deaths of persons with names beginning with C in Nova Scotia were checked for 1920, and then 1919, without result.

Mrs. Cohoon contracted influenza at some point in late 1919 or early 1920, yet lingered for between seven and eight months, severely ill, until October 5, 1920. Her death certificate shows the cause of death as flu and bronchitis. "Following a severe attack of Flu, Bronchitis set in." Secondary cause of death was listed as "an attack of Flu." Margaret Cohoon is therefore the last known Nova Scotian person—from Guysborough County, anyway—to die in the Great Influenza Epidemic of 1918–20.

HVS, Death Register, Guysborough County, Year 1920, Book 68, Page 240, states she was born in Nova Scotia, and had lived there all her life.

GUYSBOROUGH COUNTY, VITAL STATISTICS, DEATH REGISTER, BOOKS 32, 68

1918

1. Mrs. Gussie Jones, 27, d. 15 December 1918, West Cooks Cove, housewife.

2. Mrs. Laura Skinner, 32, d. 27 December 1918, Guysboro [*sic*], housewife.

3. Lester Hodgson, 22, d. 23 December 1918, Goldboro, military.

4. Acil Blakely, 19, d. 30 December 1918, Goldboro, clerk.

5. Emma Hurst, 28, d. 18 November 1918, Canso, housemaid.

6. Mrs. David Shrader, 64, d. 20 November 1918, Canso, housekeeper.

7. Jacob Manuel, 1, d. 25 November 1918, Canso.

8. Joseph Munroe, 1 year 9 months, d. 25 November 1918, Canso.

9. Augustine Hanlon, 39, d. 28 November 1918, Canso, fisherman.

10. George Rhynold, 39, d. 28 November 1918, Canso, fisherman.

11. George Smith, 19, d. 30 November 1918, Canso, fisherman.

12. Frederick Shields, 51, d. 1 December 1918, Canso, labourer.

13. Mrs. Sylvester Fanning, 22, d. 3 December 1918, Canso, housekeeper.

14. John Smith, 2, d. 3 December 1918, Canso.

15. Mrs. Robert Munroe, 34, d. 29 December 1918, Canso, housekeeper.

16. Mrs. Peter Walkins, 86, d. 9 November 1918, Hazel Hill.

17. Mrs. Joseph Bond, 48, d. 19 November 1918, Hazel Hill.

18. Clarence Armsworthy, 21, d. 24 November 1918, Philips Harbour, fisherman.

19. Mrs. Henry Mason, 23, d. 30 November, 1918, Eight Island Lake, housewife

20. *Infant* Feltmate, female, 1, d. 21 December 1918, Eight Island Lake.

21. William Jordan, 25, d. 4 December 1918, Eight Island Lake, farmer.

22. Bernadette Benoît, 30, d. 5 December 1918, Charlos Cove, housewife.

[*The number 23 had mistakenly been omitted on Dr. Marble's list, thus the present list's numbering has been adjusted.*]

23. Annie Richard, 30, d. 13 December 1918, Charlos Cove.

24. Julie Richard, 34, d. 14 December 1918, Charlos Cove, housewife.

25. David Richard, 28, d. 15 December 1918, Charlos Cove, fisherman.

26. Silvester Dorion, 19, d. 16 December 1918, Charlos Cove, labourer.

27. Joseph Anderson, 4 months, d. 18 December 1918, Mulgrave.

28. John Skidmore, 32, d. 8 December 1918, Mulgrave, railway worker.

29. Edwin Lawson, 54, d. 29 October 1918, St. Mary's, cook on a steamer.

1919

30. Mary McFhee [*McPhee*], 54, d. 15 March 1919, Upper Big Tracadie, housework.

31. Bridget Lawlor, 69, d. 11 March 1919, Ogden, housewife.

32. Margaret Rumley, 16, d. 24 March 1919, Roman Valley, student.

33. James Taylor, 72, d. 29 April 1919, Cross Roads, carpenter.

[*The following number (Number 35 on Dr. Marble's list), is a repeat of the death record for Mrs. Peter Walkins, 86, Hazel Hill. In order to arrive at an accurate count of deaths for the county, this present list has been adjusted.*]

1920

34. Florence Mason, 13, d. 19 February 1920, Cross Roads, Country Harbour.

35. John [*Jane Clarke McArthur, female*], 26, d. 23 February 1920, Guysborough. [*Her maiden name was Jane Clarke, daughter of Barbara Fenton and Isaac Clarke; she married a McArthur. Three times the original death record clearly states either that she is female or uses only the pronoun "her," yet the HVS database names her "John," and so she appears on Dr. Marble's list as John McArthur. HVS, Guysborough County Death Register, 1920, Book 68, Page 63.*]

36. Duncan McCarty, 23, d. 26 February 1920, Goldboro, labourer.

37. James McCarty, 66, d. 27 February 1920, Goldboro, labourer.

38. John W. Smith, 57, d. 9 March 1920, Cross Roads, Country Harbour, farmer.

39. Susan Fenton, 38, d. 2 March 1920, Country Harbour, housework.

40. Nicholas Sabba, 6 months, d. 11 March 1920, Canso.

41. Mrs. Percy Booth, 35, d. 11 March 1920, Hazel Hill, housewife.

42. Marg MacKenzie, 18, d. 23 March 1920, Hazel Hill.

43. Thressa Kaiser, 33, d. 8 March 1920, Indian River.

44. Sophie Jordan, 1 year 4 months, d. 26 March 1920, Upper Big Tracadie.

45. Laura Moore, 39, d. 21 April 1920, Guysboro [*sic*], housekeeper.

46. Mrs. Mary Clyke, 18, d. 30 April 1920, Guysboro [*sic*], housework.

47. *Margaret Cohoon, 78, d. 5 October 1920, Canso, housewife. [For some reason, Dr. Marble did not include her on this list, perhaps due to the late date of her death, months after she first contracted flu: "Following a severe attack of Flu, Bronchitis set in." Influenza was again emphasized, when the secondary cause of death was listed as "an attack of Flu." HVS, Death Register, Guysborough County, Year 1920, Book 68, Page 240.*]

Chapter IX

HALIFAX COUNTY

❧〰❦

HALIFAX COUNTY HAD at least 497 confirmed deaths from the Great Influenza between 1918 and 1920, with 338 in the city proper, and 159 in the rest of the county.

The Beginnings of the Disease

☞ Beechville, NS, is a community founded by War of 1812 Refugees, people formerly enslaved in the United States who were given sanctuary aboard British vessels. They were brought to Nova Scotia both during and right after the end of that war, and granted land at what became Beechville. On August 2014, Beechville descendants celebrated the two hundredth anniversary of their arrival in Nova Scotia.

Halifax, *Chronicle Herald*. 9 August 2014.

☞ The descendants of those Beechville founders would be commemorating, in September 2018, a far more tragic anniversary, a time when the Great Influenza struck the community a devastating blow. The following are the names of those who died from the flu:

- Murray Dorrington, 13 months old, was the first to die, on September 11, 1918. We don't know how many days he was ill before he died.

- Annie Henry and her sister Rachael both died of pneumonia (after whooping cough) around this time, a pneumonia perhaps created by influenza, on top of everything else, as their father, and very probably their mother, died of influenza on October 28.

- Lewis Dorrington, just 1 year old, died on September 14.

- Stella Munro, 3 months old, followed on September 25.

- Peter Munro, a 26-year-old labourer, died October 24. He had been ill for a week, starting on October 17.

- Gladys Hill, 8 months old, died on October 25, after a short illness of three days.

- Kathleen Wright, a Beechville housewife aged 20, died on the same day, October 25; she had been sick seven days.

- George Lopie, a 53-year-old widower, who worked as a labourer, died the next day, October 26.

- Clara Munro, aged 3, died October 27, after an illness of nine days.

- Zechariah Henry, a labourer aged 39, and a married man, died 28 October; he had been ill for a week. His daughters Annie and Rachael predeceased him by several weeks.

- Emma Henry, described as a widowed housewife, possibly having been married to Zechariah Henry, died on November 2, five days after Mr. Henry passed on.

- John Munroe [*sic*], only 15, died on November 3.

HVS, Death Register, Halifax County, Year 1918, Book 35.

We don't know how many other people sickened with it and survived, or who was the first to fall ill. The flu struck down whole families, like the Henrys, making it almost impossible for the sick to care for one another. We don't know when the first case appeared, but it was probably in late August or early September. Nor can we be certain when the flu finally lost its grip on Beechville, but likely sometime after the death of Mr. Munroe on November 3. We can only guess at how traumatized it must have left that very small community, especially after having to dig six graves in four days (see October 24–28).

What is also important in the story of the impact of influenza on Halifax County and the city is that the Beechville community deaths began very early on, starting with that of the Dorrington child on September 11. His was the earliest reported influenza death for the county, excluding the city.

Within the city, Dr. Marble's unpublished list of deaths titled "Vital Statistics for Halifax City, Book #21," shows three "white" children dead around that time, one on September 13, two on September 29. Adult deaths in the city, however, don't begin until October 4.

We know so little else that it is presently impossible to discover how the disease was introduced into the Beechville community. And there is not one single report in any Nova Scotia newspaper about the horrific ordeal that Beechville was experiencing. No mention, during those months, of a whole community taking ill, or mention of the eleven deaths, including those of the entire Henry family. Not one.

This was the beginning of the rollcall of the dead for Halifax County, that is, the invasion of the murderous Second Wave of the Great Influenza. It has been estimated that for every one to four deaths here, there were one hundred people ill. Using this as a general guideline, if Halifax County had almost five hundred or more deaths, then there were at least fifty thousand souls, in this one county alone, who were stricken with it.

Probable Introduction of the Disease to Halifax

☞ Halifax is a port city. In early August, according to author John Barry, "the crew of a steamship proceeding from France to New York was hit so hard with influenza 'that all of the seamen were prostrate on it and it had to put into Halifax.'" At present, the name of this steamship still has not been determined, nor whether she was a French vessel, or merely departing from France.

John M. Barry. *The Great Influenza: The Story of the Deadliest Pandemic in History.* Penguin, New York, 2009: 181.

☞ The port quarantine facility was located on Lawlor Island, east of McNabs Island, across from Fisherman's Cove on the eastern shore of Halifax Harbour. The only records of deaths there which occur in Halifax County death registers are as follows: sailor Jules Fortin, who died on September 27, 1918; Richard Olsen, "American sailor," died September 30, 1918; François Michele, sailor, died October 1, 1918; James Fell, no occupation given, died on October 6, 1918; George Taylor, no occupation given, died October 11; and Patrick Quinan, seaman, who died October 15 that same year.

HVS, Halifax County Death Register, 1918, Book 35. Page 159, Numbers 544 (Jules Fortin), 545 (Richard Olsen), 546 (François Michele, 547 (James B. Fell—the HVS search engine has it as "Fill"); Page 160, Number 553 (George Taylor); Page 161, Number 556 (Patrick Quinan).

☞ The earliest of these Lawlor Island deaths was that of Jules Fortin, a sailor from the French cable ship *Edouard L. Jeramec.* Fortin's name was at first entered into the death register as "Fortin, Francis." The first name has been crossed out in pencil, and a note of the correct first name written above it: "Jules/March 21, 1921, A.J. Campbell." As evidence for the change, Campbell appended a letter:

Station Hospital, Lawlor's Island, Feb'y 21, 1921
Mr. A. J. Campbell, Deputy Registrar General

Sir –
Among the patients admitted to this Hospital from the *S.S. Edouard Jeramec* was a man named Jules Fortin. The hospital register shows that Jules Fortin was admitted Sept. 26, 1918, and that he died Sept. 27, 1918 at 11:45 P.M.

I am, Sir,
Yours respectfully,
F. Himmelmann (Matron)

HVS, Halifax County Death Register, Book 35, Page 159, Number 544.

☞ The HVS search engine gives his surname as Fortier. The original record, as well as the letter, read "Fortin."

☞ Others on this cable ship were sick. Dr. N. E. McKay (see below) says that in late September there were at least twenty people ill with influenza aboard the *Jeramec*. One wonders if, being a French ship, they had come into contact with the crew of the ship John Barry describes as sailing from France to New York, but putting into Halifax as all their crew were down with influenza. The *Jeramec* had at least one other death, that of François Michele. He died on Lawlor Island on October 1. He was 29, described as "sailor, *Edouard L. Jeramec*, single, born at St. Quay-Portrieux [Brittany], France."

HVS, Halifax County Death Register, Book 35, Page 159, Number 546.

☞ Accounts in Halifax newspapers of the period quote health officials as blaming the arrival of influenza in the city on shipping.

DR. N. E. MACKAY WILL PROTEST TO OTTAWA AGAINST ALLOWING STEAMERS TO BE SENT HERE WITH CASES OF SPANISH INFLUENZA ON BOARD—A SERIOUS MATTER

HALIFAX, October 8. The apparent disregard of health regulations by the shipping authorities at Montreal and New York, will be reported to the Canadian director of health at Ottawa, by Dr. N. E. MacKay, Dominion government quarantine officer at Halifax. Steamers given their practique (clear bill of health) at these ports are continually reaching Halifax with large numbers of cases of Spanish influenza on board. The belief is that the disease was introduced into Halifax through this source, and a protest will be made to the Dominion director of health. Yesterday a steamer reached Halifax with a large number of influenza cases on board. The ship was from Montreal, where she had been given her practique. On a very recent occasion a steamer arrived from New York with a number of cases of the disease, even the captain being very ill with it. His temperature was 105. Dr. MacKay regards the practice of allowing steamers to come to Halifax, under the conditions referred to, as dangerous to the health of the citizens.

Other instances equally as serious, indicating an utter disregard for the health of our citizens, have been reported.

Halifax Evening Mail, 9 October 1918, 2.

Ships are still arriving in the port of Halifax with infected crews. Yesterday several more sailors were admitted as patients in hospital at Lawlor's Island. An American ship also put in with a number of cases. The introduction of Spanish influenza to Halifax is supposed to be owing to the arrival of ships whose men were suffering from the disease....DEPARTMENT OF THE PUBLIC HEALTH OF NOVA SCOTIA. Halifax, October 8.

Halifax Morning Chronicle, 10 October 1918, 5.

TWO MORE DEATHS FROM SPANISH INFLUENZA
The health authorities are using every endeavour to prevent the spread of the Disease—ships arrive in port with infected crews. Yesterday seventeen new cases of Spanish influenza among the civilian population of Halifax were reported to the Health Board, and the military authorities were obliged to care for more than this number. Two deaths occurred in the city due to disease.

Halifax Morning Chronicle, 10 October 1918, 5.

The Progress of the Disease

While influenza raged in New England, Nova Scotia in August–September 1918 had experienced only a few cases to date, yet bodies of Nova Scotians dying outside of the province were already being shipped home by train for burial.

The death occurred in Milton, Mass., on September 23rd, of Owen Harpell, son of William Harpell, of lower West Jeddore, in the thirty-third year of his age. His death was caused by pneumonia, brought on by an attack of Spanish Influenza. He leaves behind to mourn their loss a wife, daughter of Wilson and Leslie Webber, of Lakeville, Halifax County, two children, a father and mother, seven sisters and one brother....Interment was at West Jeddore on Saturday at 2.30, the Rev. Mr. Phinney preaching the funeral sermon. The remains were accompanied home [on the train] by George Harpell, of Worcester, Mass., an uncle of the deceased.

Halifax Morning Chronicle, 2 October 1918, 2.

At the first signs of influenza increasing in Nova Scotia, the authorities were cautious. The flu was downplayed, and newspaper accounts were geared toward not frightening the population.

INFLUENZA CASES ON CABLE SHIP

Dr. N. E. McKay, Chairman of the City Board of Health, when asked if an epidemic of Spanish influenza were threatening Halifax, said that there were no cases in the city proper, although there were some twenty men but mildly infected on the French cable ship, as well as a few other cases on ships now in the harbour, not exceeding a dozen. There have been no reports of an epidemic from the various Provincial centres, although some of the crew of a ship in Sydney are sick with the disease.

Halifax Morning Chronicle, 27 September 1918, 2.

Roger Marsters, Maritime Museum of the Atlantic, says, "The French cable ship was probably the Edouard Jeramec, which was a longtime fixture on the Dartmouth side of the Narrows." This is confirmed by the two death records for her crew, above.

Roger Marsters to Ruth Whitehead, personal communication, May 2018.

"No cases in the city proper." That would change in the course of the week. By September 28 or earlier, influenza was established in quite a few Nova Scotian counties (see below). By October 3, the provincial health officer was greatly concerned.

CIRCULAR TO N.S. HEALTH OFFICERS

Dr. Hattie Urges Taking of Measures of Protection Against Menace of Spanish Influenza Epidemic in This Province

There are no changes in the Spanish influenza situation throughout Halifax and Nova Scotia. In a circular addressed to Medical Health Officers, W. H. Hattie, Provincial Health Officer, says with reference to the epidemic:

"Although the menace of epidemic influenza should not be exaggerated, it would be manifestly wrong for any M.H.O. to view its appearance in several localities with other than the gravest concern. From the information thus far available, the type of influenza prevailing in the United States and central Canadian provinces is much more serious with a much larger mortality than that which recently swept over Europe. Therefore every effort should be made to check its spread upon its first appearance, and quarantine and all other means of control are strongly urged....

Such a serious menace demands prompt consideration. It is suggested that nurses and others be utilized to instruct factory employees, also that ministers and schoolteachers be requested to instruct their congregations and scholars in measures of prevention."

Dr. Hattie concludes his circular by requesting daily telegraphic reports of the distribution and number of cases developing, and also any deaths which may have occurred.

In his weekly bulletin to Medical Health Officers for the week ending September 28, Dr. Hattie states that cases of Spanish influenza have been reported in Granville, Carleton Corner, and Centrelea (Annapolis County); Liverpool, Yarmouth, Sydney, New Waterford, Arichat, Windsor, Halifax, and Port Maitland (Yarmouth County)....[P]hysicians are asked to immediately report every case to the Medical Health Officer of the district, and to act upon his instructions.

Halifax Morning Chronicle, 3 October 1918, 7.

☞ This is the earliest mention of influenza in Arichat by the provincial health officer.

NOVA SCOTIA DOCTORS AND HEALTH OFFICERS WARNED TO BE ON THEIR GUARD AGAINST THE INFLUENZA EPIDEMIC WHICH SERIOUSLY THREATENS

In another circular, Dr. Hattie says: "During the week ending September 28th cases of infectitous [*sic*] disease have been reported to this office from the following localities....Spanish Influenza—Granville, Carletons Corner and Centrelea (Annapolis Co.) Liverpool, Yarmouth, Sydney, New Waterford, Arichat, Windsor, Halifax and Port Maitland (Yarmouth Co.) Medical officers of municipalities are requested to name the localities from which infectious diseases are reported when making weekly returns."

Halifax Evening Mail, 4 October 1918, 6.

☞ Note that nothing was reported from Lockeport, even though there were people dying there by October 2.

On October 8, the *Evening Mail* published this frightening news story out of Cuba, to give Haligonians a foretaste of things to come:

NEW AND MYSTERIOUS DISEASE IN CUBA

A Cuban Port, October 7. Cuban medical authorities have not yet been able to diagnose the malady that caused twenty-four deaths on the Spanish liner Alfonso XII, which arrived here Sunday and is being held in quarantine. Nineteen persons died on the voyage and five have died since the ship reached port. Among the dead are the second officer. Two persons, crazed with suffering, committed suicide during the voyage. Sixty of the 1200 passengers on board the ship are ill, and forty are said to be in a serious condition, with very high temperatures with signs of mental derangement, characterizing the malady which was supposed to be Spanish influenza.

Halifax Evening Mail, 8 October 1918, 6.

W.H. Hattie, Provincial Health Officer, has issued the following bulletin:
Reports up to noon Monday
Sydney, 50 cases, 10 deaths (5 civilians)
Dominion, 19 cases
New Waterford, 18 cases, Oct. 5th, 29, Oct. 6th.
Windsor, 14 cases; 1 death
Ellershouse, 1 case
Chester Road, 1 case
Falmouth, several cases
Yarmouth, 3 cases
Brooklyn, Yar. Co., 1 case
Dartmouth, 5 [*for*] Oct. 6th; 1 Oct. 7th
Tufts Cove, 1 case
Halifax, 16 cases....

Halifax Morning Chronicle, 8 October 1918, 5.

☞ In a second circular (same page) addressed to Medical Health Officers, Dr. Hattie offers the following suggestion with reference to the disease: "Employees in barber shops have special opportunity for spreading infection. They should be seen daily by a competent inspector."

Halifax Morning Chronicle, 8 October 1918, 5.

☞ The above account was published in the morning, October 8. By the time the evening newspaper came out, the list had been updated to reflect cases as of noon the previous day:

 SPANISH INFLUENZA CASES IN NOVA SCOTIA
The reports up to noon yesterday were as follows:

Places	Cases
Sydney (10 deaths)	80
Dominion	10
New Waterford	38
Windsor	14
Ellershouse	03
Chester Road	01
Yarmouth	03
Brooklyn, Yarmouth Co.	01
Dartmouth, NS Hospital	56
Tufts Cove	01
Halifax	06

Halifax Evening Mail, 8 October 1918, 10.

EPIDEMIC INFLUENZA

Reports for Twenty-Four Hours Ending at Noon Tuesday.

Places	Cases	Deaths
Halifax	12	01
Chezzetcook, Halifax County	06	0
Dartmouth, NS Hospital	18	06
Stewiacke	01	0
Truro	05	06
Great Village	several	06
Central Onslow	several	0
Upper Brookside	several	0
Parrsboro	02	0
New Waterford	21	0
Rocky Bay	04	0
Lewisdale	02	0
Arichat	01	06
Lunenburg	76	0
Feltzen South	02	0
Neighbouring Com's	20	06
Middle East LaHave	08	0
Sweetland	02	0
Mahone Bay	01	0
Liverpool	05	0
Port Mouton	01	0
Newport	02	0
Bridgetown	10	0
Neighbouring Com.	15	0
Brazil Lake	01	0
Yarmouth	05	0

Halifax Morning Chronicle, 9 October 1918, 2.

Still nothing had been reported to the provincial health officer from Lockeport, Shelburne County, and nothing further from Arichat, or any other community in Richmond County, where influenza was raging unchecked.

SPANISH INFLUENZA HAS CLAIMED NO DEATHS IN DARTMOUTH

Twelve Houses are Quarantined for the Disease, Representing 25 Cases....No deaths have occurred in Dartmouth from Spanish influenza. There are at least twenty-five cases in the town, some of them of a serious nature. Dr. Payzant, town medical officer, stated last night that about twelve houses were quarantined. In some houses are five and six cases. A white placard is placed on all houses in which there exist one or more cases of the disease. It is believed that some cases have not been reported....One very fortunate thing is that it has not broken out among the reconstruction workmen [repairing the city after the Halifax Explosion of 1917]. It was at first feared that the disease would soon spread to the quarters of these men, but up to date not one case has been found there.

Halifax Evening Mail, 10 October 1918, 2.

SHIPS still continue to arrive here with many members of the crew infected. Yesterday more marine cases were cared for at Lawlor's Island....Yesterday an American destroyer reached port with a number of the crew ill with the disease.... The reports for 24 hours, ending at noon, on influenza in Nova Scotia yesterday were as below:

Place	Cases
Bedford	03
Windsor Junction	02
Gays River	01
Truro	04
Dominion	10
New Waterford	18
Newport	01
Middleton	07
Bridgetown and vicinity	10
Digby	02
Yarmouth	02
Pembroke	01
Tusket	01
Argyle Head	01
Pubnico	01
Gold River	02
Mahone	04
Rose Bay	03
Petite River	01

Amherst	07
Dartmouth	05
Nova Scotia Hospital	07
Halifax	17

Halifax Evening Mail, 10 October 1918, 7.

☞ Even by then, the health officials had received no reports from Lockeport, and nothing further from Arichat. One can see from these other reports how rapidly the influenza was spreading across the province.

The influenza reports for 24 hours ending noon Wednesday, in Nova Scotia, are as below:

Place	Cases
Halifax	19
Dartmouth	02
Milford	01
Shubenacadie	06
Stewiacke	02
South Maitland	12
Truro	12
Pictou	09
Bridgetown and vicinity	12
Annapolis Royal	02
Digby	02
Yarmouth	02
Yarmouth Bar	02
Overton	01
Wedgeport	02
Mahone	02
Rose Bay	20
Port Medway	several
Parrsboro	02

Halifax Evening Mail, 11 October 1918, 10.

Halifax, October 12. One death at Lawlor's Island, and one in Halifax occurred yesterday from Spanish Influenza. Thirteen new cases of the disease among civilians and fifty-four among the naval and military were reported to the Health Board yesterday. About seven deaths have occurred in Halifax from the disease during the past several days, and there are a large number of those admitted to hospital and [or] in their homes who are reported to be seriously ill and who may not recover.

Halifax Evening Mail, 12 October 1918, 16.

The death of George Taylor, on Lawlor Island on October 11, 1918, may be the one mentioned here. He was 37, married, an Anglican. His occupation is not given. That he died of "Spanish Influenza" is all the other personal information recorded. Dr. N. E. MacKay attended; Snow and Co. were the undertakers. His place of burial is not given.

HVS, Book 35, Page 159, Number 544.

Adequate hospital accommodation is regarded by the health officials as the only solution to prevent the spread of the disease to the epidemic stage. Several distressing cases, emphasizing the need for hospital accommodation, came to the notice of the health authorities yesterday. In one house on Tower road the husband and wife are ill with the disease. They have a family of five, and unless the mother and father can be isolated the members of the family will likely contract the disease. In a house on Market street three cases exist, and the sick and well members of this family occupy congested quarters. Several other families reside in the same place, all liable to infection. In both cases the sick are without proper treatment, and their situation is one to be deplored.

Halifax Evening Mail, 12 October 1918, 16.

Violet C. Shannon, wife of the popular postman, William Shannon, who was only stricken a few days ago, passed away at her home, 248 Tower Road, yesterday afternoon.

Halifax Morning Chronicle, 15 October 1918, 5.

Her husband, also ill from influenza, died the following day.

THE BAN ON THE THEATRES AND CHURCHES WILL NOT BE LIFTED FOR SOME DAYS: SIXTY-SEVEN NEW CASES OF INFLUENZA HERE YESTERDAY

Halifax, October 12. One death at Lawlor's Island and one in Halifax occurred yesterday from Spanish influenza. Thirteen new cases of the disease among civilians and fifty-four among the naval and military were reported to the Health Board yesterday. About seven deaths have occurred in Halifax from the disease during the past several days, and there are a large number of those admitted to hospital and in their homes who are reported to be seriously ill and who may not recover. The question of providing hospital accommodation is the most important one the Health Board is confronted with at present, and this question will be given serious consideration at a special meeting of the Board. The spread of the disease calls for immediate action on this matter. The new isolation hospital on Morris street is full to capacity and the waiting list is large enough to refill the institution or to tax the accommodation which might be available in the Victoria General Hospital.

Halifax Evening Mail, 12 October 1918, 16.

FOUR MORE DEATHS FROM SPANISH INFLUENZA

The Situation, However, Is Reported to Be More Encouraging [*in Halifax*]....

Yesterday's dead include two soldiers at the Military hospital—Private Hillbone, of Ontario, attached to the 64th Siege Battery, and Victor Grady, of Peterboro, Ont. Violet C. Shannon, wife of the popular postman, William Shannon, who was only stricken a few days ago, passed away at her home, 245 [*sic*] Tower road, yesterday afternoon. The fourth death was that of Mertie LaBlanch, who resided at 24 Hollis Street. In accordance with the order of the Health Board, all these funerals must be held within twenty-four hours after death. Although this is considerable hardship to the family of the deceased, it is considered absolutely essential to safeguard the public health.

Halifax Morning Chronicle, 15 October 1918, 5.

⟹ Mary Agnes ("Mamie") Clattenburg Gray died in Halifax of Spanish Influenza on October 16, 1918, and is listed by Dr. Allan Marble as "Gray, Mary, 29, [died] Halifax 16 OCT 1918, [days ill] not given." Garry Shutlak, Nova Scotia Archives, provided the following additional information:

✉ Mary Agnes Gray, wife of soldier John M. Gray. John Mickes Gray, soldier, married Mamie Clattenburg in 1907. In 1919, a widower, he married Ethel Clattenburg. He died in 1935. Garry D. Shutlak, Senior Reference Archivist, Reference Services, Nova Scotia Archives.

Garry Shutlak to Ruth Whitehead, email, 3 August 2018.

☞ The mixed messages between the following two newspaper accounts are unbelievable:

NO OVERCROWDING IN THE CITY OF HALIFAX CAN BE PERMITTED

The Influenza Is Now Distributed All Over Nova Scotia And The Number Of Cases Reported Is 4,000, With Sixty Deaths

While there was a further increase in the number of Spanish influenza cases reported to the Board of Health yesterday, the situation cannot be regarded as alarming.

Halifax Evening Mail, 16 October 1918, 14.

FIFTY NEW CASES OF SPANISH INFLUENZA

The Epidemic Is Spreading Throughout the Province—The Department of Public Health Issues Important Circular Regarding the Disease

In a circular issued to the medical profession of Nova Scotia, W. H. Hattie, Provincial Medical Officer, says that deaths reported from Spanish influenza in Nova Scotia now exceed 60, and there are in all more than 4,000 cases, many of them very critical....

Certain features are of the utmost importance. All influenza is infectious, and a common and disastrous mistake is to await symptoms of especial severity before adopting preventive measures. Every suspicious case should be immediately isolated and reported....The only safe place to fight influenza is in bed, and this should be impressed upon everyone. The situation is really serious....The thorough-going co-operation of every one is a prime necessity.

Since it is manifestly impracticable to place legal restraints upon travel, every physician should point out the serious result which may ensue if a person slightly ill with influenza should go from one community to another. October 14, 1918.

...During the forty-eight hours ending at noon October 14th, the cases of epidemic influenza reported from Nova Scotia to the Provincial Health Officer numbered 731. Several of these, however, are from belated returns. Recent deaths reported from this disease numbered 15."

Halifax Morning Chronicle, 16 October 1918, 2.

☞ Dr. Hattie had finally gotten word, over two weeks late, from Lockeport, and the news was appalling.

SITUATION IN NOVA SCOTIA

HALIFAX, N.S., Oct. 13. There are now, according to official records, a total of 4,000 cases of Spanish Influenza in Nova Scotia, and of these sixty have resulted in death. The situation is bad in certain localities of the province. Lockeport is in a very bad influenza condition. Dr. W.H. Hattie, provincial health officer, reports a total of 300 cases to date in that small town, four deaths from the disease, and 28 attacks which have resulted in pneumonia. Dr. Hattie has sent out an urgent call for nurses for Lockeport. Reports from Cape Breton are conflicting, but there is as yet no call from there for help. The situation in Lunenburg is bad. This does not mean that there is any epidemic in the province, for in many localities there is not a single case of flu. But it is plain that Nova Scotia is not going to escape some degree of ravage from the disease in spite of all that the provincial and local health authorities may do in the way of precautionary and curative measures.

Sydney Daily Post, 17 October 1918, 6.

HALIFAX RED CROSS SUPPLIES FOR ALL

The Red Cross workers at the Technical College, are continuing with undiminished speed to keep up the steady flow of masks, operating coats, dressing gowns, bedding and other necessities for fighting the influenza, while the Red Cross workers at the Women's Council House have worked even on Sundays, making pneumonia jackets to send to the Technical for distribution...Hundreds of masks and quantities of bedding, pneumonia jackets and other things have been sent to Windsor, Windsor Junction, Sydney, Springfield and Lockeport; samples of the masks have been sent to many other places, [on] which the Red Cross societies and auxiliary branches of those places [may] pattern their supplies; and besides all this they have kept the City Board of Health supplied, also the Nova Scotia Isolation Hospital, Cogswell Street Hospital, Royal Naval Hospital, Victorian Order of Nurses, and the King Edward Hotel.

Halifax Morning Chronicle, 18 October 1918, 9.

SEVERAL DEATHS FROM INFLUENZA

Thirty-three New Cases Among Civilians and Fifteen Among Military, Were Reported Today....Four convalescing cases were reported from Brunswick and Market streets, and several convalescing cases were reported from the north part of the city yesterday. The new cases today were from Coburg road, Fredericton avenue, North Park street, Moran street, Brunswick street, Agricola, Barrington, Mumford road, Pepperell, North Clifton, Chebucto road, Robie street and the City Home.

Halifax Evening Mail, 18 October 1918, 3.

DEATHS FROM INFLUENZA

FREDERICK DUCET [Frédéric Doucet] a seaman on the Tug *Roebling*, died yesterday at the Morris street hospital from Spanish influenza, aged 32 years. The deceased was of French nationality.

Halifax Evening Mail, 19 October 1918, 18.

Roger Marsters of the Maritime Museum of the Atlantic, wrote me the following email concerning this death:

The *F.W. Roebling* was indeed both a schooner and a tug (or a powered workboat, at least). The vessel was launched as a two-masted schooner in Milford, Delaware, in 1890. By 1916 it was fitted with a two-cylinder gas engine, and was employed by the Beaver Dredging Company of Halifax. It seems the vessel was severely damaged in the Explosion, with at least one death. No news on the post-Explosion fate, but I'll let you know if anything else turns up. (This information is from Lloyds Register for 1916/1917.)

Roger Marsters to Ruth Whitehead, personal communication, May 2018.

J.J. Ryan, an American sailor, died yesterday at the Station Hospital, of Spanish influenza. The deceased belonged to Philadelphia, and the body [illegible; possibly 'will be returned to'] Philadelphia for burial.

Halifax Evening Mail, 19 October 1918, 18.

The *Evening Mail* of October 18 announced 33 new cases in Halifax's civilian population, and fifteen among the military in the city. On October 21, the newspaper reported that there were now 500 Cases of Influenza in the city. That's a jump of 452 new cases in three days.

Halifax Evening Mail, 18 October 1918, 3; 21 October 1918, 9.

Reports of the influenza epidemic for the 24 hours up to noon yesterday, as compiled by the Nova Scotia health department, are as follows:

Halifax	28
Dartmouth	01
Hopewell	01
Foxbrook, Pictou	01
Eureka Mills	16
Stellarton	50
Cape Sable Island	06
Woods Harbor	25
Shaw Harbor	05

Barrington Passage	08
North West Harbor	05
Port Saxony	03
Grosvenor	02
Morin	01
Tracadie	01
Fairmont	11
Pictou	02
Salmon River	08
Upper Brookfield	15
Fairview	02
Great Village	01
Little Bass River	01
Tusket	01
Bells Rock	06
Wallbrook Mountain	06
Clare District	10
Glace Bay	05
Windsor	17
Hantsport	04
Mount Denison	02
Avonport	02
Lockeport and vicinity	25
Canning	04
Blomidon	01
Kingsport	03
Canard	04
Vernon Mines	05
Victoria Harbor	08
Cambridge	08
Aylesford	10
Black Rock	02
South Berwick	10
Sommerset	01
South Wentworth	04
New Waterford	04
Main a Dieu	10
Cariboo Marsh	06
Truro	07
Digby	04

Lunenburg	07
Cape North	several
Stewiacke	06
Gay's River	13
Miller's Siding	15

Halifax Evening Mail, 18 October 1918, 10.

 TWO MORE INDIANS DIE FROM SPANISH INFLUENZA

Seven Indians at Windsor Junction Have Succumbed to the Disease

Dartmouth, October 21. Two more deaths from influenza have occurred at Windsor Junction among the Indians, making seven deaths within the past few weeks. The disease among the Indians at this place appears to be of a serious kind and reports indicate that it is spreading rapidly. It has been reported that the Indians are without medical attendance or care and their unfortunate situation is believed to be the cause of the infection spreading.

A further increase in the disease has been recorded in Dartmouth and a few of the patients ill with it are on the dangerous list. The situation on the whole, however, is well in hand. An epidemic is not believed likely. While the disease continues to spread the schools will not be re-opened.

Clarence Connors is seriously ill with Spanish influenza.

Jean Campbell, child of George Campbell of the Naval Defenses, died at North Dartmouth last week. She was staying with her grandmother, Mrs. MacLean, in one of the relief tenements, her mother having died from injuries received in the explosion.

There passed away on Saturday, at the residence of his grandmother, Morris Tynes, aged 29 years, after a short illness of pneumonia. He was a valued member of the Victoria Road Baptists church, holding the office of deacon and organist.

Halifax Evening Mail, 21 October 1918, 2.

 123 NEW CASES OF INFLUENZA IN HALIFAX

This Is A Record Number, Almost Double That Of Any Day Since The Precautions Against Epidemic Began

Halifax, Oct. 22....Chairman Mackay said that R.G. Blackie, druggist, had consented to keep his store open all night for the convenience of the public. The Halifax County Retail Druggist Association has notified the board that it cannot comply with the request that three drug stores remain open all night in the city, one in the north end, in the centre, and in the south end.

Halifax Evening Mail, 23 October 1918, 18.

FRANK O'HANLEY the well-known electrician is seriously ill with influenza. C.A. HUNTER, manager of the ferry, is confined to the house by illness.

Halifax Evening Mail, 24 October 1918, 2.

 WHILE the precautionary measures enforced by the health board directly closing of all public places and restricting the hours of doing business in all the shops have had excellent results, it has not prevented many heartrending conditions among a number of the poorer families of the city. Some of the medical men have found whole families in the city down with the disease and devoid of nursing and other attention so essential in the recovery of the patient. Instances have come to the attention of the health authorities where the sick have been deserted by others residing in the same house and in one of these cases, the situation was only improved by death.

Halifax Evening Mail, 24 October 1918, 8.

A POPULAR DARTMOUTH MAN DIES FROM INFLUENZA
Frank O'Hanley, an Active Member of the AOH and an Expert Electrician, Passed Away Early This Morning

DARTMOUTH, October 25. The community was shocked this morning to hear of the death from influenza of Frank O'Hanley, at the residence of his sister, Mrs. Charles Conrad. The deceased had been ill but a short time, and while it was reported the last few days that he was seriously ill, none but those in the family were prepared for the news of his death.

Halifax Evening Mail, 25 October 1918, 2.

PLACARDING HOUSES FOR INFLUENZA TODAY. THE WORK WILL BE CONTINUED UNTIL ALL PLACES WHERE DISEASE EXISTS, ARE PLACARDED

Halifax Evening Mail, 26 October 1918, 5.

The newspaper then published a list of 105 houses to be placarded, with street name and house number, and the surname of the family living there (if known).

INFLUENZA AT PRESTON, THREE DIE
Influenza has broken out among the colored population at Preston and is taking its toll of death, three young persons succumbed to the disease this week. They are Gladys May, aged 15 years, daughter of Mr. and Mrs. Edward Beals; Paul Downey, aged 1 year, son of Mr. and Mrs. David Downey; Samuel Clayton, aged one year and two moths, son of Mr. and Mrs. John Clayton.

Peter Munroe, a colored inmate of the Nova Scotia Hospital, died from the disease on Thursday morning. Interment took place yesterday in Camp Hill cemetery.

Private James McInnes, aged 20 years, of Hollis street, Halifax, died from influenza at the Nova Scotia Military Hospital yesterday morning. The funeral took place today at 2.30 o'clock, interment in Mount Olivet.

Frances Mahar died from the disease at Wellington, Halifax county, on Thursday.

Halifax Evening Mail, 26 October 1918, 4.

 CHEBUCTO, NO. 7

When we reported in previous issue of "Forward," we were looking forward to installing our officers-elect at the next meeting. We are still looking forward, because the next meeting has not yet taken place. We acted on the instructions of the Board of Health to discontinue all gatherings until further notice, as it was the only wise thing to do under the circumstances. All Churches, Theatres, Schools, Fraternal Societies, and Commercial Societies have been closed. Two of the Churches held short services outside the Churches for two Sundays, but all other Churches were closed. All stores for trading must be closed sharp 6 p. m., Restaurants must close at 8 p. m., Drug Stores are the only establishments allowed to remain open, and they must confine their sales to medicinal goods. It is to be hoped that the prompt acting of our Board of Health may check the ravages of the 'Flu', and that the epidemic will soon die out, and the programme of regular events be in full swing again at an early date. Members of City Divisions meeting each other on the street ask the same question, "When will Division meet again?" They are all anxious to get back to the fraternal circle again. It looks now as if this drastic action of the Board of Health will be discontinued in a few days, and if so, it will enable us to get all the city Divisions together to complete arrangements for the Annual Session of Grand Division opening on Nov. 5th, so as to make it interesting and helpful. George A. McLeod.

Halifax Forward [Sons of Temperance Society news], 26 October 1918, 2.

ONE THOUSAND CASES OF SPANISH INFLUENZA REPORTED IN HALIFAX DURING THE MONTH

Imperfect Returns on Saturday and Sunday Show 77 Cases, But There Are Many More

The reports for 24 hours ending noon on Saturday were as follows:

Halifax	36
Amherst (houses)	08
Middleton	05
Chester	05
Truro	07

Hantsport	02
Lochartville	02
Parrsboro Road	25
Advocate	--
Antigonish County	07
Gardiner Mines	01
Port Maitland	03
Wedgeport	19

Halifax Evening Mail, 28 October 1918, 4.

NORMAN Walker, mate on the ferry steamer, will have the sympathy of a large number of friends in the death from influenza of his wife, Harriet, aged 28 years....Two children survive. Mr. Walker is recovering from a severe attack of the influenza....

ANOTHER tragic incident of the disease is disclosed in the death on Saturday night of James Henry Craig, aged 32 years. His wife died last week.

Halifax Evening Mail, 28 October 1918, 2.

Both of these families lived in Dartmouth.

MRS. FREDERICK BOUTILIER. The funeral of Irene Teasdale, wife of Private Frederick Boutilier of the Garrison Regiment, took place from her late residence, 75 Falkland street....She was a victim of Spanish influenza.

LILIAN RUTH HARDSTAFF. The funeral of little Lilian Ruth, daughter of Staff Sergeant and Mrs. Hardstaff...took place from the Pavilion Barracks on Monday at 3 o'clock in Fort Massey cemetery....The child had been run down from teething troubles and Spanish influenza was the immediate cause of her death.

Halifax Evening Mail, 29 October 1918, 2.

DEATH RATE HIGH

Yesterday there were five deaths from influenza or subsequent complications, and the undertaking establishments had their hands full in carrying out the funerals with the required rapidity. During the past week, the death rate has been higher than at any time since the outbreak of the disease. For Tuesday and Wednesday, the Military authorities reported forty-five new cases....Throughout the Province, exclusive of Halifax, two hundred and twelve new cases and five deaths have been reported. Three of the deaths were in Dartmouth and thirty four of the new cases in Stellarton and its vicinity. A large number of men from provincial districts, who have been working in Halifax, have become panic-stricken and have left the city for their homes, making the already serious labor shortage more acute.

Halifax Morning Chronicle, 31 October 1918, 5.

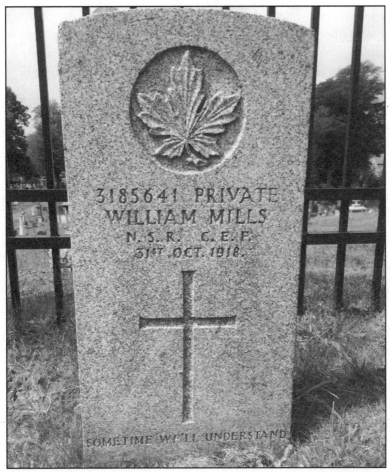

"Sometime we'll understand." William Mills's stone, Fort Massey Cemetery, Halifax. William and his brother, natives of Shulie, both died of Influenza in 1918. The quote is from a popular hymn of the period. *(Doug Pezzack)*

Mills, William, aged 32. A native of Shulie; he died in Halifax on 31 October 1918, ill 18 days with influenza and broncho pneumonia. A soldier, he was buried at Fort Massey, the military cemetery on Queen Street, Halifax. He was the brother of Charles Mills, who also died of influenza. Their parents were Enos and Prudence Ripley Mills. His religion is given as "Christian."

HVS, Halifax County Death Register, 1918, Book 21, Page 587, Number 3519.

INFLUENZA

Mayor's Office, City Hall, October 30th, 1918. All women prepared to render service of any description in influenza homes or public institutions where influenza exists are requested to register at the office of the St. John Ambulance Brigade, 20 Prince Street, or Telephone Sackville 3148. A.C. HAWKINS, Mayor.

Halifax Evening Mail, 1 November 1918, 11.

 INFLUENZA REPORTS

The reports for twenty-four hours ending yesterday were:

Place	*Cases*
Halifax	18
Dartmouth	3 houses
Truro	03
Bass River	02
Great Village	01
Stellarton and vicinity	34
Trenton	15
Antigonish	04
Pomquet	07
Cape Jack	01
Maitland	06
Noel Road	01
Rawdon Centre	07
Rawdon Gold Mines	05
Concession	15
Meteghan and vicinity	10
Wedgeport	06
East River Point	several
The Forties	epidemic
Little River	04
Thompson Station	06
River Philip	03
Northport	13
Amherst Head	03
Tidnish Bridge	02
North Wallace	*[microfilm page cut off]*

Halifax Evening Mail, 2 November 1918, 14.

SERGT. STEWART ROBSON, of the First Depot Battalion, is convalescing at his home 153 Agricola street, after an attack of influenza.

Halifax Evening Mail, 7 November 1918, 16.

☞ On Dr. Allan Marble's list of deaths from influenza, Stewart Robson is listed as dead, not as convalescing. There is no death record from any place or in any year in Nova Scotia for him, and he obviously never had a relapse of his influenza. He was born in Halifax, to Charles and Minnie Robson. Charles was employed as a "Line Man." In June of the same year that Stewart got influenza, aged 26, he married Rose George, 23, also born in Halifax. Her parents were Leonard and Amelia George, George being a salesman. It was the first marriage for each. Both bride and groom were Anglican. The wedding took place in Wolfville on June 17.

HVS, Halifax County Marriage Register, 1918, Book 33, Page 456.

 REPORTS for 24 hours ending noon yesterday were as follows:

Place	Cases
Halifax	76
Dartmouth	02
Stewiacke	02
Lower Stewiacke	02
Truro	02
Hazel Hill	03
Oxford Junction	01
Amherst	09
Hantsport	04
Kentville	03
Baxter's Harbor	01
Cunard	01
Lawrencetown	04
West Clarence	01
Upper Clements	01
Lequille	01
Middleton	02
Plympton	03
Weymouth	01
Wedgeport	06
Bridgewater	prevalent

Halifax Evening Mail, 1 November 1918, 10.

On November 13, 1918, Flossie May Tufts MacRae and her newborn son, Frank, died. Dr. Allan Marble, in his alphabetical record of victims of Spanish influenza, lists a "McCrae, Florence, 33, [died] Halifax, 13 NOV 1918, [days ill] not given." Her infant son died as well, but is not on this list, as he had no birth or death certificates. Garry Shutlak, Nova Scotia Archives, is her grandson, and provided the following additional information and corrections.

Good Morning Ruth: I checked the family bible and Vital Statistics on-line. My grandmother is listed under Florence May McCrae (sic) NSVS Halifax County 1918, Book 25, p. 5, No 26. My grandmother was Flossie May Tufts MacRae and married my grandfather in 1907. There are birth records for [their children] James Walter, Joseph Norman, Annie Irene, Mary Florence, Mildred Elizabeth and Robert Edwin MacRae. There is no birth certificate for [another child], Gerald Stanley MacRae, but there is a death certificate.

She was buried with her son Frank, born 12 November 1918 at 9 p.m. and died 9 hours later on 13 November 1918. The Tufts family plot is in St. John's Cemetery, Fairview, adjoining Fairview Lawn. She was buried in a partially glass coffin as if sleeping, her hair down with Frank nestled in her arms. You could see both mother and child when you looked through the glass. Garry D. Shutlak, Senior Reference Archivist, Reference Services, Nova Scotia Archives.

Garry Shutlak to Ruth Whitehead, email, 3 August 2018.

THREEFOLD DEATH TOLL FROM THE INFLUENZA

A host of friends will be deeply saddened by news of the death, within ten minutes of each other, of Spanish influenza, of which both had been ill for about a fortnight, of Mr. and Mrs. John MacDonald, living at 271 Agricola street. Mr. MacDonald was 27 years of age, Mrs. MacDonald was 23, the two being survived by little children.

On the same day there passed away, of the same disease, Mrs. Gorman, wife of Captain Gorman, RCNR, who also lived at 271 Agricola street, and who was a sister of Mrs. MacDonald. [They were born Sutherlands]....The case is one of the saddest in connection with the influenza epidemic. All three died at the influenza hospital.

Halifax Evening Mail, 15 November 1918, 1.

POWER. On November 20th, at Portuguese Cove, William Power, aged 28 years, of influenza. The late Mr. Power was an apprentice in the Halifax Pilot Service....Pilot Lamont Power is a brother of the deceased. Funeral took place Wednesday to Ketch Harbor.

Halifax Evening Mail, 21 November 1918, 1.

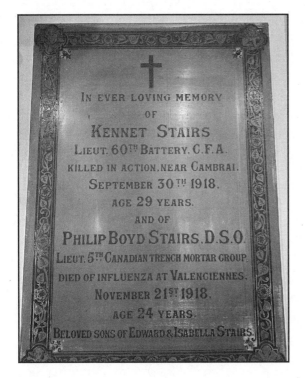

Stairs Memorial. Philip Stairs is the only Influenza victim we could find whose cause of death appears on a gravestone or church memorial. The Stairs family was from Halifax, although their soldier sons died abroad in the First World War. (*Doug Pezzack*)

 WILLIAM GARRISON. Indian Harbor, November 22. The death has occurred at Indian Harbor, of one of the most respected residents of that place, William Garrison. The deceased had been in poor health for some time, but his death was due to an attack of Spanish influenza. His funeral took place today.

Halifax Evening Mail, 25 November 1918, 6.

MRS. JOHN WHITE. Halifax, December 4. John White, 6 Smith street, motorman with the Tramway Company, will have the sympathy of many friends in the death of his wife, Mary, aged 40 years. Pneumonia, following a severe attack of influenza, was the cause of death.

Halifax Evening Mail, 4 December 1918, 16. HVS, Book 25, Page 26, Number 152, states that she was Mary Ann White, born in Cape Breton, aged 41; she died, according to the death record, on November 30, 1918.

MR. AND MRS. JAMES SIBLEY DIE OF INFLUENZA AT MEAGHER'S GRANT

There passed away at Meagher's Grant on Nov. 15, Hilda Mannette, wife of James Sibley, and just two weeks later, Nov. 29, her husband, James Kent Sibley; both had influenza and being of delicate constitutions were unable to withstand the disease.

Mrs. Sibley, who was 23 years old, was the daughter of the late W. J. and Mrs. Grant....James Kent Sibley, who was in his 32nd year, is survived by his father and mother....Altho of reserved dispositions they were well loved by relatives and intimate friends, and will be much missed.

Truro Daily News, 14 December 1918, 2. Courtesy the Colchester Historeum.

The N.S. Undertaking Co. [B. Cruikshank] offered to continue to supply an ambulance, stretcher, horse and two men for removal of patients to the influenza hospital at $1.75 per call. The offer was accepted and the company will be advised to present their bill to date for hospital removals.

Morning Chronicle, 29 November 1918, 6.

GEORGE NAUGLE, aged 41 years, died at Devil's Island, from influenza, after a brief illness. He visited Halifax on Saturday, December 7, complaining of a cold shortly after returning home the same day. This is the first death on the island in two years. Much sympathy is felt for the widow, who has a family of six small children.

Halifax Evening Mail, 17 December, 1918, 2.

Naugle died on December 13, 1918. HVS, Halifax County Death Register, 1918, Book 35, Page 168, Number 597, shows that George O. Naugle was a fisherman. He died of influenza, after an illness of five days, on December 13. His doctor was M. G. Burris; the undertaker was C. E. Guik. A Roman Catholic, Mr. Naugle was buried in Eastern Passage, the place where he was born, and where his parents still resided.

The 1911 Census shows "Naugle, George O., born March 1878, French [German?] Canadian, R. Catholic, Fisherman; Naugle, Josephine, wife, born February 1877, English Canadian, R. Catholic, Homemaker. Son, Harold, b. May 1901; daughter, Moony [sp?] b. June 1907; Son, George, b. November 1908."

1911 Census, Nova Scotia, Halifax County, Eastern Passage District.

ANDREW MOSHER. The death occurred at Giltown, of Andrew Mosher, of influenza, formerly of Musquodoboit Harbor, leaving one daughter. Besides a daughter, there survive two sisters and three brothers – John and Daniel at Musquodoboit Harbor, and Wilson, at Lower Stewiacke. The sisters are Mrs. Rhymo [Rhyno?], Sheet Harbor, and Mrs. Thomas Dooks, of Dartmouth.

Halifax Evening Mail, 12 December 1918, 3.

MRS. JOHN SHEARS. There passed away last evening under very sad circumstances, Jane H., wife of John Shears, aged 27 years. Mrs. Shears, who died in the influenza hospital, and whose infant died yesterday morning in that institution, had a wide circle of friends....The body will be taken to Newfoundland for interment.

Halifax Evening Mail, 17 December 1918, 3.

The death occurred at Preston of Louise Downey, aged thirty years, widow of Angus Downey.

Halifax Evening Mail, 17 December 1918, 2.

LUSH. On December 18, of Spanish influenza, Mabel Lush (nee Harding) darling wife of Malcolm Lush, aged 27 years. She leaves a husband, son of 6 weeks, and a very large circle of friends.

Halifax Evening Mail, 19 December 1918, 1.

BROWN. On Monday, December 23rd, Edna Grace, wife of Frank J. Brown, and daughter of the late George Burgess of this city. The deceased was ill about two weeks, influenza being the cause of her death. She was in her 20th year and a bride of but five months.

Halifax Evening Mail, 27 December 1918, 1.

"We must not again be caught unprepared."

At the end of the year 1918, an unattributed newspaper picked up a warning sparked by a report from the Surgeon General of the United States, preparing the world, and the US in particular, for a return of influenza in 1919, and perhaps a return more devastating than the world had yet seen in 1918, bad as that had been. This news item has no attribution, but the typeset decoration around the headline is something commonly used in Halifax newspapers of the period. The clipping was pasted into an old scrapbook belonging to Harriet "Hattie" Ramsey MacGougan of St. Eleanors and (latterly) Summerside, PEI; it was sent to me by her great-grandniece, Leslie Linklater Pezzack, of Halifax.

INFLUENZA A PUZZLE
It is evident that the disease which is still with us after the height of the epidemic has passed is a considerably more dangerous pest than what has hitherto been known as influenza, and requires proportionately greater efforts from the health authorities. If Surgeon-General Blue of the United States army is right in

apprehending a very serious recurrence next year, no time is to be lost in making plans and in making sure that the needful organization and equipment are ready.

On general principles such a recurrence ought to be prepared for, since it was a feature of the two previous epidemics, in 1847 and in 1889, which marked the revival of the disease after a long interim. It is a curious coincidence that the very period in which medical science was beginning to penetrate the mysteries of bacterial disease marked also the re-appearance of three pests which people had come to regard as a thing of the past so far as the western world was concerned. For a generation now influenza, plague, and cholera have been on the march, and great care must be taken not to let the ravages of war break down the defenses of civilization.

Against influenza civilization has thus far not made very serious efforts because it has been considered a minor though very pervasive disease. Bacteriology may any day find a preventive serum; meanwhile the general attitude, even of the medical profession, is one of fatalism. High contagiousness and a low death rate make a hard combination to deal with by the ordinary methods of control. But the issue may be forced by the continued tendency of the disease toward a more severe form.

This tendency is not new, for the epidemic of 1889 was markedly more severe and persisted over a longer term of years that the one of 1847. In England the death rate per million from influenza from 1847 to 1855 was 285, 460, 92, 78, 120, 76, 99, 53, 193. From 1859 to 1907, it ran: 157, 574, 534, 325, 220, 424, 122, 196, 331, 389, 504, 174, 223, 189, 163, 204, 189, 265. The average rate for nine years was 162 for the earlier epidemic, 320 for the latter, a doubling in the severity of the disease.

Those figures point to a rising wave, yet not to so extraordinary an increase as the new epidemic has brought. [On October 10, 1918, we now know there were 759 deaths in the city of Philadelphia alone. Just one day, just one city. (Barry, 2009:329).] The statistics are not yet available, but the experience of Great Britain seems to have been so terrible that they may expect a rate for the current year of from 4,000 to 5,000 deaths per million as against 574, the highest on record. So sensational a change transfers the disease to a new category and compels reconsideration of the older methods of dealing with it.

We have further to consider that in both of the nineteenth-century visitations the second year was the worst, not in the number of cases, but in the number of deaths. We do not know that this rule will hold in case of another epidemic next year, but the possibility needs to be taken into account in the organization of measures to protect the public health. A very severe epidemic attacking relatively few people would obviously have to be dealt with very differently from a mild and extremely prevalent disorder, and the public mind should be prepared for prompt and energetic measures if the need should suddenly appear. The opposite might, of course, prove true; the malignant and mysterious pest which has traveled in company with the influenza might die down, and a relatively harmless epidemic of plain grip [*La Grippe*] ensue. But the country must be ready for a danger which cannot be ignored in view of the tendency of influenza to persist over a term of years. We must not again be caught unprepared.

(Unattributed newspaper), December 1918.

☞ This was perhaps published in a Prince Edward Island paper. A similar news item was published in the *Pictou Advocate*, 6 December 1918: "The influenza epidemic is not a thing of the past by any means. In fact, leading physicians of America say it will recur in 1919, and possibly in 1920. In support of this view, they claim that on the occasions of past visitations, influenza recurred in the year following the first outbreak."

It was a story almost certainly picked up from the US Surgeon General's report. A variation occurred in the *Antigonish Casket*, which was then reprinted by the *Pictou Advocate* and published on 6 December 1918: "The influenza epidemic is not a thing of the past by any means. In fact, leading physicians of America say it will recur in 1919, and possibly in 1920. In support of this view, they claim that on the occasions of past visitations, influenza recurred in the year following the first outbreak."

☞ Heather Ludlow, Nova Scotia Legislative Library, helped clarify the source of a Spanish Flu mention in the Nova Scotia Legislature Journals, as follows.

✉ The link is to the *Hansard for the House of Assembly* for November 20, 2001. Your internet browser showed an excerpt of your search terms in context. The speaker is Dr. James Smith, speaking on Bill 95, German Settlers Day Act. Here is the full text of his speech [only an excerpt of which is shown below]:

✒ DR JAMES SMITH: It's interesting that out of tragedy comes some recognition of your own family roots sometimes. [M]y grandfather, Laurie Smith. I was thinking of him this last while, because he died a young man, coming up Halifax Harbour, 1919, suffering from, as they called it, the Spanish flu, the influenza. He left four children, the oldest, who was five, that was my father.

Hansard for the House of Assembly for November 20, published 2001, 7393–4.
Heather Ludlow, Legislative Library of Nova Scotia,
email to author, 5 March 2019.

 BREEN. On January 4th, [died at Halifax, buried] at Marie Joseph, of influenza, Calvin G. Breen, son of Mr. and Mrs. James Breen, age 17 years.

Halifax Evening Mail, 23 January 1919, 1.

☞ This newspaper account is incorrect. Calvin G. Breen, or George C. Breen, depending on whether one reads his tombstone or the newspaper, was *buried* in Marie Joseph, Guysborough County, but he died in Halifax, and his death certificate, in the registration book for Halifax County, so states: Breen died in Halifax. For details see the Guysborough County chapter.

HUBBARDS, February 11. One of the best known business men [*sic*] of Hubbards, Albert Lawson Harnish, died last evening after a brief illness. A little over a week ago he was attacked by influenza, which was followed by pneumonia. Mr. Harnish carried on a successful fish business in partnership with his brother.

Halifax Evening Mail, 11 February 1919, 3.

There has been, unfortunately, an outbreak of influenza at the School for the Deaf, one of the pupils, Annie Peters of Rollo Bay [Prince Edward Island], aged 22 years, having died of the disease. She was the oldest, apparently one of the strongest, and certainly one of the most popular of the pupils....

E. E. Parsons of the 25 Cent Store, returned this week from a trip to St. John, to find his six children ill of influenza, while on the day following, Mrs. Parsons and the nurse succumbed to the disease. However, all [the rest] are reported to be doing well.

Halifax Evening Mail, 4 March 1919, 10.

The outstanding feature of the [fiscal] year just ended [October 1, 1918– September 30, 1919] was the epidemic of influenza....Soon after the opening of the new fiscal year [1 October 1918], however, a number of other communities were almost simultaneously infected, the infection having been brought into the Province principally by sailors and fishermen from infected ports on both sides of the Atlantic.

Warning letters had already been sent out to Medical Health Officers, with instructions as to what should be done in event of an outbreak. Where there was prompt and complete compliance with these instructions, the community usually escaped an overwhelming invasion....While we suffered very severely, our experience as a whole was less disastrous than in many other places.

Our efforts to get reports of the number of cases developing met with but indifferent success, and, as the doctors were so excessively busy in ministering to the sick, the attempt to get full returns was abandoned....Doubtless, however, some deaths were not reported promptly and it may be expected that complete returns for the year will show approximately 1600 deaths attributable to this disease.

We were very ill prepared for so sudden and so serious an emergency. So large a proportion of our physicians and nurses were engaged in military duty, both overseas and at home, that many extensive districts were practically without medical or nursing assistance. Urgent appeals for such assistance could only be met to a limited extent, but the endeavor was made to allocate the doctors, medical students and nurses who were available in such a way that the districts in greatest need were afforded all the relief possible.

Dr. W. H. Hattie, Provincial Medical Officer, Annual Report of the Department of Public Health, Journals of the House of Assembly, Appendix 16, 1920.

FIFTY-SIX CASES OF FLU IN HALIFAX
The total number of influenza cases reported to the Health Board last night was fifty-six. Eighteen additional cases were reported yesterday. There was one death in a house on Poplar Grove. There are now twenty-six cases in the Isolation Hospital on Morris Street, three of which are considered to be in a very dangerous condition.

Halifax Morning Chronicle, 17 February, 1920, 7.

THIRTY SEVEN IN THE FLU HOSPITAL
Total Number Of Suspected Cases Reported To Health Board This Year Is 100. One Death Last Night

The number of influenza cases, or suspected cases, reported at the City Board of Health up to noon yesterday was 108, but there are not likely that many cases in the City as some have recovered and several families reported as having members infected have asked the Department to have placards removed from their houses, which will be done after inspection seems to warrant it. There was a death at the Morris Street Hospital Wednesday, the second fatality from the disease among domestics from a city hotel.

Halifax Morning Chronicle, 20 February 1920, 4.

☞ The death was probably that of Leone Levy, who died February 19, 1920, in Halifax, and who was described as a "domestic at Halifax Hotel." Other than noting "Female, single," there is no personal information given, not even her age. She died in the Morris Street Isolation Hospital. A doctor, whose name is illegible, saw her on February 17, and again on the next day. This is what he wrote, in answer to the requisite questions: "I last saw her alive on February 18, 1920." When he came to the Time of Death space, he scrawled: "I have no reliable information, but have been told at 4 30 am, and since this is an idiot question, why don't you drop it." Cause of death: "Influenza"; Duration: "I don't know"; secondary cause of death was "Broncho Pneumonia," and he did not know its duration, either. "Where was the Disease contracted, if not at the place of death?" "I don't know." The minimal information about this poor woman was provided by "Morris Street Isolation Hospital/ Relationship to Deceased: None." It seems likely that she was brought to the hospital in the last stages of her illness, and there was no one to give any particulars. Leone Levy was buried at Fairview Cemetery, by C. P. Snow & Co. Ltd.

HVS, 1920, Book 70, Page 429.

INFLUENZA REPORTS
The following figures given out by the Board of Health indicate fairly the 'Flu' situation in Halifax:

Reported on Saturday	29 Cases
Recovered	03
Died	01
Total number of cases in city	136
Total number of deaths to date [in 1920]	5.

Halifax Morning Chronicle, 23 February 1920, 5.

MINERVA MAY BAKER. Minerva May Baker, aged 24, a student at the Victoria General Hospital, died there yesterday, from influenza after a short illness. The remains were forwarded to Bridgewater, the home of the deceased, where interment will take place.

Halifax Morning Chronicle, 2 March 1920.

☞ Dr. Marble's lists of deaths by county gives her as "Merna Baker, 24, d. 28 February 1920. VGH nurse, influenza & pneumonia, [ill] 10 days."

☞ A cluster of nurses at the Victoria General Hospital died within three days of each other during this 1920 return of influenza: Minerva Baker (see above) on February 28, Blanche Cox, "nurse in training" on the same day, and Etta L. Clarke, a "student nurse" at the VGH two days later, on March 1. All had developed influenza, then pneumonia. Miss Clarke's was the twenty-third death in 1920 from this disease.

Last recorded deaths outside the city proper, as the epidemic came to an end in the spring of 1920, were of Clarence R. Fralic, aged 10 months, of Port Dufferin, and of Orestus O'Leary, aged 23 years, an engineer from West Quoddy. Both died on March 27. Within the city, the Great Influenza's final act took place on April 13, when the disease took both Edith E. Hughes, 32, and Grace B. Ropell, 31.

By the time the disease had run its course, Halifax County had the highest influenza death rate of any county in Nova Scotia. Within the city itself, 338 died, the rest of the county lost 159 people, making a total of 497 known dead.

HALIFAX COUNTY (CITY ONLY), VITAL STATISTICS, DEATH REGISTER, BOOKS 21, 25, 70

Please note that, in the interest of saving space, all references in this list to the death records of these individuals give only the Book, Page, and Number. All such citations refer only to the HVS, Halifax County Death Registers, 1918–20.

1918

1. Hilda Moriarity [*sic*], 6 months, d. 13 September 1918, Halifax.
2. William Moir, 13, d. 29 September 1918, Halifax.
3. Alma Lilley, 10 months, d. 29 September 1918, Halifax.
4. James Humphrey, 27, d. 4 October 1918, Halifax, engine fitter.
5. Elphege Scott, 32, d. 5 October 1918, Halifax, carpenter.
6. Chris Petropolis, 16, d. 6 October 1918, Halifax.
7. Peter Burke, 18, d. 7 October 1918, Halifax, labourer.
8. Teresa Mailman, 2, d. 9 October 1918, Halifax.
9. Ethel Rood, 25, d. 9 October 1918, Halifax, housewife.
10. Edward Scanlon, 2, d. 9 October 1918, Halifax.
11. Lillian Morrison, 25, d. 9 October 1918, Halifax, waitress. [*See essay for Cumberland County.*]
12. Lucy Cawes, 23, d. 10 October 1918, Halifax, housewife.
13. Lillian Dauphinee, 21, d. 10 October 1918, Halifax, housewife.
14. William Fitzgerald, 32, d. 11 October 1918, Halifax, traveller [*salesman*].
15. George Brock, 21, d. 12 October 1918, Halifax, soldier.
16. Richard Cahill, 24, d. 13 October 1918, Halifax, chauffeur.
17. Mertie LeBlanch, 34, d. 14 October 1918, Halifax, housewife.
18. Violet Shannon, 35, d. 14 October 1918, Halifax, housewife.
19. Victor Grady, 21, d. 14 October 1918, Halifax, soldier.
20. William Hillborn, 19, d. 14 October 1918, Halifax, soldier.
21. Alphonsis Mulloy, 36, d. 14 October 1918, Halifax, painter. [*Book 21, Page 565, Number 3388; he lived at 427 Brunswick Street.*]
22. Charles Barrett, 5, d. 15 October 1918, Halifax.
23. William Shannon, 38, d. 15 October 1918, Halifax, postman.
24. R. Sherlock, 26, d. 15 October 1918, Halifax, soldier.
25. Frank Lundy, 19, d. 15 October 1918, Halifax, soldier.
26. Mary Gray, 29, d. 16 October 1918, Halifax, housewife.
27. J. J. Ryan, male, 34, d. 16 October 1918, Halifax, soldier.
28. Lucy Noble, 34, d. 17 October 1918, Halifax.
29. George Fraser, 20, d. 17 October 1918, Halifax, soldier.
30. Gordon Stockley, 24, d. 17 October 1918, Halifax, soldier.
31. Fred Ducut [Frédéric Doucet], d. 17 October 1918, Halifax, cook. [*See essay on Halifax County. He was French and cook on board a vessel.*]
32. Howard Thomas, 20, d. 17 October 1918, Halifax, drug clerk.
33. Mary Antle, 42, d. 18 October 1918, Halifax, housewife.
34. Lloyd Mumford, 29, d. 18 October 1918, Halifax, printer.
35. Ambroze Hennessey, 26, d. 19 October 1918, Halifax, soldier.
36. Ida Burke, d. 19 October 1918, Halifax, domestic. [*HVS, Book 21, Page 570,*

Number 3419, just states "?" in the blank for her age. She had lived at 264 Barrington Street, was Catholic, born in St. Peters, Cape Breton, and died of Influenza/Pneumonia, after an illness of one week.]

37. Ruth Westburn, 11 months, d. 20 October 1918, Halifax.

38. Colin Wilson, 30, d. 20 October 1918, Halifax, soldier. *[HVS, Book 21, Page 571, Number 3425, says he was born in Ontario, son of John Wilson, and his body was returned for burial to South March, ON. Halifax Evening Mail, 21 September 1918, 9, gives his name as Lt. Calvin Wilson.]*

39. Nora Parks, 28, d. 20 October 1918, Halifax, housewife.

40. H. Madigan (male), d. 21 October 1918, at the Station Hospital, Halifax. *[Book 21, Page 572, Number 3428, says he was a soldier, a Roman Catholic, born in the United States.]*

41. Arthur Stevens, 33, d. 21 October 1918, Halifax, clerk.

42. William Harding, 26, d. 21 October 1918, Halifax, soldier.

43. Eliza Chase, 63, d. 21 October 1918, Halifax.

44. John Fraser, 8 months, d. 21 October 1918, Halifax.

45. Marion Murphy, 21 months, d. 21 October 1918, Halifax.

46. Lillian Cavanagh, 23, d. 21 October 1918, Halifax, housewife.

47. Loraine Burgoyne, 17, d. 21 October 1918, Halifax, sailor. *[Book 21, Page 572, Number 3428, says he was male, had been born in Mahone Bay, resided there at time of death, was buried there. He was Presbyterian.]*

48. Florence Todd, 22, d. 21 October 1918, Halifax.

49. William Russell, 1, d. 22 October 1918, Halifax.

50. Alfred Brightman, 45, d. 22 October 1918, Halifax, labourer.

51. Elsie Hilchey, 19, d. 22 October 1918, Halifax, housework.

52. Sidney Leach, 37, d. 22 October 1918, Halifax, salesman.

53. Michael Hannon, 31, d. 22 October 1918, Halifax.

54. Sarah Billard, 27, d. 23 October 1918, Halifax, housewife.

55. John Moore, 56, d. 23 October 1918, Halifax, merchant.

56. Walter White, 25, d. 23 October 1918, Halifax, soldier.

57. Thomas Adams, 16, d. 23 October 1918, Halifax.

58. Helen Hann, 9 months, d. 23 October 1918, Halifax.

59. Margaret Burchell, 24, d. 24 October 1918, Halifax, housewife.

60. Peter Tobin Jr., 26, d. 24 October 1918, Halifax, book keeper.

61. James Carter, 31, d. 24 October 1918, Halifax, railway employee.

62. Melissa Barrie, 54, d. 24 October 1918, Halifax, housework.

63. Catherine Marshall, 47, d. 25 October 1918, Halifax, housewife.

64. Harold Batty, 21, d. 25 October 1918, Halifax.

65. William Caldwell, 72, d. 25 October 1918, Halifax, City Home.

66. William Rogers, 67, d. 25 October 1918, Halifax, City Home, labourer.

67. John Murphy, 64, d. 25 October 1918, Halifax, City Home, labourer.

68. Margaret Rangell, 26, d. 25 October 1918, Halifax, housewife.

69. Joseph Crawley, 9, d. 26 October 1918, Halifax, student.

70. George Barber, 49, d. 26 October 1918, Halifax, City Home.

71. John Bradley, 27, d. 26 October 1918, Halifax, City Home.

72. Lillian Hardstaff, 11 months, d. 27 October 1918, Halifax.

73. Alexander Moxon, 29, d. 27 October 1918, Halifax, teamster.

74. Joseph Manette, 23, d. 27 October 1918, Halifax, soldier.

75. James Cleary, 32, d. 27 October 1918, Halifax, soldier.

76. Elizabeth Lannigan, 24, d. 27 October 1918, Halifax, housewife.

77. Irene Boutilier, 35, d. 27 October 1918, Halifax, housewife.

78. Catherine Slauenwhite, 20, d. 28 October 1918, Halifax, housewife.

79. Edward Thompson, 40, d. 28 October 1918, City Home, Halifax, labourer.

80. Edward DeYoung, 50, d. 28 October 1918, Halifax.

81. Lottie Flick, 27, d. 28 October 1918, Halifax, nurse.

82. Muriel Blinis, 22, d. 28 October 1918, Halifax, domestic.

83. George Farish, 37, d. 28 October 1918, Halifax, army officer.

84. Thomas Dillman, 35, d. 28 October 1918, Halifax, dockyard employee.

85. Kathleen Hanrahan, 7 months, d. 29 October 1918, Halifax.

86. Margaret Bennett, 23, d. 29 October 1918, Halifax, housewife.

87. Carl Levi, 25, d. 29 October 1918, Halifax, painter.

88. Anthony MacMillan, 41, d. 29 October 1918, Halifax, Pine Hill Hospital, sergeant.

89. Katherine Shanlea, 60, d. 29 October 1918, Halifax.

90. Mary D. McDonald, 26, d. 29 October 1918, Halifax, domestic.

91. Elizabeth Schultz, 75, d. 29 October 1918, Halifax, City Home, cook.

92. Thomas Smith, 77, d. 29 October 1918, Halifax, City Home, watchman.

93. John Moore, 19, d. 29 October 1918, Halifax, student.

94. Thomas Rogers, 45, d. 29 October 1918, Halifax, carpenter.

95. Thomas Mowbray, 80, [no date], died Halifax, retired.

96. Emerie Bourque, 9 months, d. 29 October 1918, Halifax.

97. Sarah Carmichael, 4, d. 29 October 1918, Halifax.

98. August Buideksson, 40, d. 29 October 1918, Halifax, steward.

99. Cyril Clancy, 5, d. 30 October 1918, Halifax.

100. Frank Naylor, 22, d. 30 October 1918, Halifax.

101. Harry McKenzie, 29, d. 30 October 1918, Halifax, carpenter.

102. L. Durant, 23, d. 30 October 1918, Halifax, soldier.

103. William Mills, 32, d. 31 October 1918, Halifax, soldier.

104. Mary Mountain, 26, d. 31 October 1918, Halifax, housewife.

105. Margaret Allander, 47, d. 1 November 1918, Halifax, house duties.

106. William Lemieux, 20, d. 1 November 1918, Halifax, Morris Street Hospital, labourer.

107. Mary Byrne, 70, d. 1 November 1918, house duties.

108. Eliza Arnold, 58, d. 1 November 1918, Halifax, house duties.

109. Alfred McDonough, 35, d. 1 November 1918, Halifax, soldier.

110. George Adams, 8, d. 2 November 1918, Halifax.

111. Ung Gong [An Long Gong], 50, d. 2 November 1918, Halifax, laundryman.

112. Joseph O'Connell, 2, d. 2 November 1918, Halifax.

113. Mary Hemming, 25, d. 2 November 1918, Halifax, housewife.

114. Frank Purdy, 3, d. 2 November 1918, Halifax.

115. Mary Copan, 8 days, d. 3 November 1918, Halifax.

116. Hercules La Belle, 27, d. 3 November 1918, Halifax, painter.

117. B. F. Cooper, 31, d. 4 November 1918, Halifax, soldier.

118. Jeu On [*Jeu (or Jen) Ao On*], 28, d. 4 November 1918, Halifax, laundry man.

119. Jammes [*sic*] Boudreau, 19, d. 5 November 1918, Halifax, soldier. [*HVS, Book 21, Page 592, Number 3550, shows a largely illegible first name; the HVS Search Engine gives it as Jammies.*]

120. William Davidson, 28, d. 5 November 1918, Halifax, carpenter.

121. Stephen O'Brian, 39, d. 5 November 1918, Halifax, teamster.

122. Charles Moxon, 37, d. 6 November 1918, Halifax, engineer.

123. Marjorie Fox, 13, d. 6 November 1918, Halifax, student.

124. Allan Pirie, 18 months, d. 6 November 1918, Halifax.

125. George Cruise, 65, d. 7 November 1918, Halifax, shoemaker.

126. Thomas Chason, 34, d. 7 November 1918, Halifax, plasterer.

127. Margaret MacDonald, 23, d. 8 November 1918, Halifax, housewife.

128. Lena Petitpas, 27, d. 8 November 1918, Halifax, housewife.

129. George Andrews, 22, d. 8 November 1918, Halifax, teamster.

130. Louise Graham, 31, d. 8 November 1918, Halifax, housewife.

131. John MacDonald, 24, d. 8 November 1918, Halifax, labourer.

132. Margaret MacDonald, 20, d. 8 November 1918, Halifax, housemaid.

133. Frank Barrett, 30, d. 8 November 1918, Halifax, labourer.

134. Kate Romana, 39, d. 8 November 1918, Halifax, housewife.

135. Frederick Bryan, 30, d.8 November 1918, Halifax, chief, E.R.A.

136. Jennie Ellis, 58, d. 8 November 1918, Halifax, housewife.

137. Francis Fewer, 7 months, d. 9 November 1918, Halifax.

138. Soo Chung [*Soo Lee Chung*], 38, d. 9 November 1918, Halifax, laundry man. [*Book 25, Page 1, Number 3. Born in China, lived at 176 Lower Water Street, was unmarried, Presbyterian, and buried in St. John's cemetery. Death Register, 1918, Book 25, Page 1, Number 3, has "Soo Lee Chung," but the HVS Search Engine gives him as "Sou Moo Ching."*]

139. Charles Falt, 21, d. 9 November 1918, Halifax, labourer.

140. Gordon Forsyth, 14 months, d. 10 November 1918, Halifax.

141. Louise Stimers, 35, d. 10 November 1918, Halifax, housewife.

142. Mendel Whitzman, 34, d. 10 November 1918, Halifax, junk dealer.

143. Edward Smith, 7, d. 12 November 1918, Halifax.

[*Next number in Dr. Marble's list skips to "148"; corrected here.*]

144. William Greenwood, 39, d. 12 November 1918, Halifax, soldier.

145. Ella Fertham, 42, d. 14 November 1918, Halifax, housewife.

146. Maud White, 27, d. 14 November 1918, Halifax, housewife.

147. Terence Daley, 41, d. 14 November 1918, Halifax, soldier.

148. Henry Ryan, 7 days [*sic; 67 years old*], d. 14 November 1918, Halifax, labourer. [*HVS, 1918, Book 25, Page 8, Number 43, his death record, states he was born in England, a Roman Catholic, buried at Mount Olivet.*]

149. Luke Flinn, 37, d. 15 November 1918, Halifax, longshoreman.

150. Margaret Beckford, 35, d. 15 November 1918, Halifax, housewife.

151. Florence Walker, 42, d. 15 November 1918, Halifax.

152. Thomas Connolly, 38, d. 15 November 1918, Halifax, checker.

153. Eric Clemens, 27, d. 15 November 1918, Halifax, seaman.

154. William Minn, 28, d. 15 November 1918, Halifax, fireman [*stoker?*]

155. William Adams, 2, d. 16 November 1918, Halifax.

156. Sam Fong, 33, d. 17 November 1918, Halifax, laundryman.

157. Thomas Healey, 14 months, d. 17 November 1918, Halifax.

158. Donald McIver, 26, d. 17 November 1918, Halifax, sailor.

159. Lilian Douglas, 6, d. 17 November 1918, Halifax.

160. Margaret De Young, 44, d. 18 November 1918, Halifax, housewife.

161. Beatrice Wambolt, 26, d. 18 November 1918, Halifax, housewife.

162. Oriah Sound, 18 months, d. 19 November 1918, Halifax.

163. Allen Landry, 29, d. 20 November 1918, [*8 Birmingham Street,*] Halifax. [*Book 25, Page 14, Number 83.*]

164. Florence Monk, 26, d. 21 November 1918, Halifax, housewife.

165. Alexander Cotter, 19, d. 22 November 1918, Halifax, signaller, C.E.F.

166. Percy Mathias, 17, d. 22 November 1918, Halifax, seaman.

167. Elmer Sevigne, 1 year, d. 22 November 1918, Halifax.

168. Victor Levy, 12, d. 23 November 1918, Halifax.

169. Annie Gibson, 24, d. 23 November 1918, Halifax, housewife.

170. David W. Vaughan, 38, d. 23 November 1918, Halifax, labourer.

171. James Roven, 31, d. 24 November 1918, Halifax, Petty Officer.

172. Margaret Arthur, 23, d. 24 November 1918, Halifax, housewife.

173. Arthur Munroe, 2, d. 24 November 1918, Halifax.

174. Wilbert Phillips, 32, d. 24 November 1918, Halifax, cook.

175. William Murphy, 27, d. 24 November 1918, Halifax, chauffeur.

176. Herman Lurie, 23, d. 26 November 1918, Halifax, agent.

177. Rita Wier, 7, d. 27 November 1918, Halifax.

178. Marie Dooley, 3, d. 28 November 1918, Halifax.

179. Daniel Hauser, 54, d. 28 November 1918, Halifax, labourer.

180. Thomas Ward, 28, d. 28 November 1918, Halifax, soldier.

181. Eleanor Etter, 33, d. 29 November 1918, Halifax.

182. Ellen Cordo, 21, d. 29 November 1918, Halifax, domestic.

183. Margaret Breach, d. 30 November 1918, Halifax, housewife.

184. Josephine Penny, 22, d. 30 November 1918, Halifax, housewife.

185. Mary White, 41, d. 30 November 1918, Halifax, housewife.

186. Catherine Cohoon, 23, d. 26 November 1918, Halifax, social worker.

187. Joseph Yetman, 28, d. 1 December 1918, Halifax, barber.

188. Ethel Hotchkiss, 19, d. 2 December 1918, Halifax.

189. John Longard, 37, d. 4 December 1918, Halifax, employee Moirs [*Chocolate Factory*].

190. Gustave Larson, 28, d. 4 December 1918, Halifax, soldier.

191. Frank Cleveland, 26, d. 4 December 1918, Halifax, soldier.

192. Anastatia Brown, 28, d. 4 December 1918, housewife.

193. Beatrice Shatford, 18, d. 5 December 1918, Halifax, domestic.

194. Daisy Hays, 31, d. 5 December 1918, Halifax.

195. Glena Robinson, 28, d. 5 December 1918, Halifax. [*Book 25, Page 29, Number 174: she was Mrs. William Robinson, Roman Catholic, resided at 61 Rhode Island Avenue, buried at Mount Olivet.*]

196. Dora Foyle, 25, d. 5 December 1918, Halifax, stenographer.

197. Jennie Mason, 23, d. 5 December 1918, Halifax, housewife.

198. Daniel Martin, 4, d. 5 December 1918, Halifax.

199. Edith Laidlaw, 17, d. 6 December 1918, Halifax.

200. Walter McDonald, 49, d. 6 December 1918, Halifax, labourer.

201. Margaret Leahey, 38, d. 6 December 1918, Halifax, housewife.

202. Thecla Julien, 16, d. 6 December 1918, Halifax, domestic. [*Book 25, Page 31, Number 185; she was Mrs. Ephraim Julien. HVS Search Engine lists her as "Theola Julien."*]

203. Thomas Hubley, 39, d. 7 December 1918, Halifax, agent.

204. Hilda Power, 3, d. 8 December 1918, Halifax.

205. Myrtle Clark, 25, d. 8 December 1918, Halifax, housewife.

206. Firman Kennedy, 16, d. 9 December 1918, Halifax, soldier.

207. Elizabeth Turner, 42, d. 9 December 1918, Halifax, housewife.

208. David Nichols, 25, d. 10 December 1918, Halifax, seaman.

209. Josephine Curry, 24, d. 10 December 1918, Halifax.

210. Malcolm Magee, 30, d. 11 December 1918, Halifax, soldier.

211. William Lawson, 38, d. 11 December 1918, Halifax, soldier.

212. Donald Cummings, 30, d. 12 December 1918, Halifax, plumber.

213. Charles Lively, 20, d. 12 December 1918, Halifax, painter.

214. Lena Jackson, 23, d. 12 December 1918, Halifax, City Home, domestic.

215. Bridget Steele, 18, d. 12 December 1918, Halifax.

216. Ellen Wimpers, 5 months, d. 12 December 1918, Halifax.

217. Michael McNeil, 26, d. 13 December 1918, Halifax, soldier.

218. Elizabeth Knowlton, 37, d. 13 December 1918, Halifax, housewife.

219. James Rabbie, 18, d. 15 December 1918, Halifax, soldier.

220. William Power, 45, d. 15 December 1918, Halifax, painter.

221. Jean Forbes, 2, d. 16 December 1918, Halifax.

222. William Newell, 50, d. 16 December 1918, Halifax.

223. Bradis Levy, 12, d. 18 December 1918, Halifax.

224. William McCaul, 33, d. 18 December 1918, Station Hospital, Halifax, soldier.

225. Mabel Lush, 27, d. 18 December 1918, Halifax, housewife.

226. Ward Neys, 20, d. 19 December 1918, Station Hospital, Halifax, stoker.

227. Clarence Cadmon, 25, d. 20 December 1918, Halifax, carpenter.

228. Ida Kraft, 52, d. 20 December 1918, Almon Street Hospital, Halifax, domestic.

229. Alonzo De Guist, 30, d. 20 December 1918, Halifax, sailor.

230. William Saulnier, 29, d. 21 December 1918, Halifax, skipper.

231. Charles Coulter, 52, d. 21 December 1918, Halifax, painter.

232. Matsutaro Matsusaki, 34, d. 21 December 1918, Halifax, sailor.

233. Arthur Brisson, 18, d. 22 December 1918, Halifax, soldier.

234. Osborne Lucas, 35, d. 23 December 1918, Halifax, porter.

235. Lester Hodgson, 22, d. 23 December 1918, Halifax, soldier.

236. Edith Steadman, 42, d. 23 December 1918, Halifax, housewife.

237. Edna Brown, 20, d. 23 December 1918, Halifax, housewife.

238. Joseph Francis, 1, d. 24 December 1918, Halifax.

239. Martin Fogarty, 17, d. 25 December 1918, Station Hospital, Halifax, soldier.

240. Harry Carney, 38, d. 28 December 1918, Halifax, machinist.

241. Stella Nearing, 22, d. 29 December 1918, Almon Street Hospital, Halifax, domestic.

242. Bridget Myette, 21, d. 29 December 1918, Halifax, cook.

243. Dora Rooker, 26, d. 30 December 1918, Halifax, domestic.

244. Acile Blakeley, 19, d. 30 December 1918, Halifax, clerk.

245. Matilda De Young, 18, d. 31 December 1918, Halifax.

246. Ada Baker, 26, d. 31 December 1918, Halifax, domestic.

247. Pauline Johnson, 17, d. 21 December 1918, Halifax, housework.

248. Annie Ehman, 16, d. 31 December 1918, Halifax.

249. Alice Day, 29, d. 31 December 1918, Halifax, housewife.

250. Bella Heptidge, 18, d. 31 December 1918, Halifax.

251. Willard Boomer, d. 19 December 1918, Influenza Hospital, Halifax.

252. George Boutilier, 21, d. 19 December 1918, Halifax, labourer.

1919

253. Arthur Gray, 11 months, d. 2 January 1919, Halifax.

254. Bessie MacDonald, 23, d. 2 January 1919, Halifax, nurse.

255. Calvin Breen, 17, d. 4 January 1919, Halifax. [*He was buried in Guysborough County.*]

256. George Dimeule, 7, d. 5 January 1919, Halifax, student.

257. Maria Deigan, 33, d. 6 January 1919, Halifax, housewife.

258. Eliza Boutilier, 27, d. 6 January 1919, Halifax, housewife.

259. Lizzie Flannigan, 35, d. 7 January 1919, Halifax, housewife.

260. Charles Briand, 27, d. 10 January 1919, Halifax, labourer.

261. Stella Pyke, 19, d. 14 January 1919, Halifax.

262. Helen Arab, 2 months, d. 16 January 1919, Halifax.

263. Victor Hanna, 21, d. 17 January 1919, Halifax, soldier.

264. George McGrath, 27, d. 19 January 1919, Halifax.

265. Ellen Lanigan, 64, d. 20 January 1919, Halifax.

266. Thomas Holmes, 27, d. 23 January 1919, Military Hospital, Halifax, soldier.

267. George Sargent, 33, d. 23 January 1919, Military Hospital, Halifax, soldier.

268. Henry Gordon, 23, d. 24 January 1919, Military Hospital, Halifax, soldier.

269. J. De Battista, 17, d. 26 January 1919, Military Hospital, Halifax, seaman.

270. Thomas Speakman, 28, d. 26 January 1919, Military Hospital, Halifax, soldier.

271. Laurie Smith, 27, d. 27 January 1919, Halifax, fireman.

272. D. Farnam, 21, d. 29 January 1919, Halifax, soldier.

273. George McAulay, 33, d. 12 February 1919, Halifax, soldier.

274. Charles Laba, 1, d. 14 February 1919, Halifax.

275. Weston Newberry, 29, d. 15 February 1919, Halifax, stoker in Navy.

276. Helen Shaffelburg, 16, d. 17 February 1919, Halifax.

277. Alva Baglole, male, 22, d. 20 February 1919, Halifax, soldier. [*He was from PEI.*]

278. Isabella Graham, 76, d. 23 February 1919, Halifax, housework.

279. Ernest Cleveland, 9 months, d. 23 February 1919, Halifax.

280. Andrew McKenna, 21, d. 26 February 1919, Halifax, soldier.

281. Annie Peters, 22, d. 28 February 1919, Halifax, School for the Deaf.

282. Eric Malanda, d. 3 March 1919, Halifax, janitor.

283. Mary Malanda, 42, d. 5 March 1919, Halifax, housework.

284. James Waldron, 57, d. 10 March 1919, Halifax, goldsmith.

285. Virginia Martell, 20, d. 10 March 1919, Halifax.

286. Gordon Brown, 14, d. 10 March 1919, Halifax, student.

287. Catherine Gregory, 27, d. 11 March 1919, Halifax, housewife.

288. Margaret Armsworthy, 26, d. 12 March 1919, Halifax.

289. Ruine Walker, 10 months, d. 16 March 1919, Halifax.

290. Harry Holden, 32, d. 20 March 1919, Halifax.

291. Robert Jackson, 28, d. 21 March 1919, Lawlor's [sic] Island, 2nd mate. [HVS, Halifax County Death Register, 1919, Book 25, Page 98, Number 587.]

292. D'Arcy Spencer, 68, d. 11 May 1919 in Halifax, fisherman. [Formerly listed in Digby County.]

"Checked register from 17 December 1919–2 May 1920." [Allan Marble Note.]

1920

293. Georgina Muriel Campbell, 13, d. 25 January 1920, Halifax, school student.

294. Sie Ching Ga [sic; HVS search engine shows nothing resembling this name], 30, d. 30 January 1920, Rockhead Hospital, Halifax, soldier.

295. Beatrice Luddington, 18, d. 15 February 1920, Morris Street Hospital, Halifax.

296. Elizabeth Madden, 49, d. 17 February 1920, Halifax, housewife.

297. Austen Dixon, 1 year 4 months, d. 19 February 1920, Africville, Halifax.

298. Leone Levy, d. 19 February 1920, Halifax, domestic. [HVS, Halifax County Death Register, 1920, Book 70, Page 429.]

299. Vincent Dereskevice, 36, d. 20 February 1920, Morris Street Hospital, Halifax, tailor.

300. Margaret McGinn, 1 year 5 months, d. 22 February 1920, Halifax.

301. Alva Edison Wingate, 31, d. 22 February 1920, Halifax, Captain.

302. Fenwick W. Collen, 49, d. 22 February 1920, Halifax, labourer.

303. Florence Bower, 54, d. 22 February 1920, Isolation Hospital, Halifax, housewife.

304. Catherine Bezanson, 29, d. 24 February 1920, Halifax.

305. Clyde Riggs, 19, d. 22 February 1920, Morris Street Hospital, Halifax, labourer.

306. Nettie Coussins, 24, d. 27 February 1920, Morris Street Hospital, Halifax. housewife.

307. Charles D. Glenister, 23, d. 27 February 1920, Halifax, mail clerk.

308. Merna [Minerva May] Baker, 24, d. 28 February 1920, Victoria General Hospital, Halifax, nurse.

309. Annie E. Power, 48, d. 28 February 1920, Halifax, housewife.

310. Blanch Cox, 35, d. 28 February 1920, Halifax, nurse in training, Victoria General Hospital, Halifax.

311. Charles Wallace Lohnes, 43, d. 28 February 1920, Halifax, labourer.

312. Sarah J. Bobbitt, 59, d. 29 February 1920, Halifax, housewife.

313. Robert Howard, 10 months, d. 29 February 1920, Halifax.

314. Etta L. Clarke, 33, d. 1 March 1920, Halifax, student nurse, Victoria General Hospital, Halifax.

315. Lila Purcell, 23, d. March 1920, Halifax, housewife. [*Cause of death: "influenza & pneumonia, pregnant." HVS, Book 70, Page 1.*]

316. Arthur Anderssen, 22, d. 2 March 1920, Halifax, clerk.

317. Lillian Richardson, 22, d. 2 March 1920, Isolation Hospital, Halifax, servant.

318. Margaret Slaunwhite, 29, d. 3 March 1920, Halifax, housewife.

319. Winnifred M. Mayne, 23, d. 3 March 1920, Halifax, housewife.

320. Leona Shupe, 21, d. 4 March 1920, Isolation Hospital, Halifax, worked in candy factory [*Moirs?*].

321. Emily M. Johnson, 12, d. 5 March 1920, Halifax, Victoria General Hospital, student. [*Neither Annapolis nor Halifax have a death record shown for her in the HVS database. Dr. Marble found her in the Annapolis death records, original ledger, and recorded it in his list for Annapolis County. Likely her home was in Annapolis County, but she died in the VG Hospital, Halifax. She may even have two death records, the second being in the Halifax original ledger. Since she died in Halifax, her entry has been transferred to this present list for Halifax County.*]

322. Arthur W. Taylor, 25, d. 6 March 1920, Halifax, clerk.

323. Emmeline McLean, 70, d. 7 March 1920, Halifax.

324. Annie Hulme, 22, d. 8 March 1920, Halifax.

325. William Russell, 40, d. 9 March 1920, Isolation Hospital, Halifax, seafarer.

326. Mary C. Flannigan, 33, d. 9 March 1920, Halifax, housewife.

327. Mrs. Maude Hilton, 30, d. 12 March 1920, Halifax, housework.

328. Frances Burke, 6 months, d. 14 March 1920, Halifax.

329. Elizabeth Sampson, 21, d. 17 March 1920, Morris Street Hospital, Halifax, housework.

330. Frank Sampson, 45, d. 17 March 1920, Morris Street Hospital, Halifax, stevedore.

331. Desneige Laura LeClair, 1 year 6 months, d. 19 March 1920, Halifax [*no date of death given on Marble list. Death Register, 1920, Book 70, Page 612, states that she was French, born in Halifax, and that the primary cause of death was tuberculosis, aggravated by measles and influenza. Again, no date of death shown on the original.*]

332. Mary Moriarity, 58, d. 19 March 1920, Halifax, housewife.

333. Edgar D. Blair, 67, d. 21 March 1920, Halifax, wine merchant.

334. William Dalton, 33, d. 22 March 1920, Halifax, labourer.

335. Percy E. Moore, 1 year 8 months, d. 23 March 1920, Halifax.

336. Minnie Nowes, 27, d. 31 March 1920, Halifax, housework.

337. Edith E. Hughes, 32, d. 13 April 1920, Halifax.

338. Grace B. Ropell, 31, d. 13 April 1920, Halifax, housewife.

"Records searched to 1 May 1920, for Halifax City." [Allan Marble Note.]

HALIFAX COUNTY (EXCLUDING THE CITY), VITAL STATISTICS, DEATH REGISTER, BOOKS 35, 70

1918

1. Murray Dorrington, 13 months, d. 11 September 1918, Beechville.
2. Lewis Dorrington, 1 year, d. 14 September 1918, Beechville.
3. Christine McIsaac, 37, d. 19 September 1918, Chocolate Lake.
4. Stella Munro, 3 months, d. 25 September 1918, Beechville.
5. Jonas Paul, 64, d. 11 October 1918, Herring Cove Road, guide.
6. Peter Munro, 26, d. 24 October 1918, Beechville, labourer.
7. Gladys Hill, 8 months, d. 25 October 1918, Beechville.
8. Kathleen Wright, 20, d. 25 October 1918, Beechville, housewife.
9. George Lopie, 53, d. 26 October 1918, Beechville, labourer.
10. Clara Munro, 3, d. 27 October 1918, Beechville.
11. Annie Greening, 42, d. 27 October 1918, Melville Island, housewife.
12. Zeckariah Henry, 39, d. 28 October 1918, Beechville, labourer.
13. Emma Henry, 34, d. 2 November 1918, Beechville, housewife.
14. John Munroe, 15, d. 3 November 1918, Beechville.
15. Jerome Burke, 26, d. 6 November 1918, Portuguese Cove, fisherman.
16. Gladys Hart, 18, d. 9 December 1918, Sambro.
17. Alice Hart, 10, d. 13 December 1918, Sambro.
18. Mary Gray, 67, d. 13 December 1918, Sambro.
19. Annie Slauenwhite, 24, d. 21 December 1918, Terence Bay, housewife.
20. Doria Boutilier, 2, d. 6 November 1918, Tantallon.
21. Douglas Jennings, 3 months, d. 21 November 1918, French Village.
22. Elizabeth Richardson, 57, d. 4 November 1918, Indian Harbour, housewife.
23. Francie Frederick, 29, d. 25 November 1918, French Village, housewife.
24. Louis Fraser, 43, d. 30 November 1918, Glen Margaret.
25. Janet Fraser, 42, d. 1 December 1918, Glen Margaret, housewife.
26. Mary Johnston, 15, d. 5 December 1918, Glen Margaret, housemaid.
27. Bulah Fraser, 10, d. 8 December 1918, Glen Margaret.
28. Wallace Brigley, 14, d. 20 December 1918, Black Point.
29. _____ Miller, 26, d. 21 December 1918, Hubbards, housewife.
30. Kitchener Snair, 3, d. 19 December 1918, Black Point.
31. Edmund B. Norwood, 42, d. 30 December 1918, Hubbards, physician.
32. Malcolm McLean, 20, d. 13 November 1918, Hubbards, fireman.
33. Wilbert Phillips, 23, d. 24 November 1918, Ingramport, cook.
34. Ester Johnson, 18, d. 23 November 1918, Ingramport, housewife.
35. Franklin Vogler, 3 months, d. 2 December 1918, Ingramport.
36. Annie Cope, 1, d. 8 October 1918, Windsor Junction.
37. Sarah Cope, 38, d. 13 October 1918, Windsor Junction, housewife.
38. Joseph Paul, 78, d. 13 October 1918, Windsor Junction.
39. Sarah Paul, 73, d. 19 October 1918, Windsor Junction, housewife.
40. Katie Paul, 28, d. 20 October 1918, Windsor Junction, housewife.

41. Mary MacNeil, 11, d. 19 November 1918, Rockingham.

42. Gordon Boutilier, 27, d. 10 December 1918, Bedford, labourer.

43. James Sibley, 30, d. 29 November 1918, Meaghers Grant, railway worker.

44. Mrs. Hilda Sibley, 23, d. 15 November 1918, Meaghers Grant, housewife.

45. Helen Leslie, 17, d. 26 October 1918, Upper Musquodoboit, housewife.

46. Mary Burgess, 4, d. 31 October 1918, Upper Musquodoboit.

47. Mary Burgess, 43, d. 8 November 1918, Upper Musquodoboit, housewife.

48. Daniel Farnell, 13, d. 16 November 1918, Sheet Harbour Road, student.

49. Earl McIvoy, 22, d. 3 November 1918, Dartmouth, fireman.

50. John O'Hearn, 30, d. 3 November 1918, Dartmouth, plumber.

51. Robert Shephard, 26, d. 13 November 1918, Dartmouth.

52. Minnie Bayley, 10, d. 21 November 1918, Dartmouth.

53. Maud Cohoon, 24, d. 28 November 1918, Dartmouth.

54. Gladys Maxner, 28, d. 5 December 1918, Dartmouth, housewife.

55. Ethel Montague, 34, d. 11 December 1918, Dartmouth, housewife.

56. Archibald Gregorie, 26, d. 14 October 1918, Dartmouth, carpenter.

57. Thomas Motte, d. 15 October 1918, Dartmouth.

58. Ada Morgan, 2, d. 15 October 1918, Dartmouth.

59. Josephine McGrath, 35, d. 16 October 1918, Dartmouth.

60. Susan Craig, 32, d. 21 October 1918, Dartmouth, housewife.

61. Mary O'Brian, 25, d. 21 October 1918, Dartmouth.

62. Thomas Connors, 24, d, 22 October 1918, Dartmouth, labourer.

63. Joseph Graham, 36, d. 24 October 1918, Dartmouth, labourer.

64. Frank O'Hanley, 37, d. 25 October 1918, Dartmouth, electrician.

65. Harriet Walker, 28, d. 26 October 1918, Dartmouth, housewife.

66. Elizabeth Brown, 31, d. 28 October 1918, Dartmouth.

67. Joseph Roach, 2, d. 31 October 1918, Dartmouth.

68. Rufus Zwicker, 32, d. 31 October 1918, Dartmouth, machinist.

69. Mable Powell, 24, d. October 1918, Dartmouth, housewife.

70. Nellie Miller, 23, d. 2 November 1918, Dartmouth.

71. Jules Fortin, d. 27 September 1918, Station Hospital, Lawlor's [*sic*] Island, sailor.

72. Richard Olsen, d. 30 September 1918, Lawlor's [*sic*] Island, American sailor.

73. François Michels, 29, d. 1 October 1918, Lawlor's [*sic*] Island, sailor.

74. James Fell, 24, d. 6 October 1918, Lawlor's [*sic*] Island.

75. George Taylor, 37, d. 11 October 1918, Lawlor's [*sic*] Island.

76. Patrick Quinan, 25, 15 October 1918, Lawlor's [*sic*] Island, seaman.

77. Gladys Beale, 15, d. 23 October 1918, Preston.

78. Alfred Downey, 2, d. 25 October 1918, Preston.

79. Lillie Downey, 1, d. 25 October 1918, Preston.

80. Daniel Chisholm, 25, d. 26 October 1918, N. S. Hospital, Dartmouth, coal miner.

81. Nicholas Boylan, 37, d. 27 October 1918, N. S. Hospital, Dartmouth, farmer.

82. Rita Lovett, 9, d. 1 November 1918, Tufts Cove.

83. Hilda Wyatt, 29, d. 5 November 1918, Tufts Cove, housework.

84. Mary Hayward, 40, d. 10 November 1918, Woodside.

85. Alice Naugle, 35, d. 11 November 1918, Eastern Passage.

86. John Richards, 41, d. 16 November 1918, Woodside.

87. George Naugle, 41, d. 13 December 1918, Devil's [*sic*] Island. [*He was a fisherman. See chapter above for further details.*]

88. Henry Murphy, 3 months, d. 11 December 1918, Mineville.

89. Joseph Roma, 21, d. 19 October 1918, West Chezzetcook, farmer.

90. Rita Gaetz, 16, d. 28 October 1918, Seaforth.

91. Mary Julien, 21, d. 31 October 1918, Middle Porter's [*sic*] Lake.

92. Alvin Gaetz, 24, d. 3 Novembeer 1918, Head Chezzetcook, farmer.

93. Gertrude Conrod, 19, d. 8 November 1918, East Chezzetcook.

94. Evangelina Roma, 46, d. 9 November 1918, West Chezzetcook.

95. Herbert Myette, 19, d. 25 November 1918, Grand Desert, fisherman.

96. Alexander McInnis, 77, d. 4 December 1918, Musquodoboit Harbour, carpenter.

97. Arthur Baker, 21, 30 October 1918, East Jeddore, fisherman.

98. Gladys Hartling, 29, d. 2 November 1918, Jeddore, housewife.

99. Anna Young, 18, d. 2 November 1918, Bayers Settlement, housewife.

[*100. This name was voided from Dr. Marble's list as it was a repeat registration, in the original ledger, of Number 51, Elsie Hilchey's death in Halifax city. The list has been corrected to show an accurate death count.*]

100. Howard De Wolfe, 7 months, d. 25 November 1918, Lower Ship Harbour.

101. Harold O'Brien, 22, d. 9 December 1918, Murphy's [*sic*] Cove.

102. William Weeks, 25, d. 1 November 1918, Ship Harbour.

103. Ray DeBay, 6 months, d. 26 November 1918, DeBay's [*sic*] Cove.

104. Edward Hartling, 21, d. 28 November 1918, Quoddy, labourer.

1919

105. Edith White, 27, d. 22 January 1919, North West Arm, housewife.

106. John Christopher, 29, d. 13 March 1919, Ketch Harbour, fisherman.

107. Eva Buchanan, 30, d. 19 March 1919, Ketch Harbour, housewife.

108. Margaret Harnish, 35, d. 7 January 1919, East Dover, housewife.

109. Daisy Hubley, 9, d. 16 February 1919, French Village.

110. Warren Boutilier, 8 months, d. 29 January 1919, Boutilier's [*sic*] Point.

111. Madge Snair, 1, d. 5 February 1919, Black Point. [*Madge Cyndeline Snair, wife of Alvin Snair. HVS, Death Register, 1919, Book 35, Page 191, Number 689.*]

112. Albert Harnish, 31, d. 10 February 1919, Hubbards, fish merchant.

113. F. Roy (male), 17, 15 February 1919, Mill Cove.

114. Ruth Jollymore, 12, d. 22 February 1919, Mill Cove.

115. Ella Boutilier, 26, d. 25 February 1919, Mill Cove.

116. Annie Pulsiver, 13, d. 21 January 1919, Beaver Bank.

117. Kathleen Webber, 35, d. 1 March 1919, Middle Sackville, schoolteacher.

118. Lucy Anderson, 54, d. 8 November 1919, Hammonds Plains, housework.

119. Howard Carroll, 20, d. 7 January 1919, Lantz Siding.

120. William Isenor, 20, d. 12 January 1919, Lantz Siding, lumberman.

121. Elias Isenor, 2 months, d. 14 January 1919, Lantz Siding.

122. Edith Horobin, 20, d. 12 January 1919, Dartmouth.

123. Charles Jackson, 17 months, d. 27 February 1919, Dartmouth.

124. Mabel Mitchell, 19, d. 24 February 1919, Dartmouth.

125. Eldred Ham, 30, d. 15 February 1919, Dartmouth, blacksmith.

126. Matilda De Young, 18, d. 1 January1919, Eastern Passage.

127. James Grant, 5, d. 10 March 1919, Preston.

128. Robert Williams, 59, d. 19 February 1919, Fall River, farmer.

129. Judith Lapierre, 45, d. 21 March 1919, Grand Desert, housewife.

130. Flora Lapierre, 16, d. 23 March 1919, Grand Desert.

131. John Chittick, 3 months, d. 7 March 1919, Sheet Harbour.

132. Harold Grono, 21, d. 16 April 1919, Glen Haven, fisherman.

133. Rosa Taunt, 33, d. 13 May 1919, West Dover.

134. Albert Gerrard, 4 months, d. 24 December 1919, Tangier.

1920

135. John J. Cornell, 45 d. 27 February 1920, Rockingham, wheelwright.

136. Colin J. McDonald, 31, d. 27 February 1920, N. S. Hospital, Dartmouth, printer.

137. Dorothy May Lueder [*also spelled Luidee, Luedes, Lueden*], 8 months, d. 28 February 1920, Eastern Passage. [*Father, John Lueder, born in Newfoundland. Mother's name, blank. Halifax County Death Register, Book 82, Page 210. HVS shows her surname as Luidee*]

138. Ethel Brunt, 19, d. 8 March 1920 in the Victoria General Hospital, Halifax, but was from Harrietsfield.

139. Florence M. Edmonds, 28, d. 9 March 1920, North West Arm, Halifax.

140. Morgan E. Christian, 39, d. 27 March 1920, Upper Prospect, fisherman.

141. Albert L. Fralick, 2 months, d. 10 March 1920, Glen Margaret.

142. Sarah Fralick, 73, d. 12 March 1920, Glen Margaret.

143. Sarah Fralick, 72, d. 19 March 1920, Hacketts Cove, housewife; "different people with different parents" [*Dr. Allan Marble, list marginalia, regarding the two Sarah Fralicks*].

144. Vella Tulloch, 32, d. 4 March 1920, Dartmouth, housewife.

145. Victor Henderson, 32, d. 17 March 1920, Dartmouth, machinist

146. Evangeline Croak, 47, d. 23 March 1920, Dartmouth, housewife.

147. Peter D. MacIntyre, 56, d. 5 March 1920, Nova Scotia Hospital, Dartmouth, coal miner.

148. Jessie MacLellan, 44, d. 6 March 1920, Nova Scotia Hospital, Dartmouth.

149. Elsie Brown, 24, d. 17 March 1920, Nova Scotia Hospital, Dartmouth.

150. Wilfred G. Lunn, 25, d. 18 March 1920, Nova Scotia Hospital, Dartmouth, chauffeur.

151. Lilla Jones, 29, d. 18 March 1920, Nova Scotia Hospital, Dartmouth.

152. Clara M. Maxim, 46, d. 19 March 1920, Nova Scotia Hospital, Dartmouth.

153. George Conrad, 32, d. 12 March 1920, Porters Lake, farmer.

154. Basil Ogilvie, 16, d. 20 March 1920, Porters Lake, labourer.

155. Charles Dahr, 12, d. 6 March 1920, Port Dufferin, student.

156. Joseph Malay Sr., 76, d. 12 March 1920, Lochaber Mines, labourer.

157. Mariah Malay, 75, d. 19 March 1920, Lochaber Mines, housewife.

158. Clarence R. Fralic, 10 months, d. 27 March 1920, Port Dufferin.

159. Orestus O'Leary, 24, d. 27 March 1920, West Quoddy, engineer.

Chapter X

HANTS COUNTY

IN HANTS COUNTY, there are at least fifty-eight confirmed deaths from the Great Influenza: forty-nine in the 1918–19 period, and nine more deaths in 1920. Dr. Allan Marble, while making a list from death registers of the Hants County dead, assumes there are others, some perhaps overlooked in the registers, as well as persons who never had death certificates returned to the registrar for their county. I have identified more potential victims, all British Expeditionary Forces soldiers, who died while training in Windsor. Only one of these military men—Edwin Albury—is on the Marble list of Hants County influenza victims. He and the other seven soldiers are all in the Hants County Death Register as pneumonia victims (see below for the evidence.) All Hants County victims' names are given at the end of this essay.

␥ In the three years of this influenza epidemic, Hants County had only minimal local newspaper reports of deaths from this disease, although at least sixty-five people would die in the county. On Dr. Marble's list of newspaper articles from the *Hants Journal*, he jotted, "NOTE: Nothing about epidemic in the Province or how severe it was in Hants County."

Most of this rather short essay, therefore, comes from modern research. The first section deals with the passing of the British Expeditionary Force soldiers who were taken by the flu during their training at Fort Edward. While seven of these early eight victims of "Spanish Influenza" (see below) don't appear on Dr. Allan Marble's lists, the West Hants Historical Society has a website which indicates they were all taken by influenza.

WEST HANTS HISTORICAL SOCIETY / POSTED ON DECEMBER 14, 2015.
␥ This post is in conjunction with our December newsletter and our upcoming June 2016 symposium on Nova Scotia Communities in the First World War....

It is well known that individuals trained at Fort Edward during the First World War but did you know that not all these soldiers survived to fight in Europe? Here is some information on some of those individuals....In October of 1918 Windsor was visited by the Spanish Influenza. It took many lives amongst the civilian population along with several soldiers, killing 9 recruits of the B.E.F. [British Expeditionary Force] in six weeks. The deaths as they were listed in the Hants Journal of that year [see that newspaper article, below]:

- October 1—Private A. Abraham Aronovitch, age 29, of Montreal, died [*sic*]. His body was shipped to Montreal for burial.
- October 1—Private Frank Kidd, age 35, born in Westham, London, England, died. He was buried in Maplewood Cemetery.
- October 4—Private Cecil Lewis, age 19, a native of Barbados, died in Payzant Memorial Hospital. He is buried at Maplewood Cemetery.
- October 15—John J. Galway, a native of Ireland, died. He is buried in St. John's Roman Catholic Cemetery.
- October 19—Private William Campbell Richardson died at the Military Hospital, age 33. He was from Jacksonville, Florida. He was buried at Maplewood Cemetery.
- October 26—Edwin Hartley Aubrey [Albury], age 18, a native of Nassau, British West Indies, succumbed to the Flu. He is buried in St. John's Roman Catholic Cemetery.
- October 26 [*sic*]—Vivian Ashley Dodd, age 20, a native of Australia, who had resided in Stockton, California, died on October 29. He is buried in Maplewood Cemetery in the Strangers lot.
- October 21—Thomas Hope died and is buried in the Strangers lot, Maplewood Cemetery.
- November 18 – James, Smith, of Vancouver, died. He is buried in Maplewood Cemetery. His death is the last recorded at Fort Edward during World War One.

West Hants Historical Society website; westhantshistoricalsociety.ca
posted December 14, 2015.

THE NECROLOGY LIST. COMPILED ESPECIALLY FOR THE *HANTS JOURNAL*.

Town of Windsor—For Six Months, Ending December 31st, 1918.

- 20. Abraham Aronovitch, B.E.F. soldier, 29, Jewish, Oct. 1

- 21. Frank Kidd, B.E.F. soldier, 35, Methodist, Oct. 1

- 24. Cecil Lewis, B.E.F. soldier, coloured, 19, C. of R. [Church of Rome], Oct. 7

- 30. John J. Galway, B.E.F. soldier, 36, R. C., Oct. 16

- 32. William Campbell Richardson, B.E.F. soldier, 33, C. of E. [Church of England, Anglican], Oct. 20

- 33. Thomas Hope, B.E.F. soldier, 19, C. of E., Oct. 22

- 34. Edwin Hartley Aubrey [Albury], B.E.F. soldier, 18 yrs. 2 mos., R. C., Oct. 27

- 36. Vivian Ashley Dodd, B.E.F. soldier, 20 yrs. 2 mo., C. of E., Oct. 29

> *Hants Journal*, Windsor, 1 January 1919, 1. [The numbers indicate their place in the overall necrology list of Hants County dead for the previous quarter year.]

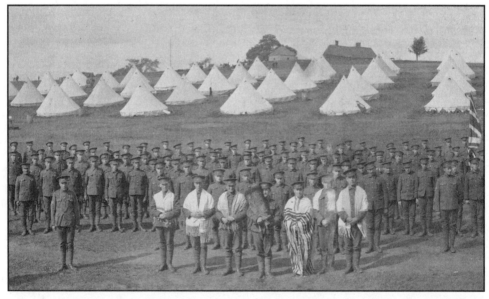

Jewish Legion "Draft" Imperial Recruit Depot—Yom Kippur 5679. New recruits' training encampment, Ft. Edward, Windsor. The year would be 1918. Thanks to Eli Diamond for the year conversion. (*The Army Museum Halifax Citadel*)

☞ No cause of death is given in this published necrology list, perhaps to protect the families' privacy. There is no entry for a James Smith in this list, either. In order to clarify information on these B. E. F. soldiers, recorded as influenza victims on the West Hants website, I searched other sources, primarily the death registers, for more detail.

- Abraham Aronovitch [or Aaronovich?]. The Hants County Death Register, 1918, Book 35, Page 505, Number 423, says he died at 'P. M. Hospital' (Payzant Memorial), Windsor. Cause of death: "Double Lobar Pneumonia, Heart Failure." The HVS Search Engine calls him 'Aronoditch, Abraham,' but the original death record, in cursive, is clearly 'Aronovich, Abraham.' I don't know where the website got the name "A. Abraham Aronovitch."

  Abraham Aronovitch was a member of the Jewish Legion: "The Jewish Legion (1917–1921) is an unofficial name used to refer to five battalions of Jewish volunteers, the 38th to 42nd (Service) Battalions of the Royal Fusiliers, raised in the British Army to fight against the Ottoman Empire during the First World War."
  en.wikipedia.org/wiki/Jewish_Legion

- A more famous member of this legion was a man named David Green. David Ben-Gurion (born David Green), Israel's first prime minister, trained with hundreds of other members of the Jewish Legion at Fort Edward "in the Annapolis Valley" [in Windsor] in preparation for the British Army's plan to liberate Israel from Turkish rule during the First World War. At right [refers to a photo in the original article], the 39th Battalion of the Jewish Legion at Fort Edward in Windsor (Army Museum, Halifax Citadel). "In Windsor, one of the great dreams of my life—to serve as a soldier in a Jewish Unit to fight for the liberation of the Land of Israel (as we always called Palestine)—became a reality," Ben-Gurion wrote in a letter to Windsor's mayor three years after he left the prime minister's job. "I will never forget Windsor where I received my first training as a soldier and where I became a corporal."
  Halifax Chronicle Herald online: thechronicleherald.ca/thegreatwar/1236057-nova-scotia-and-the-jews-of-the-firstworldwar#.Wvu2MaTRXX4 [link now inactive].

- Private Frank Kidd was born in Westham, London, England. Hants County Death Register, 1918, Book 35, Page 505, Number 424, gives cause of death as "Double Lobar Pneumonia, Heart Failure."

- Private Cecil Lewis, born in Barbados, died in Payzant Memorial Hospital. Hants County Death Register, 1918, Book 35, Page 505, Number 427, gives cause of death as "Pneumonia, Heart Failure."

- John J. Galway was born in County Cork, Ireland. Hants County Death Register, 1918, Book 35, Page 506, Number 433, gives cause of death as "Pneumonia, Heart Failure."

- Private William Campbell Richardson had lived in Jacksonville, Florida; a married soldier, born in Jamaica, he died in Fort Edward Barracks, 20 October. Return of death by Sgt. Harris B. Weinstein. Doctor: O. B. Kelly. Hants County Death Register, 1918, Book 35, Page 507, Number 435, gives cause of death yet again as "Pneumonia, Heart Failure."

- Edwin Hartley Albury, only 18, was born in Nassau, British West Indies. Hants County Death Register, 1918, Book 35, Page 505, Number 437, gives his cause of death as "Influenza & Pneumonia, Heart Failure."

- Vivian Ashley Dodd, born in Australia, then residing in Stockton, California, was only 20 when he died. Hants County Death Register, 1918, Book 35, Page 507, Number 439, gives his cause of death as "Pneumonia, Heart-Failure."

- Thomas Hope was born in Eleuthra, Bahamas. Hants County Death Register, 1918, Book 35, Page 507, Number 436, gives his cause of death as "Pneumonia, Enteritis."

☞ One of these eight soldiers died of "Double Lobar Pneumonia, Heart Failure," six of them from simple "Pneumonia, Heart Failure," and one of "Pneumonia, Enteritis." Only one single person has "Influenza" as a cause of death included with the ubiquitous "Pneumonia, Heart Failure." So where did the West Hants website get its information that all these deaths were a result of the influenza pandemic? I haven't been able to find out. Nor could I find any trace of the final death at Fort Edward during the First World War, that of a "James Smith of Vancouver...buried in Maplewood Cemetery." While he appears on the West Hants website list as an influenza victim, this man has no death record accessible through the HVS database; nor does he appear on Dr. Marble's list of Hants County influenza victims, extracted from the original records. He is not in the necrology list of the period, leaving us another website mystery yet to be solved.

TWO B. E. F. RECRUITS DIED OF PNEUMONIA

Pte John J. Galaway [*sic*], a native of Ireland, and stationed at the Depot here, died of pneumonia on Wednesday last, following an attack of influenza....

Pte. Wm. Richardson, colored, aged 33 years 4 months, and whose home is in Jacksonville, Florida, passed away at 4 o'clock on Sunday, at the Military Hospital on Gerrish St. Pte. Richardson's funeral took place at 2 p.m. on Tuesday.

Hants Journal, 23 October 1918, 1.

Other Hants County Deaths

William Faulkner McLellan, aged 85 years, 1 month; widower, farmer, Cambridge, Hants County, NS.
Born: Tennecape, NS. Died 8 October 1918, in Halifax, NS.

Information from Linda Littlejohn, Parrsborough Shore Historical Society.

SITUATION STILL SERIOUS

Various rumors in circulation on our streets re the influenza situation led us to enquire of Health Officer Bissett on Monday, as to whether or not public meetings of any kind would be permitted during the coming week. Dr. Bissett emphatically stated that no public meetings would be permitted this week. The situation still remains serious, and every precaution should be taken to safe-guard the health of the people. The Health Officer's report covering a period from Saturday a. m. to Sunday evening, showed that twenty-one new cases had developed; (6 military and 15 civilians), and one death was reported on Sunday.

Hants Journal, Windsor, 23 October 1918, 4.

OBITUARY.

On October 21st, there passed away at Eastern Passage, Halifax, Alfred Brightman, in his forty fifth year. While working with the Nova Scotia Construction Company, Mr. Brightman was seized with Spanish Influenza, which caused his death. His brother, Mr. James Brightman, Maple Grove, Hants, Co. with whom he made his home, was with him during his last hours. He leaves a sorrowing mother, two brothers, and one sister of Andover, Mass, besides James, already mentioned.

Truro Daily News, 15 November 1918, 11. Courtesy the Colchester Historeum.

DEATH OF PTE. HENRY G. ALLISON

The death occurred at Vancouver, Oct. 28th of Pte. Henry Gordon Allison in the thirty-eighth year of his age. Pte. Allison was born at Upper Kennetcook, Hants County, N.S., being the eldest son the late John Allison. When about eighteen years of age, Gordon Allison went West, and for a time worked in the lumbering woods, for W.S. Cook, lumberman, of Vancouver. He was then appointed foreman, for the Mainland Transfer Co. of Vancouver, which position he retained until he enlisted in a British Columbia battalion of overseas service. He served in France for about two years, being wounded nine times and gassed once. Becoming physically unfit for military service, he was sent back to Vancouver, and discharged. He was studying engineering when he contracted influenza, of which he died. The body was buried in Vancouver.

Truro Daily News, 21 December 1918, 2. Courtesy the Colchester Historeum, Truro.

DETH [*sic*] OF FRANK MACAULAY AT TRURO NOV. 23RD

The deth of Frank MacAuley, aged 32 years, occurred at the Emergency Hospital, Willow Street, on November 23rd. His home was in East Noel, Hants Co. where the remains were forwarded Monday afternoon for burial. Mr. MacAuley was attack with "Flu" which later develop into pneumonia.

Truro Daily News, 25 November 1918, 4. Transcribed exactly as printed.

POPLAR GROVE

We are called upon to record the sad death of Mrs. Charles Burke, which shocked the community on Tuesday evening, Jan. 7th, 1919. Leaving six small children—one baby just two weeks old, and a loving husband to mourn their loss. The deceased was 37 years of age, a woman of sterling character, and faithful mother to her children. Mr. Burke has the sympathy of every living soul in the neighbourhood in which he resides. Also among friends and relatives in other places. Mrs. Burke died of Influenza, followed by pneumonia. The funeral took place on Thursday, interment at the Presbyterian cemetery. The floral offerings were very numerous.

The schools here opened on Tuesday, Jan. 14th.

All cases of influenza are gone—we trust forever.

Churches all opened on Sunday, Jan. 12th.

Hants Journal, 15 January 1919, 1. Transcribed exactly as printed.

J.A. FRASER, FORMERLY OF ELMSDALE, DIED IN SEATTLE, DEC. 10TH, OF INFLUENZA

The Vancouver Daily Province states that after having escaped death by cancelling his reservation on the ill-fated Princess Sophia, J. Austin Fraser, a porminent [*sic*] lawyer of Dawson and formerly a member of the Yukon legislature, deid [*sic*] on the morning of December 10th at the home of his sister-in-law, Mrs. J. N. McLean, of pneumonia, following influenza, now prevailing in Seattle, and of very severe type. Mr. Fraser had come to Seattle to take his family to Vancouver where he proposed to practise law. He was 32 years of age. Mr. Fraser has many friends and relatives in Nova Scotia. He was formerly a student at the Halifax Academy. He left his old home at Elmsdale, Hants Co., 14 years ago, and had achieved much distinction as a lawyer in the Yukon since his admission to the bar in 1914.

Hants Journal, 15 January 1919, 1.

A LIFE OF SERVICE
The following tribute is paid the late Mrs. Meek, a native of Hants Co., who lately passed away in Alberta. Mrs. Meek was the wife of Rev. J. G. Meek, a former pastor of Noel Presbyterian church:

Mrs. Meek, wife of Rev. J. G. Meek, of Willowdale, Alberta, died last month [December 1918], deeply regretted by a host of friends. Mrs. Meek was born in Centre Burlington, Hants Co. She began teaching when seventeen years old, and taught steadily until, as she naively put it, 'she entered the ministry.' For ten years she was the wife, companion and trusted counsellor of her husband, who now misses her sorely as he tries to carry on alone. In April 1911, Mr. and Mrs. Meek came to Acme, where they passed twenty strenuous months on that difficult mission field. Then came the call from Willowdale, Edwell, and Hill End, in November 1918. In this new change, Mrs. Meek made use of her gifts as a teacher to carry on the education of a number of girls who had completed the public school course, but for whom the way was not open to continue through high school. During the first three years in Willowdale, she led the 'Whatever' class of young ladies, and helped to develop a missionary spirit which will doubtless continue through life. She was also a central figure in everything that made for a better community life. This work was carried on under the strain of increasing ill health. Patiently and courageously she bore with pain and weariness and kept up her interest in the world movements. She was constant in her correspondence with the boys at the front, many of whom were her loyal friends. She died a victim of influenza. –Toronto Presbyterian.

Hants Journal, 29 January 1919, 8.

DEATH IN A LUMBER CAMP AT ELMSDALE
On Tuesday, Jan. 21st, word was received by Mr. and Mrs. Charles Graves, Nicholsville, that their son, Abner, was very ill of influenza in the camp at Elmsdale, Hants County, where he had been working. His father left on the first train from Kentville, but arrived too late, his son having passed away but a few hours previous. On Friday the body was brought to Aylesford, where the funeral took place after the arrival of the morning express. Rev. Mr. Hicken conducted a short service at the grave.

Truro Daily News, 19 February 1919, 2. Courtesy the Colchester Historeum, Truro.

INFLUENZA DEATHS AT WALTON, HANTS CO.

CHEVERIE, March 31. The death took place at Walton, on the 26th, of Mrs. Howard Lake, due to influenza. At one o'clock the following morning, her husband also died. He was seized with illness at his brother's funeral, in Brookville, a week previous. Dr. Hennigar, of Cheverie, has been attending over 100 cases of influenza in Walton, the first case coming from Halifax. Mrs. Lake's mother was also dangerously ill.

Halifax Evening Mail, 31 March 1919, 3.

REMAINS OF MAN AND WIFE OCCUPY ONE GRAVE

As an unusually sad circumstance of the 'Flu' epidemic at Walton was the death on the same day, March 26 [Howard Lake died in the very early hours of the following day], of Mr. and Mrs. Howard Lake. The death occurred within two hours of each other, and both were laid away in a double grave on March 27th. The Rev. Mr. Rebinson [*sic*] officiated at the funeral services.

Truro Daily News, April 1919, 2. Courtesy the Colchester Historeum, Truro.

DEATH OF MRS. ELLEN WEBB

The death of Mrs. Ellen Webb, wife of Robt. Webb, Noel, Hants Co., occurred on Saturday, March 6th. Influenza followed by pneumonia was the cause of her death. The deceased was 60 years of age, and is survived by a sorrowing husband, seven sons and four daughters—all of whom were present at the funeral. Two brothers, and four sisters also survive.

Hants Journal, Windsor, 17 March 1920, 4.

OBITUARY. Clarence Fox. There passed away at his home here early Saturday afternoon, March 20th, Clarence, only son of Mr. and Mrs. Edward Fox, aged 18 years. Clarence had been a great sufferer since he was four years old. He was patient through all his affliction, surrounded by tender and ceaseless care through all the years. About two weeks ago, he was the victim of 'flu' and gradually grew weaker until death released him from his sufferings. The death of Clarence is a blow to the father and mother and sister Luella and half-sister Mrs. Frank Pugsley, who, while mourning the loss of their loved one, feel he is so much better off, away from all pain.

Hants Journal, 24 March 1920, 5.

So Hants County had fifty-eight confirmed deaths from the Great Influenza. But what about the seven soldiers who died from "pneumonia" at Fort Edward? It would seem likely that influenza *was* the root cause of all their deaths, as they were all young, fit, and ill only a short while. We know that influenzas, then and now, kill by triggering pneumonias. We know that there was at least one case of influenza at the fort; there were others in the town of Windsor outside the fort. There were no other illnesses listed as killing anyone else at Fort Edward during this short time period, between October 1 and November 18. If influenza *had* become pneumonia and thereby killed these seven men, it would bring the death total for Hants County to sixty-five.

HANTS COUNTY VITAL STATISTICS, DEATH REGISTER, BOOKS 35, 86

1918

1. Edwin Albury, 18, d. 27 October 1918, Windsor, soldier.

2. Kenneth Wynott, 22, d. 11 December 1918, Windsor, labourer.

3. Charles Underwood, 37, d. 20 October 1918, Mapleton, Hants Co., quarryman.

4. Mary Vaughan, 14, d. 2 December 1918, Windsor Forks, student.

5. Theresa O'Leary, 45, d. 4 December 1918, Windsor Forks, domestic.

6. Catherine Flemming, 1 yr., d. 24 December 1918, Hantsport.

7. Alonzo Coburn, 41, d. 29 September 1918, Summerville, sea captain.

8. Mary Crossley, 32, d. 2 November 1918, Cheverie, housewife.

9. Beulah Lake, 24, d. 7 November 1918, Kempt Shore, housewife.

10. Perry Brown, 16, d. 6 November 1918, Cheverie.

11. Wilson Mills, 2, d. 13 November 1918, Bramber.

12. Juaneta Lake, 1 month, d. 15 November 1918, Cheverie.

13. Madge Brown, 3, d. 20 November 1918, Bramber.

14. Jennie McLellan, 17, d. 10 December 1918, Cambridge, Hants County, housework.

15. Frank Davis, 36, d. 20 December 1918, Newport, farmer.

16. Francis Chambers, 68, d. 26 December 1918, Newport, farmer.

17. Frederick Maxner, 54, d. 23 October 1918, Windsor, farmer.

18. Mrs. Florence Gray, 36, d. 23 October 1918, Newport Station, housewife.

19. Sadie Kelly, 8 months, d. 28 October 1918, Wentworth.

20. Lillie Kelly, 3, d. 29 October 1918, Wentworth.

21. Ralph Kelly, 2, d. 30 October 1918, Wentworth.

22. Brenton Clements, 22, d. 11 November 1918, Mapleton, labourer.

23. Lavenia Riley, 1, d. 24 November 1918, Mapleton.

24. Helen McPhee, 14, d. 19 November 1918, West Cove, student.

25. Minnie Wheadon, 1, d. 16 November 1918, Walton.

26. Maggie McCulloch, 16, d. 25 October 1918, Noel Road, student.

1919

27. Mary Fudge, 88, d. 1 March 1919, Windsor, domestic.

28. Louise MacDonald, 23, d. 2 January 1919, West Gore, nurse.

29. Eva Lake, 34, d. 26 March 1919, Walton, housewife.

30. Howard Lake, 34, d. 27 March 1919, Walton, labourer.

31. Matilda Sanford, 75, d. 30 March 1919, Walton, housekeeper.

32. Frank MacAuleay, 32, d. 21 November 1918, East Noel, farmer.

33. Eral Miller, 3, d. 22 December 1918, Northfield.

34. Fred Allison, 15, d. 3 February 1919, Five Mile River.

35. Rodney Moody, 25, d. 4 February 1919, Wallace, Cumberland County, teamster. [*Recorded in the Hants County Death Register, Book 35, Page 567, Number 592, listed as born and residing in "Wallace, Cumberland County." No place of death given. HVS search engine lists him as dying in "Wallace, Cumberland, Hants County," which is erroneous. There is no record in the Cumberland County Death Register for a Rodney Moody, so he must*

have died while in Hants County.]

36. Emily Cook, 60, d. 12 February 1919, Five Mile River, housewife.

37. John L. MacDonald, 32, d. 27 January 1919, Indian Reserve, Shubenacadie, [*axe?*] handle maker.

38. John Cleary, 75, d. 5 January 1918 [*sic; 1919*], Enfield, farmer. [*Recorded in the Hants County Death Register, Book 35, Page 571, Number 602, as born in Antrim, Halifax County, residence Enfield. There is no mention in the original death record as to where he died, but the date on the original return is given as 1919. The HVS search engine headlines him as dying in Windsor, but there is no evidence for it in the original register, and this could be merely that he died in Windsor District.*]

39. Abner Graves, 20, d. 22 January 1919, Nicholsville, Kings County, lumberman. [*Recorded in the Hants County Death Register for 1919 as born in Nicholsville, residing in Nicholsville, Kings County. He was buried in Aylesford. There is no mention in the original document as to where he died. The HVS search engine headlines him as dying in Windsor (District), but there is no evidence for it in the original register. Abner Graves has two death records. One was issued in Hants County (see above). Record 2 was issued in Kings County (Book 40, Page 489, Number 1465). All the details are the same, with the exception of his occupation being given as a farmer in Record 2, and the undertaker's name as S. J. Ray (Hants), as opposed to Jas. Logan (Kings). On both records, his father is Charles Graves. The doctor's name, R. D. MacLellan, is the same. Obviously, Abner died in Hants County, and one undertaker prepared his body to be shipped home to Kings County, then another undertaker took over for the Aylesford burial, and both filed returns of his death to their respective county registries. For clarification, see the newspaper*

account of his death, above.] *HVS, Hants County Death Register, 1919, Book 35, Page 571, Number 605.*

40. Annie Aylward, 27, d. 31 May 1919, Falmouth, domestic.

41. Stella Lake, 8, d. 21 May 1919, Summerville.

42. Viola Lake, 6, d. 22 May 1919, Summerville.

43. Elsie Dimock [*Dimmock?*], 14, d. 10 April 1919, Scotch Village.

44. Gerald Lake, 4 months, d. 8 April 1919, Walton.

45. Frances Porter, 87, d. 1 May 1919, Upper Selma, housewife.

46. Henry Miller, 87, d. 9 May 1919, Upper Kennetcook, farmer.

47. Nicholas Singer, 75, d. 5 April 1919, Kennetcook, farmer.

48. Anthony Barron, 43, d. 26 May 1919, Rawdon Gold Mine, farmer.

49. Morris Young, 11, d. 5 June 1919, Burlington.

1920

50. Marjorie Levy, 5 months, d. 27 February 1920, Windsor.

51. George Kilcup, 1 year 8 months, d. 1 March 1920, Windsor.

52. Ada Stabb, 52, d. 3 March 1920, Windsor, domestic.

53. Charlotte Anderson, 4, d. 3 March 1920, Windsor.

54. Reuben Porter, 74, d. 5 March 1920, Windsor, carpenter.

55. Harold S. Ross, 2, d. 8 March 1920, Windsor.

56. Allie Bacon, 49, d. 11 March 1920, Windsor, domestic.

57. Dorothy M. Bell, 3, d. 11 March 1920, Windsor.

58. Ellen Webb, 60, d. 6 March 1920, Noel, housekeeper. [*HVS, Death Register, Book 86, Page 154, gives her cause of death*

as "Double Broncho Pneumonia and Pleurisy," with contributory cause of death "Influenza (epidemic)."]

Taken from Dr. Allan Marble's list of deaths made using the originals in the county death registers. This list does not include the following (possible) influenza deaths of British Expeditionary Force soldiers dying of Spanish Influenza/Pneumonia at Fort Edward, Windsor, Hants County (as follows).

Necrology List. Compiled Especially for the *Hants Journal.* Town of Windsor—For Six Months, Ending December 31st, 1918.

1. Abraham Aronovitch, B.E.F. soldier, 29, Jewish, Oct. 1.
2. Frank Kidd, B.E.F. soldier, 35, Methodist, Oct. 1.
3. Cecil Lewis, B.E.F. soldier, coloured, 19, C. of R. [*Church of Rome*], Oct. 7
4. John J. Galway, B.E.F. soldier, 36, R. C., Oct. 16.
5. William Campbell Richardson, B.E.F. soldier, 33, C. of E. [*Church of England*], Oct. 20.
6. Thomas Hope, B.E.F. soldier, 19, C. of E., Oct. 22.
7. Vivian Ashley Dodd, B.E.F. soldier, 20 yrs. 2 mo., C. of E., Oct. 29.

Hants Journal, Windsor, 1 January 1919, 1. See above, for their Hants Death Register records. Their deaths from pneumonia, if accepted as an influenza-triggered pneumonia, would give a total of sixty-five influenza deaths in Hants County.

Chapter XI

INVERNESS COUNTY

THERE WERE NINETY-THREE confirmed deaths in Inverness County from the Great Influenza of 1918–20.

 EPIDEMIC NOW UNDER CONTROL

Hundred Cases of Influenza In Inverness County

The inhabitants of the Cape Breton coast in the vicinity of Point Tupper have been seriously alarmed over an epidemic of influenza in Inverness. At their urgent request, Dr. Hattie, the provincial medical officer, personally investigated the

	DEATHS		
Form H.	District No.	County of	
	No. 1149	Nr. 1150	No. 1151
	Surname first	Surname first	Surname first
Name of Deceased	McDonald John	McDonald Mrs John	McIsaac Flora
Sex	Male	Female	Female
Date of Death	Dec 26th 1918	Jan 17th 1919	Feb 12th
Age	24 years	71 years	56 years
Residence Street and No. or P.O. Address	Little Judique in Inverness Co NS	Little Judique Inverness Co NS	Judique Inverness Co
Occupation	Labourer	Housewife	Domestic
Single, Married or Widowed	Single	Widow	Single
If Single give Name of Father / If Married give Name of Husband	McDonald James		
Where Born	Little Judique NS	P.E. Island	Judique NS
Cause of Death Primary / Immediate	Epidemic Influenza Broncho Pneumonia	Dropsey	Dropsey
Length of Illness	6 days		one year
Religious Denomination	Catholic	Catholic	Catholic
Race of Deceased	White	White	White
Name of Physician in attendance	D McChisholm MD	D McChisholm MD	C S Campbell
Name of Undertaker			
Place of Burial Cemetery / at	St Peters Port Hood	St Andrews Port Hood	St Andrews Judique
Name of Person making Return	McDonald James	McDonald Daniel A	McDougall Alex
Date of Return	Jan 1st 1919	Apr 4th 1919	Feb 15th
REMARKS	3	3	3

Death record for John McDonald, 24, a labourer from Little Judique. (*Nova Scotia Archives*)

situation. Last night he received a message from the three principal doctors of the afflicted district, stating that, while there had been 100 cases of influenza in the past two weeks, only four deaths had resulted, and that the epidemic was now under control, and rapidly waning. Although it is popularly supposed to be Spanish influenza, Dr. Hattie says that there is as yet no evidence to prove that such is the case, and that the plain or garden influenza is at present very prevalent throughout various sections of Nova Scotia.

Halifax Morning Chronicle, 9 September 1918, 2.

☞ Note the really early date. Dr. Marble felt that Inverness likely had been infected in late August or early September, by a soldier, Murdo M. Kennedy, perhaps returning from Europe or the United States. Kennedy died September 3 of influenza, after an illness of seven days. Wherever he had caught it, he came down with influenza on August 28. John D. McLellan died of pneumonia on September 11, 1918, after an illness of twelve days, possibly triggered by influenza. He fell sick on August 31. Marjorie McDonald died two days prior to Murdo's death. She too is listed as dying of influenza, and had been ill only thirty-six hours, becoming sick around September 1. These three people are clustered on the same page, one right after another, in the death register. All lived in the town of Inverness; all were Roman Catholic. All were young adults who died fairly swiftly—in Marjorie's cases, after only thirty-six hours. It's possible they caught it from Murdo, perhaps at church.

HVS, Death Register, Inverness County, Year 1918, Book 43 Page 290, Number 931 (Kennedy), 932 (McDonald), and 933 (McLellan).

☞ Inverness County lost many more people to this influenza, when a stronger form began raging in late November. One only has to see these extracts from Dr. Allan Marble's list, covering a few communities around the Margaree, to see the extent of the tragedy. Families lost not one, not two, but often way more members within a few days or weeks:

Arsenault, Dimian	09	East Margaree	18 DEC 1918	days ill: 05
Arsenault, Mrs. Simon	72	East Margaree	30 DEC 1918	days ill: 14
Arseneau, Joseph	8m	East Margaree	20 DEC 1918	days ill: 08
Arsenault, Leo	04	Belle Cote	28 DEC 1918	days ill: 07
Chaisson, Alexander	30	Margaree Harbour	26 DEC 1918	days ill: 03
Chaisson, Annie	02	Belle Cote	14 DEC 1918	days ill: 14
Chaisson, Beatrice	07	Belle Cote	31 DEC 1918	days ill: 21
Chaisson, Florence	8m	Belle Cote	11 DEC 1918	days ill: 07
Chaisson, John	03	Belle Cote	13 DEC 1918	days ill: 07
Chaisson, Lillie	06	Belle Cote	13 DEC 1918	days ill: 14
Chaisson, Lucy	6m	Belle Cote	14 DEC 1918	days ill: 07
Chaisson, Lucy Ann	04	Belle Cote	16 DEC 1918	days ill: 07

Chaisson, Mary	18m	Belle Cote	14 DEC 1918	days ill: 07
Cormier, Catherine	12	Belle Cote	21 DEC 1918	days ill: 04
Doucet, Mrs. Simon	46	Belle Cote	22 DEC 1918	days ill: n/a
Gallant, Margaret	7m	Belle Cote	13 FEB 1919	days ill: 14
Gillis, Dougald	17	Upper Margaree	30 OCT 1918	days ill: 05
Gillis, John	15	Upper Margaree	19 JAN 1919	days ill: 3m
Gillis, Minnie	19	Upper Margaree	17 JAN 1919	days ill: 05
LeBlanc, Amelia	38	Belle Cote	17 DEC 1918	days ill: 07
LeBlanc, Caroline	74	Belle Cote	25 DEC 1918	days ill: 14
LeBlanc, Flora	57	Margaree Forks	15 MAR 1920	days ill: 15
LeBlanc, Germain	03	Belle Cote	19 DEC 1918	days ill: 07
LeBlanc, Margaret	17	Belle Cote	16 DEC 1918	days ill: 07
LeBlanc, Mrs. Patrick	31	East Margaree	26 DEC 1918	days ill: 09
LeBlanc, Placide	80	Belle Cote	17 DEC 1918	days ill: 07
LeBlanc, Mrs. Thomas	45	Margaree Harbour	13 DEC 1918	days ill: 07
LeBlanc, Wilfred	03	Margaree Harbour	14 DEC 1918	days ill: 07
McDonald, Agnes	31	Little Judique	24 DEC 1918	days ill: 07
McDonald, Daniel	14	Little Judique	27 DEC 1918	days ill: 06
McDonald, John	24	Little Judique	26 DEC 1918	days ill: 06
McDougall, Sarah	23	Margaree Forks	29 NOV 1918	days ill: 14
McKinnon, Mary	30	Margaree Harbor	29 Dec. 1918	days ill: 03
McLelland, Mary Ann	25	Southwest Margaree	10 Oct. 1918	days ill: 10
McLeod, Flora	21	Upper Southwest M.	18 January 1919	days ill: 09
Murray, Mrs. Malcolm	69	N.E. Margaree	1 January 1920	days ill: 08
Stubbart, Germain	70	Belle Cote	22 DEC 1918	days ill: 07
Timmons, Douglas	08	Margaree Forks	05 April 1920	days ill: 10

Compiled from Dr. Allan Marble's list of Inverness County deaths; used by permission.

☞ Just look at the Chaissons of Belle Côte alone: between the December 11 and the end of that month, 1918, they lost nine relatives, including three in one day (December 14).

☞ This kind of list is extremely telling. Since newspaper coverage of the flu's progress in Inverness County is almost nonexistent and all we have was published elsewhere, we are somewhat hindered in tracking the progress of this disease through the county. There is at least one account, however, that describes a mere three of the ninety-three tragedies that took place during this time. As it is truly in stories of individuals that this period in Nova Scotia's history becomes real, we are exceedingly lucky to have the tragic and yet very dramatic memoir by Rannie Gillis, about the time when "Spanish flu" took three of the eighteen Gillis children from Gillisdale. It shows the horror of the influenza epidemic so much more clearly than mere statistics or lists ever could.

Rannie Gillis Website Article

She was young, still only a teenager, and appeared to be in the best of health. Had she lived she would have been my aunt Minnie, but she died suddenly of the flu, in a private home in Inverness, on the west coast of Cape Breton. She was only 19 years old.

Mary (Minnie) Gillis was born on July 31, 1899, on my father's family farm in Gillisdale, Upper Margaree, Inverness County. It was a large family, with eight girls and 10 boys. Out of the 18 children, aunt Minnie was No. 8, while my father was the second youngest. When she died, my father, Ambrose James, was only six years old.

Aunt Minnie was teaching school in rural Saskatchewan when she was called home at the end of Dec. 1918, because her younger brother Dougald had died of the flu. He was only 17. Another younger brother, Alex, was also sick. Minnie, who was travelling by train, fell ill in Montreal, and was very sick when she arrived in Inverness. She was taken to a hotel, placed in a room with no heat, and word was sent to the family farm in Upper Margaree.

My uncle Jack and my grandmother Margaret took five hours to travel by horse and sleigh from the farm to the town of Inverness (20 miles) in heavy snow. They took aunt Minnie from the hotel to a cousin's home in the town, where she died the next day. She was buried the following morning in south-west Margaree. One hour after the family returned home from her funeral, a younger brother named John Joseph died, also as a result of the flu. He was only 15....In less than one month, two brothers and a sister had died from the flu. My uncle Dougald was 17, aunt Minnie was 19, while my uncle John Joseph was 15. All three had been in excellent health, when they suddenly, and without warning, started to feel sick. None of the three lasted longer than five days after the onset of their illness, and all died from severe respiratory problems. According to older relatives, they had trouble breathing, and more than likely died from pneumonia, or related conditions.

Surprisingly, my uncle Alex survived his near-death experience. He was 18 when he suddenly became very sick, in early Dec. 1918. Although he later lived in "The Boston States," he and I got to know each other in the late 1960s, after I graduated from Saint Francis Xavier University. Once I had my own car, I went up to the Boston area quite frequently, but he would never talk about his survival from perhaps the most deadly plague in the history of mankind.

My uncle Alex had survived the Spanish flu, a worldwide pandemic that killed an estimated 21 million people in 1918–1919. (Some estimates go as high as 50 million fatalities!) [Some say 50 to 100 million.] A shocking statistic, especially when you consider that the total number of dead and wounded from the First World War only came to about 15 million.

It is believed that at least 50,000 Canadians died from the Spanish flu. It seems that the virus was brought back to Canada by troops returning from the First World War, and made its way into even the remotest communities. A number of isolated villages in Quebec and Labrador were almost totally exterminated by the disease. It got its name, so the story goes, because it killed several million people in Spain, in one month.

Cape Breton Post, website article by Rannie Gillis, published Feb 18, 2010 at midnight; updated Oct 02, 2017 at 11:03 A.M.

THE LATE DAN C . MCLEAN
Promising Young East Lake Ainslie Man Passes Away (From a Correspondent)

The community of East Lake Ainslie was saddened when the news went around of the death of Dan C. McLean Jr., son of John J. McLean, elder. It felt the blow keenly because he was at the threshold of life, being but 18 years, 10 months when the call came. Our young friend had always been at home with his parents. He attended the public schools at his home and was looking forward to a professional career…. He died on Nov. 8th from pneumonia following influenza. Rev. M. McKillop conducted the funeral service. To his father and mother, his three older brothers (who are on active service in the American army) and three young sisters at home, the whole community of Lake Ainslie and the many friends of the family elsewhere extends its heart felt sympathy.

Sydney Daily Post, 10 December 1918, 1.

INFLUENZA AT MARBLE MOUNTAIN
There are about 100 cases of influenza in Marble Mountain [Inverness County], it is reported, and a plea for outside medical assistance has been made. Medical Officer MacAuley [of Sydney] had been requested to go to the community, but he was unable to leave the city.

Sydney Daily Post, 16 December 1918, 5.

WILLIAM YOUNG, L'ARDOISE, JANUARY 7

A death occurred at Marble Mountain which was particularly sad. William Young of Sydney Mines, employed by the Dominion Coal company, and who was nursing influenza patients at Marble Mountain, contracted the disease and succumbed after a few days' illness. Only three months ago he had married Miss Lillian Sampson, youngest daughter of George J. Sampson at Lower L'Ardoise. His young bride was notified of his illness and hastened to his bedside. All that medical aid could do was done but he passed away. His father and grandfather were also present at the last and with Mrs. Young accompanied the remains to Sydney Mines where interment took place.

Halifax Evening Mail, 8 January 1919, 2.

☞ The Second Wave of the Great Influenza hit Inverness County sometime in late summer. Alexander LeBlanc, a 6-year-old, became ill on July 22, 1918. His was the earliest death, taking place on August 12. Naturally, we do not know how many people may have taken ill before Alexander did, and who survived. In Inverness County, this Second Wave lasted slightly over a year. Two people died in July 1919: Louise LeBlanc of Eastern Harbour, and Donald McDonald, an elderly inmate of the Inverness County Asylum. The final death of this wave came on August 22, 1919, when Alex McLean, 71, a married farmer in Scotsville, finally died of "Influenza"; he had been ill with it for "six months." The record also shows he was Presbyterian, buried in East Lake Ainslie. His return of death was sent in by a J. Morris McLean, so his name was definitely McLean, even thought the HVS search engine has it as McLeon.

HVS, Inverness County Death Register, 1919, Book 43, Page 457, Number 1330,

☞ Dr. Jim St. Clair, a teacher and storyteller, a genealogist and champion of Cape Breton heritage, has sent in this wonderful information about some of the souls on Dr. Allan Marble's Inverness County list. Without his research, this would have been a very sparse county essay indeed. The following twenty-one paragraphs were submitted to this project by Dr. St. Clair:

✉ Mrs. Donald Campbell, Catherine (Beaton) Campbell, aged 70, Mabou Mines. She was the daughter of Alexander Beaton of the "Mason" Beatons of Mabou Mines, and Mary (Campbell) Beaton. Her husband, Donald Campbell, was the son of Darby and Ann (MacNeil) Campbell of Jamesville, Iona. He came to the Mabou Mines area to work in the gypsum mining operation, and operated a farm as well, located on the hill overlooking the wharf at Finlay Point. Donald and Catherine Campbell had three children, from whom there are descendants in the Mabou area today. It is a tradition in the family that Catherine was infected with the bug when she went to assist her daughter who was married at West Mabou, as she came down with the illness only several days after her return home. They were speakers of Gaelic and were Roman Catholic.

✉ Dan Campbell McLean/MacLean of East Lake [Ainsley] died at age 18. He was the son of John and Catherine MacLean. It is a tradition that people would not go into the MacLean house at the time of the wake in fear of being infected, but viewed the remains through a window, outside of which they stood. The family was a farming family and Gaelic was their preferred language. The family were Presbyterians.

✉ Catherine "Katie" MacLean, who died at age 35, was born in 1883 in Stewartdale, Whycocomagh. Her parents were Hugh and Jane MacLean. Her father died before she did, between 1901 and 1911. The family had at least three children and adopted three or four children. They attended the MacLean Church of Stewartdale and were proficient in Gaelic. It appears that Katie had worked away for several years in "the Boston States" where she had several friends, also from the Stewartdale section of Whycocomagh. But she is at home on the 1911 census, perhaps to be supportive of her widowed mother.

✉ Alexander McDonell, born April 1892, the son of Dan (Donald) and Catherine (Gillis) McDonell, of S.W. Mabou Ridge. According to the census record, he did not have siblings, at least at home. Gaelic speaking, they were members of a large family from Lochaber, Scotland, and were Roman Catholic. The family lived on a remote farm which has had not residents for more than sixty years. The area where they lived would be called Alpine Ridge today.

✉ Frank Smith of Smithville, Mabou, a community between Hillsborough (Mabou) and Lake Ainslie. He was the second of eight children of Thomas and Minnie (aka Melinda) (Burton) Smith. His mother was from Margaree, and his father was a descendant of the first immigrant settlers on Port Hood Island. They were from Cape Cod area, Massachusetts and arrived in Cape Breton in 1786 or 1787. He was 29 years old. The family had a large farm and were members of the Baptist Church, located on the border between Glendyer and Hillsborough. He is buried in the small cemetery near the location of the former church.

✉ Hannah Smith, Smithville, age ca. 78, was unmarried and lived at the time of her death in the house of her brother, Benjamin Smith, and his wife Margaret (McEffery) Smith. She was the daughter of Benjamin and Jennie (McDougall) Smith. Jennie was from Musquodoboit, N. S. Benjamin was the son of Lewis and Christiana (Worth) Smith. Lewis was the son of Capt. David and

Rebecca (Lombard) Smith of Cape Cod, Massachusetts and Port Hood Island. Christian was the eldest child of Capt. Benjamin Worth, loyalist settler from New Jersey and the first year-round immigrant settler in Mabou area. The family had a large farm. They were members of the Mabou-Hillsborough Presbyterian Church and she is buried in the Pioneer/First Settlers Cemetery in Hillsborough.

✉ Horace Smith, Smithville, son of Benjamin and Margaret (McEffery) Smith was born in 1875. He was a nephew to Hannah Smith, above, and they resided in the same house. He married Florence MacKinnon. They had four children, who were ages 9, 6, 5, and 4 years at the time of his death. His widow married a second time to Dan MacLean of East Lake Ainslie, but died soon thereafter, in 1921. After her death, the children of Horace and Florence were raised at the home of their grandparents. They did not remain in the area when they were grown—victims, in a way, of the influenza bug.

✉ Angus Smyth, age 29, Judique, died December 1919, son of Raymond Smyth and Mary (MacIsaac) Smyth, merchant and farmer, several siblings. Grandparents: Peter and Ellen (Keating) Smyth of Port Hood. Peter was a native of Ireland and came to be a prominent merchant of the area and an M. L. A. The family was Roman Catholic and has many descendants today in other places.

✉ Effie McRury (her first name was really Euphemia in English, but was common in Gaelic as Oighrig [see *Oirigh* below], which is what the family would have used generally). Age 19, born on Skye Mountain, outside of Whycocomagh, above Stewartdale. Her parents were Angus and Mary. There were three other siblings. The name is unusual and is found almost only in the Island of North Uist, Scotland, from where these MacRurys came in the 1830s. There were four separate families with this last name on Skye Mountain on the 1911 Census. The family was Presbyterian. Effie is buried in Stewartdale Cemetery near the site where the MacLean Church once stood. There was a steep walking trail down from Skye Mountain to the church where services were held in both Gaelic and English during Effie's life time. [Dr. Allan Marble lists her as Effie McRory, Skye Mountain, died 22 January, 1919.]

✉ Albert Rankin, 18 Dec. 1918, age 23, Scotch Hill; this is not Scotch Hill, Inverness County, but Pictou Co. Single, Presbyterian, born Magdalen Islands, not the same as Mabou area Rankins—do not find him on 1901 or 1911 census records in that area. [Transferred to Pictou County chapter.]

Mary McKinnon, Margaree Harbour—daughter of Murdoch and Mary MacKinnon—Roman Catholic, has siblings.

John Young, Strathlorne, Inverness County, son of Edward and Ann (MacDougall)Young; mother Annie age 45 is listed as divorced on 1901 census. The father of John, Edward Young, lived in Sydney, where John was born. John is listed as a labourer, born in Sydney. Family is Presbyterian. Father Edward is of a family which came to Cape Breton in early 1800s and settled in Mabou—not apparently Loyalist. Mother Annie is listed as housekeeper and is a daughter of Allan MacDougall, a merchant of the area. John had three siblings. Buried in Strathlorne Presbyterian Cemetery.

Effie McKay, West Bay, (Mrs M. H.) Her name was properly Euphemia, or Oirigh [see Oighrig, above] in Gaelic which was the language of the household. Wife of Malcolm H. McKay/MacKay, who was a medical doctor in West Bay. Effie was the daughter of John and Mary (Calder) MacInnis of West Bay, and granddaughter of Alexander and Euphemia (MacFarlane) MacInnis, of Isle of Skye and Isle of Mull, Scotland, and of Mull River and West Bay, Cape Breton. She was born in West Bay in 1882. Euphemia was a graduate of Dalhousie University. She left seven children all under twelve years of age.

Hugh McDonald, West Bay, son of Donald and Ann MacDonald. The family was Presbyterian. The father, Donald, was a time-keeper/clerk at the Marble Mountain Quarry.

Agnes Taylor, died 23 Dec. 1918, age 23, in Margaree Harbour. She was a trained nurse who lived elsewhere, but she died at the home of her parents, Alfred (A.A.) Taylor, merchant, and Annie (Gillis) Taylor. Agnes was Roman Catholic and buried in East Margaree Roman Catholic Cemetery; her mother was Roman Catholic and her father was Presbyterian, on one record, but is listed as Church of England as well. According to the 1911 census, her brother Alfred lived at home and was employed by their father. Perhaps she had contracted the disease while nursing and came home to recover, but died there.

George Livingstone of Westville was the son of Duncan and Sadie (Craig) Livingstone. His father was a miner. He had at least two siblings, according to the 1911 census. The family was Presbyterian and descended from the Livingstones of Isle of Mull, Scotland, and Mull River, Inverness County, NS. They were related to Dr. David Livingstone.

✉ Charles Hawley, died 20 Oct. 1918. The Doctor who signed the death certificate is listed as being of Sydney. Charles is listed as living in Ingonish and was buried in Ingonish. He is stated to be Roman Catholic and a fisherman. The census records are unclear about him and his death record seems to suggest he was in his eighties. But Charles J. Hawley of Ingonish on the 1901 census was then 17. His father is listed as Isaac. The Ingonish Hawleys are descended from Capt. Matthew Hawley and his partner Abigail Squires. Capt. Matthew was a Loyalist immigrant from Connecticut in the late 1700s. He settled in Mabou after being in Guysborough County, and then Port Hood briefly. Some of his descendants moved to Ingonish to fish in the 1850s. Although most of his descendants are Presbyterian, those who went to Ingonish are Roman Catholic, probably to follow Matthew's partner, Abigail Squires, who was of Irish ancestry and was Roman Catholic. If the death listed is Charles, son of Isaac, he was sixteen or seventeen at the time of his death. Charles seems not to be in Ingonish at the time of the 1911 census.

✉ Mrs J. C Cadegan/aka Cadgen, died in Marble Mt., Inverness County, 23 December 1918, where she had gone to volunteer her nursing skills. She is listed as a nurse on 1911 census—her husband is Dr. John C. Cadegan of Glace Bay, a graduate of Bellevue Hospital, New York City. She was a MacNeil by birth and born in Nova Scotia. They had one son, Paul. She was born in 1868. The Cadegans were early Irish immigrants to Glace Bay coal mining industry. In 2018, there are still Drs. Cadegan in Glace Bay.

✉ Mrs Simon Arseneault of East Margaree was born in 1846, as Mary Deagle, the daughter of Robert and Mary (Gallant) Deagle of East Margaree. The Deagles arrived from France at Port Royal in 1643. The name has been variously spelled. The Deagles and the Arsenaults are listed as farmers at East Margaree. Mary's husband, Simon, died between 1901 and 1911, for she is listed on the 1911 census as a widow in the home of her daughter Marguerite (Daigle) LeBlanc, the wife of William LeBlanc, with four grandchildren in the house. She was the mother of at least three other children, born in 1873, 1879 and 1881. Her marriage to Simon Arseneault (the name is spelled in several ways) took place in 1868, when she was 21 and he was 23. Her name is also given as Marie on the 1911 Census. Her descendants still live in the area. There are four households with this surname on the census records in that area of Margaree. The family is Roman Catholic and the burials are at St. Michael's Cemetery at East Margaree.

Angus H. McMillan (MacMillan) of East Lake Ainslie died 7 Nov. 1918. He was unmarried, a son of Peter and Catherine (MacInnis) MacMillan. He was born at East Lake 6 October 1879. He is the eldest of nine brothers and one sister in the family. They are farmers and Presbyterian. One of his brothers, Duncan A., was an ordained Presbyterian Minister. The family farmed and were quite prominent in the community. The ancestor arrived in 1822 from the Isle of Muck in the Hebrides. Members of the MacMillan family still reside in Lake Ainslie. Angus was listed on the 1911 Census as the head of the household, with his mother identified as a widow.

Dr. Jim St. Clair to Ruth Whitehead; all of the above sent to Ruth Whitehead as various texts, throughout May 2018.

The only newspaper obituary for Inverness County in 1920 was published in another county, as follows:

At Brookline, Mass, Feb. 10th, 1920, after 3 days illness of influenza, Mary Jessie McLellan, daughter of the late Malcolm McLellan, South West Margaree. The deceased was much esteemed for her kind, gentle and cheerful disposition. Fortified by the consoling rites of the Church she passed calmly and hopefully away. She is survived by her aged mother; four brothers, three of whom, Simon, Joe and Peter are in the far West and John at home; four sisters, Mrs. Dan Gillis, South West Margaree, Mrs. Neil Gillis, Broad Cove Chapel, Mrs. Dan Campbell, Mabou, and Mrs. Allan McLellan South West Margaree. Her remains were accompanied home by her cousin, John McLellan. R.I.P.

Antigonish Casket, 10 February 1920. Courtesy the Antigonish Heritage Museum.

The final death recorded from the Great Influenza epidemic in Inverness County was that of Murdena MacQuarrie, 18, of Valley Mills. She died on April 1, 1920, after an illness of three days.

INVERNESS COUNTY, VITAL STATISTICS, DEATH REGISTER, BOOKS 43, 89

1918

1. Murdo Kennedy, 37, d. 3 September 1918, Inverness, soldier.

2. Marjory McDonald, 26, d. 1 September 1918, Inverness, housework.

3. Hattie Leforte, 23, d. 2 September 1918, Inverness, housework.

4. Alexander Le Blanc, 6, d. 12 September 1918, Inverness.

5. Charles Leforte, 3 months, d. 14 September 1918, Inverness.

6. John Kennedy, 30, d. 13 September 1918, Inverness, mining.

7. John McIsaac, 33, d. 7 September 1918, Inverness, railway manager.

8. James McEachern, 52, d. 4 September 1918, Inverness, merchant.

9. Mary Chiasson, 31, d. 12 September 1918, Little River, housekeeper.

10. Rose McCuish, 16, d. 24 December 1918, Port Hood, housekeeper.

11. Ida Embrie, 34, d. 5 October 1918, Port Hawkesbury, housework.

12. John McQuarrie, 42, d. 26 December 1918, Port Hastings, farmer. [*Dr. Allan Marble wrote*: *"(Note attached stating it is doubtful that he died from influenza. Author does state there are a lot of influenza cases near Port Hastings but they are mild cases as no deaths so far.)" The actual note, Book 43, Page 335, Number 1028, reads: "we have a lot of Influenza all round hear, but very mild cases so far no deaths but this one which I think is doubtfull." The signature is illegible, but is in the same handwriting as the registrar doing the rest of the record, and with the same thick pen nib.*]

13. Alexander McEachern, 27, d. 27 November 1918, Port Hood, labourer.

14. Angus Smyth, 29, d. 11 December 1918, Judique, clerk.

15. Alexander McEachern, 26, d. 14 December 1918, Judique, farmer.

16. Dennis Chiasson, 13, d. 8 December 1918, Grand Etang [*sic*].

17. Mary Ann McLellan, 25, d. 10 October 1918, Southwest Margaree, housemaid.

18. William McDaniel, 25, d. 7 November 1918, Margaree Forks, farmer.

19. Sarah McDougall, 23, d. 29 November 1918, Margaree Forks, postmistress.

20. Rachael McInnes, 78, d. 8 December 1918, McInnes Mountain, "old maid."

21. Dimian Arsenault, 9, d. 18 December 1918, East Margaree.

22. John McInnes, 83, d. 29 December 1918, McInnes Mountain, farmer.

23. Elise Des Veaux, 28, 16 November 1918, Belle Marche, housekeeper.

24. Celeste Des Veaux, 12, d. 18 November 1918, Little River.

25. Marguerite Aucoin, 42, d. 6 October 1918, Cape Rouge, housekeeper.

26. Malthulde [*Mathilde*] Chiasson, 33, d. 23 October 1918, Eastern Harbour, housekeeper. [*Book 42, Page 352, Number 1072.*]

27. Mrs. Donald Campbell, 70, d. 13 December 1918 1918, Mabou Mines, farmer [*sic*].

28. Mary Chaisson, 18 months, d. 14 December 1918, Belle Côte.

29. Annie Chaisson, 2, d. 14 December 1918, Belle Côte.

30. Lucy Chaisson, 6 months, d. 14 December 1918, Belle Côte.

31. Lucy Ann Chiasson, 4, d. 16 December 1918, Belle Côte.

32. Margaret LeBlanc, 17, d. 16 December 1918, Belle Côte.

33. Amelia LeBlanc, 38, d. 17 December 1918, Belle Côte, invalid.

34. Placide LeBlanc, 80, d. 17 December 1918, Belle Côte, farmer.

35. Germain LeBlanc, 3, d. 19 December 1918, Belle Côte.

36. Mary McKinnon, 30, d. 29 December 1918, Margaree Harbour, housewife.

37. Agnes Taylor, 23, d. 20 December 1918, Margaree harbour, nurse (trained).

38. Joseph Arseneau, 8 months, d. 20 December 1918, East Margaree.

39. Catherine Cormier, 12, d. 21 December 1918, Belle Côte.

40. Mrs. Simon Doucet, 46, d. 22 December 1918, Belle Côte, housewife.

41. Germain Stubbart, 70, d. 22 December 1918, Belle Côte, harnessmaker.

42. Caroline LeBlanc, 74, d. 25 December 1918, Belle Côte, housewife.

43. Alexander Chaisson, 30, d. 26 December 1918, Margaree Harbour, labourer.

44. Florence Chaisson, 8 months, d. 11 December 1918, Belle Côte.

45. John Chaisson, 3, d. 13 December 1918, Belle Côte.

46. Mrs. Thomas LeBlanc, 45, d. 13 December 1918, Margaree Harbour, housewife.

47. Lillie Chaisson, 6, d. 13 December 1918, Belle Côte.

48. Wilfred LeBlanc, 3, d. 14 December 1918, Margaree Harbour.

49. Catherine Morrison, 28, d. 12 January 1919, Port Hastings, housework.

50. Florence McQuarrie, 30, d. 15 January 1919, Port Hastings, housework.

51. Raymond Smythe, 4, d. 16 December 1918, Judique.

52. Mary Coady, 60, d. 22 December 1918, Harbour View.

53. Mrs. Annie McDougall, 62, d. 21 December 1918, Centennial, housewife.

54. Agnes McDonald, 31, 24 December 1918, Little Judique.

55. John McDonald, 24, d. 26 December 1918, Little Judique, labourer.

56. Dan McDonald, 14, d. 27 December 1918, Little Judique.

57. Mrs. M. H. McKay, 37, d. 2 January 1919, West Bay.

58. Hugh McDonald, 18, d. 23 February 1919, West Bay, farmer.

59. John McDonald, 20, d. 28 February 1919, West Bay, farmer.

60. Frank Smith, 29, d. 30 January 1919, Smithville, farmer.

61. Hannah Smith, 86, d. 12 January 1919, Smithville.

62. Horace Smith, 43, d. 19 January 1919, Smithville, farmer.

63. Mary McDonald, 50, d. 26 February 1919, Black River.

64. Michael Croat, 6, d. 8 February 1919, Deepdale.

65. Allan McIsaac, 6, d. 28 March 1918, Dunvegan.

66. John Young, 20, d. 11 March 1919, Strathlorne, labourer.

67. Louise Doucet, 87, d. 5 March 1919, Friar's [*sic*] Head.

68. Minnie Gillis, 19, d. 17 January 1919, Upper Margaree.

69. Dougal Gillis, 17, d. 30 October 1918, Upper Margaree.

70. John Gillis, 15, d. 19 January 1919, Upper Margaree, student.

71. Katie McLean, 35, d. 3 January 1919, Whycocomagh, domestic.

72. *Infant* McRory, male, 10 days old, d. 15 January 1919, Skye Mountain. [*HVS, Book 43, Page 395, Number 1207, shows his name was McRury; his father's name was Angus McRury. This infant's sister, Effie McRury (same page, Number 1209), died a week later.*]

73. Effie McRory, 19, d. 22 January 1919, Skye Mountain, domestic. [*She was the daughter of Angus McRury, and the sister of the baby McRury who died a week previous (see above).*]

74. Flora McLeod, 21, d. 18 January 1919, Upper South West.

75. Mrs. Patrick LeBlanc, 31, d. 26 December 1918, East Margaree, housewife.

76. Leo Arsenault, 4, d. 28 December 1918, Belle Côte.

77. Beatrice Chaisson, 7, d. 31 December 1918, Belle Côte.

78. Mrs. Simon Arsenault, 72, d. 30 December 1918, East Margaree, housewife.

79. Margaret Gallant, 7 months, d. 13 February 1919, Belle Côte.

80. Alex McEachern, 8, d. 26 April 1919, Port Hood.

81. Marie Boudreau, 9, d. 17 April 1919, Eastern Harbour. [*HVS search engine has her name as "Marie Annie," but the death record, Book 43, Page 430, Number 1284, shows it to be "Marie Anne." She died of "Spanish Influenza."*]

82. Alex McDonnell, 24, d. 15 May 1919, South West Ridge, farmer.

83. Alex McLean, 71, d. 22 August 1919, Scotsville, farmer.

84. Louise LeBlanc, 28, d. 28 July 1919, Eastern Harbour, housekeeper.

85. Donald McDonald, 68, d. 13 July 1919, Inverness County Asylum, inmate.

86. Mrs. Malcolm Murray, 69, d. 1 January 1920, North East Margaree, ill 8 days.

87. Alexander C. McArthur, 57, d. 4 March 1920, mill man, ill 10 days.

88. Flora LeBlanc, 57, d. 15 March 1920, Margaree Forks, housework, ill 15 days.

89. Catherine McDougall, 43, d. 15 April 1920, Port Hood, housewife, time ill not given. [*HVS, Book 89, Page 171, gives her full name as Catherine Cameron McDougall.*]

90. Margaret McKinnon, 80, d. 10 April 1920, Hays River, housework, ill 13 days.

91. Daniel Arseneau, 2, d. 3 April 1920, Friars head, time ill not given.

92. Douglas Timmons, 8, d. 5 April 1920, Margaree Forks, ill 10 days

93. Murdena MacQuarrie, 18, d. 1 April 1920, Valley Mills, ill 3 days.

Chapter XII

KINGS COUNTY

THERE WERE AT least seventy-two confirmed deaths from the Great Influenza between 1918 and 1920, with a possibility of two more from the First Wave of this epidemic. Newspaper records for influenza in Kings County are sadly lacking. In spite of all these known deaths, there are only a few obituaries. Many of the Kings County news items—obituaries, or influenza information within and without the county—are therefore from newspapers published elsewhere, or from family histories. One interesting situation was reported by Ross Baker, in a family memoir.

Ross Hardy Baker Memoir

   Ross Hardy Baker wrote a family-tree memoir for his granddaughter, Elizabeth Peirce. The title was "The Long Trail," he being from the Long family of King's County. He noted that his relative Henrietta Mahailly Long (Mrs. Holton Atwell) and her husband had both died of "Spanish Flu" in May 1918, leaving nine orphan children. This date is borne out by the Kings County Death Registration for 1918, but given that their deaths are so early in the year (May 11, 1918 and May 20, 1918), was the influenza that killed these two people really "Spanish flu"? It sounds like it, because it killed them fast: Holton was only ill for seven days, Henrietta lasted nine days, and they both died within nine days of each other. Dr. Allan Marble was consulted, told of the memoir and that the family insisted it was Spanish flu. They would certainly have remembered this event vividly, as there remained nine children for whom extended-family homes had to be found. The other reason Ross Baker's tradition was likely to be accurate is that his own father, James, sent in the return for the death of Holton Atwell, his neighbour and relation by marriage.

Dr. Marble agreed the Atwell deaths should go on the list of Great Influenza Victims, and we discussed the First Wave of a milder form of this Great Influenza, which appeared in the spring of 1918. It was the autumn's Second Wave that proved really harsh, lasting into 1919, after which came a Third Wave in 1920, winter into spring. Therefore, the Atwell couple were considered two of the first reasonably-confirmed victims of the First Wave. In typing Dr. Marble's list of Kings County deaths, at the end of this chapter, the Atwells were added at the end of his entries. He was focused on Second and Third Wave victims and perhaps did not examine death records as early as May, especially if the cause of death did not say "influenza."

Dr. Janet Baker, daughter of Ross Hardy Baker, to Ruth Whitehead, personal communication, March 2018. Dr. Allan Marble to Ruth Whitehead, personal communication, April 2018.

☞ Holton Atwell, according to his death record, died May 11, 1918, of "Pleuro Pneumonia / Oedema of Lungs." He was 65, and a farmer at Newtonville, Kings County.

Died: 11 May 1918. He had been born at Black River in that county, was a Baptist, and his body was apparently returned to the Black River cemetery for burial. He had only been ill for a week. Dr. J. W. Reid attended, probably only after things took a turn for the worse. "Name of Person Making Return" was the aforementioned James Baker, his relative by marriage, and his neighbour while growing up in Black River. James Baker sent it in the very day Holton died, and perhaps was helping out there.

HVS, Kings County Death Register, 1918, Book 35, Page 444, Number 291.

☞ Henrietta Mahailly Long Atwell, Holton's wife, was 43 at the time of her death, being 22 years younger than her husband. She died at Newtonville on 20 May 1918. She had been born in Black River as well, and is buried in the cemetery there. Her name appears as "Henrietta M." on the reverse of her parents' tombstone. The cause of death was given as "Pleuro Pnemonia / Pericarditis," after an illness of nine days. Strangely, she had a different doctor: M. N. Elliott, and a different undertaker: A. J. Inndiman [sp?]. Her oldest son, Roslyn Atwell, sent in the return of death the same day.

HVS, Kings County Death Register, 1918, Book 40, Page 416, Number 1185.

Henrietta Mahailly Long (10 May 1875–20 May 1918) [date of birth typed as 1878, but changed by hand to 1875] m. Holton Watson Atwell (2 Nov 1853–11 May 1918).

Children: Roslyn Grove; Evelyn Araline; Bartley Leverett; Warren Watson; Stoessel Byran [Byron]; Lulu Gertrude; Lena Henrietta; Ella Arabella; Neva Regina.

Ross Hardy Baker, unpublished manuscript The Long Trail, collection of Elizabeth Peirce, Halifax.

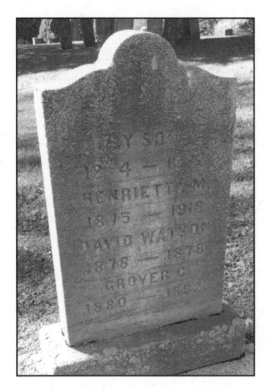

Black River Cemetery, Kings County, where Henrietta M. Long Atwell and her husband, Holton Atwell, are buried. Her name appears on the reverse of her Long parents' tombstone as "Henrietta M.," with no Atwell surname mentioned. (*R. H. Whitehead*)

MRS. JESSE WOTTEN. The death of Mrs. Hannah Wotton, wife of Jesse C. Wotton, of Aylesford Mountain, took place, under peculiarly sad circumstances, on October 15th. Influenza, followed by pneumonia in its most severe form was the cause of her death. An aged father, Mr. James Parks, who has passed his eightieth year, a sorrowing husband, and three small children, mourn the loss of a dutiful daughter, a faithful wife, a loving mother.

Berwick Register, 13 November 1918, 2.

There entered into rest on Saturday, October 19th, after two years illness, followed by an attack of influenza, Amelia, wife of John Burns, of Berwick West. Mrs. Burns, who was formerly Miss Amelia Sullivan, was born in Granville, Annapolis County, fifty-four years ago. She removed from there to Springfield, where she made her home with her uncle. Besides her husband, she leaves four daughters and two grandchildren. The daughters are Mrs. Earle Congdon, of St. John; Gertrude, wife of Pte. Arthur Gelinas, now in Scotland; Maggie, wife of Pte. Lloyd Durling, Somewhere in France [*sic*], and Katherine, at home.

Berwick Register, 30 October 1918, 2.

MRS. JOHN N. WOTTON. Mrs. Anna Baltzer Wotton, mother of the above named Jesse C. Wotton, and widow of the late John N. Wotton, passed away at her home in Aylesford, on Monday October 28th. She was also a victim of Spanish Influenza. One brother, John Baltzer, of Hasley Mountain, and two sons, Jesse and Charles, mourn her loss. She was seventy-four years of age.

Berwick Register, 13 November 1918, 2.

 A very sudden and unexpected sorrow came to the house of Ainsley B. Chute, South Berwick, on Wednesday, October 30th, when his beloved wife was taken away by the dread disease, influenza. The maiden name of Mrs. Chute was Annie E. Doucette. She was the daughter of Mr. and Mrs. Patrick Doucette, of Norwood, Yarmouth County....[and mother of] two little girls: Laura E. and Dora Mary.

Berwick Register, 13 November 1918, 2.

 MRS. LESTER ROBINSON. Mrs. Lester Robinson, of Waterville, entered into rest at 3 a.m. on Saturday Nov. 23rd. From the health and strength of her young womanhood, the influenza and pneumonia in a few days laid her low. Florence was a general favourite.

Berwick Register, 27 November 1918, 2.

 Miss Eagles, of the Telephone Central at Kentville, passed away on Monday morning, after a brief illness from influenza.

Berwick Register, 18 December 1918, 3.

☞ Her name was Nellie Eagles, aged 27; she was born in Wolfville, resided in Kentville, single, and was a bookkeeper. Her father, Ernest W. Eagles of Wolfville, filled out her death record. A Baptist, she was buried in Wolfville.

HVS, Kings County Death Register, 1918, Book 40, Page 442, Number 1290. (She has two other death records in the register.)

 Death of Mrs. Leslie R. Fairn. Her many friends in Bridgetown and elsewhere regret to learn of the death of Bessie, wife of Mr. Leslie R. Fairn, which occurred at her home in Aylesford at an early hour Tuesday morning, Dec. 17.....She was a native of Bridgetown, being a daughter of the late Mr. and Mrs. William Tupper, and a grand-daughter of the late Minard Tupper. Besides her grief-stricken husband, who has the sympathy of a host of friends (for few are better or more favourably known than Architect Fairn) she leaves two daughters: Alice, who was in Toronto, and a younger one at home.

Bridgetown Monitor, 25 December 1918, 4.

Aylesford mourns the loss of one of its most highly esteemed residents, Mrs. Fairn, wife of Mr. Leslie R. Fairn the wellknown architect, who passed away Tuesday [December 17] morning from Influenza. Her daughter, Miss Alice, who was in Toronto, was notified by telegraph of her mother's illness, but was unable to reach her home before the end came. She arrived in Aylesford yesterday....(Kentville Chronicle, 19th)

Annapolis Spectator, 2 January 1919, 1.

 Mrs. John Taylor [Sophie, 61] died at her home in Medford, Kings Co., Jan. 6th; after the funeral which was held the 8th, the husband passed away after a few hours illness. They leave a large family of which Capt. Robt. Taylor, of the Tug "Chester" is a son.

Hants Journal, 15 January 1919, 1.

 A SAD CASE AT LOCKHARTVILLE
Four in One Family, Dead

Mr. and Mrs. John Carly and daughter, residing at Lockhartville, died on Thursday last, of pneumonia, and the son succumbed on the following day. The mother had been ill for some weeks, and the father, who was exceedingly ill, struggled quite a distance to the home of a neighbour, who immediately summoned Dr. Shankel, of Hantsport. The doctor hurried to the scene, and found all in a dying condition. The four members of the home passed away as stated above. Mr. E. L. Gertridge assisted the undertaker, Mr. Borden, in conveying the remains of father, mother and two children to the undertaking rooms, from which the funerals took place on the following day. Rev. Mr. Crandall conducted the burial services.

Hants Journal, 15 January 1919, 1.

☞ This newspaper account has errors. First of all, the family name is Carty, not Carly.

Death records for Kings County show four Cartys, three of whom died on January 10, 1919, in Lockhartville, and one who died the next day, on the eleventh. It's their family relationships that are a little confusing. All four were Baptists, and buried at Riverbank Cemetery, Hantsport.

Emmeline S. Carty, aged 84, was the first to die. The wife of John M. Carty, she was born in Kellyville, Kings County, and was a Baptist, buried in Riverbank Cemetery, Hantsport.

HVS, Death Register, Kings County, 1919, Book 40, Page 477, Number 1425.

☞ John M. Carty, husband of Emmeline, aged 75, was the second of the three deaths on 10 January. He was a farmer at Lockhartville, and had been born at Canard. Because his wife predeceased him, even if just by a few hours, John Carty was recorded as a widower.

HVS, Death Register, Kings County, 1919, Book 40, Page 480, Number 1440.

☞ Minnie E. Carty, who worked as a needlewoman, aged 43, unmarried, was almost certainly their daughter. She appears in the HVS search engine as "Carty, Maurice E. / female." Minnie was born at "Hants Border."

HVS, Death Register, Kings County, 1919, Book 40, Page 480, Number 1439.

☞ Theodore Carty, aged 16, whose death was recorded before the other three family members, was the "son" who died on the eleventh, but Emmeline is too old to have been his mother, and his death record says that a "Wm. E. Carty" was his father. He is either a grandson or other family member, taken in by John and Emmeline.

HVS, Death Register, Kings County, 1919, Book 40, Page 707, Number 1424.

☞ To make things even more complicated, a Halifax newspaper picked up the story of the tragedy, but called the family the Carters.

FOUR DEATHS FROM INFLUENZA IN ONE FAMILY
Kentville, Jan. 22. The epidemic of influenza has been very serious at Lockhartville. The Carter home has been especially afflicted. Four members of this family have died. Three were buried on Saturday and one on Sunday—father, mother, daughter and son.

Halifax Evening Mail, 23 January 1919, 11.

SAD NEWS TO A TRURO HOME
Mrs. Mosher, Prince Street West, has just received news of the deth [*sic*] from Spanish Influenza on the 4th of her daughter, Mrs. Arthur Morine, at her home, Church Street, Cornwallis, Kings Co. Mrs. Morine leaves a husband and four children all down with this terrible disease.

Truro Daily News, 5 December 1918, 2.

MRS. ARTHUR MORINE DIED FEB. 15 AT THE FAMILY RESIDENCE, CHURCH STREET, CORNWALLIS
Particularly sad has been the deplorable [in]roads by Influenza in the family of Mr. Arthur Morine, Church Street, Cornwallis, Kings County, within the past six or seven weeks. Early in January Mrs. Morine, formerly Edith Wright, daughter of

Mrs. Mosher, Prince Street West, Truro, was taken down with Spanish influenza and in a short time she succubmed [*sic*] to the epidemic and past away, leaving husband, two daughters and two sons. Then this epidemic seized one of the boys, Robie—with youth and strength on his side—and with expert medical attention and in the hands of professional nurses; but all were unavailing and on Jan'y 15, he past on to the spirit land. Now the three left in this little family, two daughters and son, are in deep sorrow over a triple affliction as the father, Mr. Arthur Morine, after but a short illness from influenza meningitis, has joined his loved ones in the Great Beyond.

Truro Daily News, 17 February 1919, 2.

⟜ Edith Morine and her son Robie Wilfred, aged 20, a farmer, both died of influenza and were buried in Canard. Arthur Morine's record not found.

HVS, Death Register, Kings County, 1918, Book 40, Page 443, Number 1293 (Edith), 1295 (Robie).

⟜ Dr. Marble found no newspaper accounts at all from 1920, when six people died between January 5 and March 16. The final death from the Great Influenza for Kings County was that of Abbie M. Bowles, 46, who died on March 16, 1920, of influenza and pneumonia. She was born in Coldbrook, Kings County, the daughter of Henry Marchant and Ruby Porter Marchant; her "racial origin" was given as "French," she was married to Aubrey L. Bowles (whose address was given as "Waterville Hospital"), a housewife, ill only nine days. The space for undertaker's name, cemetery or cemetery location was left blank on her death record.

HVS, Death Register, Kings County, 1920, Book 92, Page 183.

KINGS COUNTY, VITAL STATISTICS, DEATH REGISTER, BOOKS 40, 92

1918

1. Nellie Gray, 28, d. 28 October 1918, Kentville, nurse.

2. Nellie Eagles, 27, d. 14 December 1918, Kentville, bookkeeper.

3. Kathlyn Collins, 26, b. 25 December 1918, Kentville, housewife.

4. Edith Morine, 42, d. 2 December 1918, Church Street, Kentville.

5. Robie Morine, 20 d. 16 December 1918, Church Street, Kentville, farmer.

6. Wilfred Snow, 21, d. 26 October 1918, Canard.

7. Alfred Ells, 50, d. 10 November 1918, Canning, soldier.

8. Owen Huntley, 38, d. 31 December 1918, Medford.

9. Grace Barkhouse, 37, d. 2 January 1919, Canning, housewife.

10. William B. Tully, 38, d. 23 October 1918, Kentville, farmer.

11. Martha Guptell, 14, d. 23 October 1918, Wallbrook, housework.

12. Leslie Smith, 24, d. 23 October 1918, Grand Pre, farmer.

13. Sydney Mosher, 21, d. 29 October 1918, Hantsport, ship carpenter.

14. Gertrude Pinch, 14, d. 31 October 1918, Wallbrook.

15. Gladys Pinch, 6, d. 11 November 1918, Wallbrook.

16. David Bambrick, 43, d. 10 November 1918, Melanson, cooper.

17. David Pinch, 43, d. 7 December 1918, Wallbrook, farmer.

[*Number 18 on Dr. Marble's list proves to be a repeat (one of three!) of the death record for Nellie Eagles (See Number 2, above); this list has been adjusted in order to give an accurate number of deaths for the county.*]

18. Kenneth Curry, 28, d. 15 December 1918, Hortonville, railway employee.

19. Edith Kelly, d. 16 December 1918, Hortonville, housewife.

20. Irvine Gaetz, 3, d. 5 December 1918, Grafton.

21. Anthony Langille, 58, d. 15 October 1918, Centreville, farmer.

22. Lloyd Coulter, 18 days, d. 17 October 1918, Berwick.

23. Frank Cleveland, 19, d. 29 October 1918, Berwick, labourer.

24. Lucy Ramey, 5 months, d. 5 November 1918, South Berwick.

25. Florence Robinson, 20, d. 23 November 1918, Waterville, clerk.

26. Annie Watton, 74, d. 29 October 1918, [*place name illegible; possibly "Fairview" (Street), Kentville," Kings County, widowed housekeeper, name of husband was John Wotton. Book 40, Page 463, Number 1372.*]

27. Hannah Watton, 38, d. 15 October 1918, Victoria, housekeeper. [*Book 40, Page 463, Number 1373, gives her as married to Jas. Wotton.*]

28. Nora Palmer, 30, d. 2 October 1918, Morristown, "wife." [*Book 40, Page 463, Number 1374. She was born in Owen Sound, Ontario, and was married to Carol Palmer. They were living in "Morristown, N.S."*]

29. David Bent, 25, d. 24 October 1918, Victoria, farmer.

30. Bessie Fairn, 39, d. 17 December 1918, Aylesford, housekeeper.

1919

31. Frank Moore, 30, d. 4 February 1919, Kentville, farmer.

32. Etta Bishop, 22, d. 4 January 1919, Greenwich, clerk.

33. Annette Manson, 54, d. 25 January 1919, Centreville, housewife.

34. Freeman Walton, 45, d. 4 February 1919, New Ross Road, farmer.

35. John Sullivan, 28, d. 26 March 1919, Kentville, farmer.

36. Sophie Taylor, 61, d. 6 January 1919, Medford, housewife.

37. William Bennett, 2, d. 13 January 1919, Canning.

38. Jessie Pearl, female, 16, d. 19 January 1919, Arlington, domestic.

39. Theodore Carty, 16, d. 11 January 1919, Lockhartville.

40. Emmeline Carty, 84, d. 9 January 1919, Lockhartville.

41. Dennison Atwell, 20 months, d. 2 March 1919, Morine Mountain.

42. Kathleen Woodworth, 2, d. 8 January 1919, Lockhartville.

43. Albert Atwell, 16, d. 23 February 1919, Melanson.

44. Eva Davison, 1, d. 10 February 1919, Gaspereaux.

45. Minnie Carty, 43, d. 10 January 1919, Lockhartville, needlewoman.

46. John M. Carty, 75, d. 10 January 1919, Lockhartville, farmer.

47. Bessie Lyman, 65, d. 1 January 1919, Cambridge, housewife.

48. Bessie Lutz, d. 10 January 1919, Lake George, housewife.

49. Margaret Swindell, 66, d. 2 February 1919, Burlington, housewife.

50. Lorne Young, 29, d. 14 January 1919, Lake Paul, farmer.

51. Robert Munro, 2, d. 8 May 1919, Kentville.

52. Mary Williams, 56, d. 5 April 1919, Kentville, housewife.

53. John Smith, 18, d. 9 May 1919, Aldershot, labourer.

54. Eugena Kilcup, 8 months, d. 10 May 1919, Aldershot. [*Book 40, Page 494, Number 1490, "Female."*]

55. Ellen Borden, 53, d. 11 January 1919, Sheffield Mills, housewife. [*Buried at Upper Canard.*]

56. Vincent Gaum, 78, d. 7 April 1919, Blomidon, farmer.

57. Mildred Cox, 38, d. 4 May 1919, Medford, housewife.

58. Wellington Walsh, 42, d. 4 May 1919, Avonport, labourer.

59. Selina Weagle, 30, d. 14 May 1919, Avonport, housewife.

60. Arnold Selby, 5, d. 13 May 1919, Avonport.

61. Ethel Henderson, 20, d. 7 May 1919, Avonport, schoolteacher.

62. James Henderson, 48, d. 18 May 1919, Avonport, merchant.

63. Amelia Illsley, 66, d. 2 April, 1919, Halls Harbour.

64. Freeman Eisnor, 34, d. 12 April 1919, Lakeville, carpenter.

65. John Dorman, 51, d. 6 May 1919, Billtown, merchant.

66. William Rand, 83, d. 27 May 1919, Sheffield Mills, farmer.

1920

67. Mabel Murphy, 31, d. 5 January 1920, Auburn, "Epidemic influenza & T.B."

68. Nellie Rockwell, 20 months, d. 2 March 1920, Upper Canard.

69. Alice H. Davison, 53, d. 9 March 1920, Grand Pré.

70. Burton Algee, 23, d. 17 March 1920, White's Corner, farmer.

71. Pauline Reiss, 5 months, d. 14 March 1920, Waterville.

72. Abbie M. Bowles, 46, d. 16 March 1920, Waterville, housewife.

Possible but Unconfirmed First Wave Victims
1. Holton Atwell, d. 11 May 1918,
   Newtonville, farmer; time ill 7 days.
2. Henrietta Atwell, d. 20 May 1918,
   Newtonville; time ill 9 days.

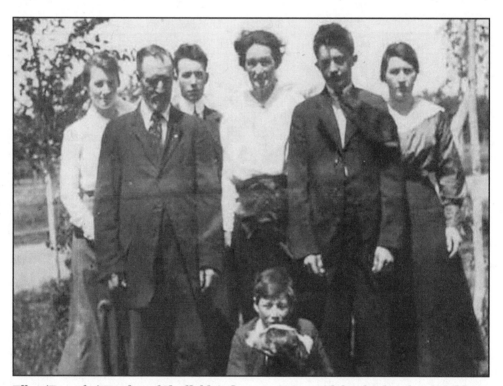

Ellen (Forsythe) Borden of Sheffield, influenza victim, with her husband and children: L–R: Helena Borden, John Nelson Borden (Ellen's husband), Harry, Ellen herself, Clarence, Mary, and Carl (kneeling, with Spot the dog). Ruth Legge, her great-grandchild, says, "My grandfather Wilfred and his brother David are not in the photo, so we think it was taken during the War years." Ellen died 11 January, 1919. She and John are buried in Upper Canard, in what was then the Presbyterian cemetery, and is now the Canard Community Church, Kings County. *(Courtesy of the Borden Family descendants; photographer unknown)*

Chapter XIII

LUNENBURG COUNTY

LUNENBURG COUNTY HAD at least 139 confirmed deaths from the Great Influenza epidemic. This sort of situation was common: whole families falling ill at once, and the sick nursing the even sicker. The number of children left orphaned, or with only one parent, was appalling. The Lunenburg victims included fishermen, master carpenters, ice dealers, machinists, ship builders, a boatbuilder, clerks, cooks, mechanics, traders, coopers, a male nurse, labourers, an electrician, a pauper, a clergyman and a blacksmith, as well as trained nurses, housekeepers, housemaids, domestics, teachers, housewives, and children of all ages.

Death record for Ivan Winters, 27, of the Ovens, a fisherman who died of Influenza and Bronchial Pneumonia on 6 October 1918—the first death in the Second Wave of the Great Influenza in Lunenburg County. (*Nova Scotia Archives*)

How did influenza come to the county, and when did it taper off? Here are some examples from Dr. Marble's list by county, showing the extent of the epidemic through those who were among the first to die, and those among the last to die. Supplemental information is from the Historical Vital Statistics (HVS) database, and the few extant few newspaper obituaries:

- "Ivan Winters, 27, single, fisherman, resided Ovens; died 6 October 1918, Spanish Influenza." He fell ill on September 30, 1918. The death record says his father was Gabriel Winters, who sent in the return of death to the registrar. Ivan was a Methodist, born at Ovens, and was buried at Middle South. Doctor was H. G. Grant, undertaker A. L. Sweeny.

  HVS, 1918, Book 43, Page 87, Number 288.

- "Leslie Tanner, 16, single, Lunenburg; died 10 October 1918, influenza & pneumonia." The death record says his father, W. B. Tanner, sent in his death return. He was ill only five days, falling sick October 5th. Leslie was born at Blue Rocks, and resided in Lunenburg. Episcopalian, he was buried in Lunenburg. Undertaker was A. L. Sweeny. Dr. Forbes attended him.

  HVS, 1918, Book 43, Page 91, Number 298.

TANNER. Leslie Tanner, eldest son of William and Sevilla Tanner, passed away on Thursday after a short illness of bronchial pneumonia following Spanish Influenza. The funeral was held on Friday morning.

  Lunenburg Progress Enterprise, 16 October 1918, 1.

"Maud Mack, 50, married, Lunenburg; died 11 October 1918, influenza and pneumonia." She fell ill on September 29, 1918. The record in the register gives her name as Maud C. Mack, born in Newfoundland, married to Darius Mack; Episcopalian, buried at Lunenburg. Doctors were Forbes and McLellan. Undertaker was A. Sweeny.

  HVS, Year 1918, Book 43, Page 91, Number 301.

- "John F. Chesley, 76, widower, New Germany; died 7 April 1920, influenza and pneumonia." The record gives him as John F. Chesley, born in Nova Scotia 4 February 1844; parents were Elizabeth (Young) and Nelson Chesley. He was a farmer, and had lived in New Germany "all his life." Doctor was W. H. Cole, undertaker J. W. Langille. He was buried in New Germany, and his son, Horton P. Chesley, sent in the return.

  HVS, Year 1918, Book 95, Page 268.

- "Amy Bezanson, 37, housewife, New Ross; died 28 April 1920, influenza and pneumonia." The death record says she was the daughter of James Keddy and Martha (Veinot) Keddy, born and resided at Lake Ramsay, New Ross, had been a domestic when single; died at New Ross from "Influenza, Lobar Pneumonia and Parturition w Influenza." She was pregnant, and Influenza precipitated the labour. The return was made by Harden Keddy, Lake Ramsay, "no relation." Buried at New Ross; undertaker A. L. Lohnes. Husband's name not given.

HVS, 1918, Book 95, Page 281.

CROUSE. The death of Florrie, wife of Edmund Crouse, occurred on Tuesday last, after a short illness of Spanish Influenza. The deceased was a daughter of Charles Crouse and a sister of Mrs. Steadman Corkum. She is survived by her husband and a family of seven children, most of whom are quite young, who will sadly miss the care of a devoted mother.

Lunenburg Progress Enterprise, 23 October 1918, 1.

The sad death of Morris Mason, son of Francis Mason of Eastern Points, occurred on Wednesday last at the age of 23 years. Death was due to Spanish Influenza.

Among the many sorrowful incidents attendant upon the prevailing epidemic of Spanish Influenza are the deaths of the young wife and sister of Captain Frank Whynacht of Newtown. Probably no one in this community has been harder hit than Captain Whynacht. He was married for the second time, in the first week of January of this year, to Hilda, only daughter of Hudson Mason of Eastern Points. During the past week Mrs. Whynacht contracted the dread disease, on Sunday succumbed to pneumonia, leaving a heartbroken husband and an infant son which was born on Saturday.

Captain Whynacht's sister Florence, wife of Angus Mason, was also especially dear to him. She contracted the disease last week and…passed away on Saturday.

Lunenburg Progress Enterprise, 23 October 1918, 1.

The home of Francis Mason of Eastern Points has again been saddened by the death of his young son, Philip Morris, who was the second of the family to succumb to Influenza within a week. The boy was 10 years of age.

Lunenburg Progress Enterprise, 30 October 1918, 1.

The death took place this morning at Bridgewater, of Madora May, wife of Huston Wynacht, aged 38 years. Deceased had been ill but a few days with influenza. She leaves besides her husband seven children to mourn their loss. Interment will take place in Trinity Church cemetery tomorrow afternoon.

Liverpool Advance, 6 November 1918, 2.

The very sad death of Olive, wife of Harris Naas, of Centre Range, occurred on Monday, Oct. 28, from pneumonia, following influenza....The death is the ninth to occur in Mr. Naas' family in the past four months: three men, three women and three children.

Lunenburg Progress Enterprise, 6 November 1918, 5.

Nova Scotia was not only receiving those sick with flu, she was also exporting them, as this Lunenburg County newspaper article shows: "Norman Cxner [Coxner?], of Lower La Have, a member of the crew of the schooner General Haig, was landed at Turk's Island suffering from Spanish Influenza." Turks Island, in the Caribbean, was a commercial source of salt for Nova Scotia.

Lunenburg Progress Enterprise, 6 November 1918, 8.

Funeral ceremonies were being held outside, after quarantine regulations closed churches.

J. Wilfrid Mossman of Rose Bay passed into eternal rest on October 16, 1918, after a brief illness of ten days from Spanish Influenza and pleuro pneumonia. The deceased was 35 years old....He leaves a wife, Lavinia (nee) Himmellman, two small children, an aged father and mother....The deceased was a loyal and devoted member of St. Matthews Ev. Lutheran Church of Rose Bay.... An open air funeral was held in front of his late residence by his pastor the Rev. S. W. Hirtle, and interment was made in the Rose Bay Cemetery on Thursday afternoon Oct. 17th.

Lunenburg Progress Enterprise, 23 October 1918, 1.

Mrs. Wilfrid Mossman has been appointed Registrar of Births and Deaths.

Lunenburg Progress Enterprise, 6 November 1918, 8.

 Lunenburg Progress: Influenza had again visited this district and claimed two victims in one family, in the persons of George and Melbourne Lohnes, sons of the late Capt. Obediah Lohnes, of Riverport. On Friday, George, who lived at home with his mother, succumbed to the disease and on Sunday; Melbourne, aged 30, Secretary-Treasurer of the Acadia Gas Engines Limited, of Bridgewater, died at that town.

Yarmouth Telegram, 13 December 1918, 1.

"I could not begin to do what was needing to be done."

⟾ The following account by a nurse on duty in an unnamed Canadian emergency hospital [Vancouver] during the worst months of 1918 will show you the horror of this epidemic, and why the doctors and nurses quickly became exhausted and, even more, susceptible. It was sent in by her mother, Mary R. Chesley of Lunenburg County, to the *Lunenburg Progress Enterprise*, and headlined "Trying Experiences of Mary A. Chesley in Hospital." An excerpt appears in the Cape Breton County chapter.

Dear Editor of the Progress-Enterprise: Perhaps the subjoined excerpts from recent letters of Mary A. Chesley who last month offered as night nurse in an improvised "Flu" hospital may be of interest to your readers as giving a glimpse of the sad occurrences that have transpired in numberless hospitals all over this Dominion and the United States during the past two or three months. MRC.

⟾ Mary Chesley's letter:

Now I will tell you some of my experiences as night nurse. The first night I was placed, one of two helpers, on a women's ward with seventeen patients. Matters were not too bad at that time. The other helper was Isabel Thomas, the Methodist minister's daughter and she knew no more about nursing than I did. I had not met her before but we saw a good deal of each other during the first four nights, for though we were never in the same ward again, we took our lunch and breakfast together, and I missed her greatly when, after the fourth night, she came down with the "flue." I performed some very unpleasant tasks (which I learned later properly should have been done by the orderlies) that night and was feeling quite sick when a nurse took me into the women's worst ward to help her give a cold sponge bath to a woman who seemed to be dying. Imagine my feelings when she said she wanted me to [be] able to do that the next night alone. However, I guess I was broken in that night, for the close air, smell of new drugs, etc. never made me so sick again.

The next night the awful shortness of help began. One nurse who had only had two wards and three helpers the night before now had four wards with the same number of helpers. She told us at breakfast that she did not discover till morning that one woman had a temperature of 105 and then she had no time to do anything. Is it any wonder the people died off as they did?

That night I was put alone, on a ward that had twenty men patients – two of them delirious. One of them was continually sitting up in bed and I would have to make him lie down. The poor fellow died a few nights later. The other man would strip off his shirt whenever I left the room and the patient in the next bed would call 'Nurse, that man's got his shirt off again' and I would have to go and put it on him. The following night I had the same ward but they had taken away my two delirious patients, and I found time to do what seemed to me badly needed to be done, that was to put paper shade over the lamps and to tie the doors so they would not bang and wake everyone up. Some of the trained nurses would come in during the night banging the door and switching on the lights needlessly, so, as far as I could, I saw that these things were in all the wards on my floor.

The next night I was put on ward 21, the worst men's ward. It was not a hard night as far as the work was concerned, for there were only twelve beds, and there was another helper and we had two orderlies. Besides that, the nurses came in off and on. But there were things happening that took your heart-strength. One man was dying a slow death—just gasping—for five hours, while his wife—the sweetest little woman—who was brought in from another ward lay beside him. She was so brave; though she was quite sick, she wanted nothing for herself, but would ask us to do something to relieve his suffering. They had been married but three years and had been in the city only two months. Then there was one poor boy of seventeen, in just the next bed, who was quite sane [not delirious], and with proper care, I think might have recovered, but there he was right beside the poor man gasping for breath for hours while another fine looking young fellow was talking nonsense all night long, and another screaming and fighting with the orderlies. Poor fellow, he [the boy] would say 'Nurse it scares me,' and it seemed to comfort him to have me hold his hand. Well—the next night poor Milford died, and five others out of the twelve, the eight hours I was on duty. It was an awful night....

The next night, the fifth one, I felt obliged to take a rest but the sixth night I was feeling fine and went on duty again in one of the women's pneumonia wards. There were others there most of the time, and there were only seven patients, so I had a fairly easy night. The only troublesome patient was a poor Italian girl, who was so wild and strong that they had been obliged to tie her down to the bed.

The seventh night I was again alone with three pneumonia patients, women, one of them my dear little Mrs. Aitkens, whom I mentioned in my last letter, and another an old lady who was dying. She and the third one, also a young married woman, both died the next day.

The next night I went early, so that I might be put on the ward where Mrs. Aitkens was, and I felt repaid when, on recognizing my voice (of course I had my gown and mask on) she said 'Oh here's my dear night nurse.' They had moved five other pneumonia cases in, that night.

But it was the next night—the ninth—that took all there was of me, that night they moved in four new patients, two women and two little children, about seven and nine years; altogether there were nine. Both women were delirious, one wanting continually to know when she was going home, and the other, poor thing, was always asking for the doctor. I got him for her once, and he ordered a prescription. When, after some time, the medicine hadn't come, and she was continually asking for the doctor, I went to see about the prescription, only to find that the nurse to whom the doctor sent it had been too rushed to see about getting it made up. The poor woman had a baby girl at home and she used to say, 'Will I live, nurse?' I tried to comfort her and quiet her. I learned the next day that she had died. I was almost distracted that night. I would just start to rub one woman's chest with olive oil when another would call me. I could not begin to do what was needing to be done. I felt my ignorance, and there was no one to help.

The next night I was on the same ward, but it was somewhat easier, as there were only seven patients, but two of them were pretty sick. My little Mrs. Aitkens said to me that night 'Oh nurse, I dread the day—I wish you were twins so that one of you could be with me during the day.' Poor little woman, I learned later that she died in less than a week from that night.

I had the satisfaction that night of seeing one woman pass the crisis—or so it seemed to me. She was terribly sick all the first few hours. I applied plasters, put an ice bag to her head, fanned her, etc. and she seemed decidedly better when I went off duty late in the morning.

Before I finished my breakfast, I felt that I was coming down with the 'flu', and when my temperature was taken by one of the nurses it proved to be 101. The next day I was taken to another hospital—the one for nurses in training. Of my experiences there, I will write you another time.

Lunenburg Progress Enterprise, 25 December 1918, 1.

⇨ After only nine nights on duty, Mary Chesley herself contracted influenza. The 1901 Census for Lunenburg County shows Mary's parents, Samuel and Mary R., living in the town of Lunenburg. They were both 51, having been born in 1849. Little Mary A., 9 years old, born 30 July 1891, was the only child still at home. Thus by 1918, when she heroically volunteered at the flu hospital, Mary Albee Chesley was 26. Some of the above information was provided by researcher Sharon MacDonald, who is writing a book about Mary Chesley.

⇨ Sharon MacDonald provided additional material:

✉ "Mary Albee Chesley (known familiarly as Polly) lived and taught high school in Vancouver from 1918 to 1921. During the flu epidemic, schools were closed and Polly volunteered as a night nurse. This was published in the Lunenburg Progress Enterprise newspaper on Christmas Day, Wednesday 25, 1918. M.R.C. was Polly's mother."

Sharon MacDonald to Ruth Whitehead, email, May 31, 2018.

DIED OF INFLUENZA

BRIDGEWATER, Feb. 23. Influenza has again broken out here, and 180 residents are ill with the disease. There were two deaths today. In both cases pneumonia, following influenza, caused death. Rev. John D. MacIntosh, pastor of St. John's Presbyterian Church, and Morris Hebb, town electrician, died to-day.

Liverpool Advance, 26 February 1919, 3.

 OBITUARY. Mrs. Edgar Hume. At her home in East Chester, Thursday, Feb. 20th, at the early hour of 2.15 a. m. there passed away to her eternal rest, in her thirty-fourth year, Irene Henrietta, beloved wife of Mr. Edgar Hume. Her death occurred from pneumonia, following Spanish influenza. Although in a critical condition since Saturday, Feb. 13th, yet she did not go to her bed until Sunday, because all in her home, including her father-in-law, husband and five children were stricken down, at one time with the Flu, and in administering to their wants, she forgot her own sufferings. Such a good wife, mother and friend was she, that even when her temperature was at 104, she went about caring for those whom she loved....During her illness she used to say that she did not expect to get better. She thought if she had gone to her bed before she did, there might have been a chance.

Hants Journal, 12 March 1919, 6.

 FLU SPREADING IN LUNENBURG CO.

Mahone Bay Has Closed Its School and Churches

The flu...is spreading rapidly to all parts of the Country; at New Dublin, Parks Creek and Riverport, there are numerous cases, and the health boards are busily engaged taking measures to combat the disease. Quite a lot of houses are placarded. From all parts of the municipality have come rush demands for placards, and the municipal clerk is kept busy sending out supplies to the sanitary inspector.

Halifax Morning Chronicle, 28 February 1920, 1.

☞ This Third Wave hit Lunenburg harder than in many other counties—34 people died. When it finally tapered off, the Great Influenza had killed a total of 139 souls in the county. Others, who survived, would having lasting health problems.

LUNENBURG COUNTY, VITAL STATISTICS, DEATH REGISTER, BOOKS 43, 93

1918

1. Ivan Winters, 27, d. 6 October 1918, Ovens, fisherman.
2. Leslie Tanner, 16, d. 10 October 1918, Lunenburg.
3. Maud Meck, 50, d. 11 October 1918, Lunenburg, housewife.
4. Archibald Demone, 38, d. 17 October 1918, Lunenburg.
5. Florence Mason, 39, d. 19 October 1918, Lunenburg, housewife.
6. Hilda Wynacht, 21, d. 20 October 1918, Lunenburg, housewife.
7. Rosabella Himmelman, 45, d. 27 October 1918, Lunenburg, housewife.
8. Harry Oxner, 17, d. 3 November 1918, Lunenburg.
9. Mable Jackson, 28, d. 7 November 1918, Lunenburg, housewife.
10. Elida Prince, 59, d. 9 November 1918, Lunenburg, housewife, "widower" [*sic*].
11. Mary Langille, 45, d. 30 November 1918, Lunenburg, housewife.
12. Henry Deal, 61, d. 12 October 1918, Sentry, fisherman.
13. Maggie Wentzell, 27, d. 16 October 1918, Sentry, housewife.
14. Morris Mason, 24, d. 18 October 1918, Eastern Points, fisherman.
15. Mary Tanner, 20, d. 21 October 1918, Blue Rocks.
16. Philip Mason, 9, d. 25 October, 1918, Eastern Points.
17. Jervois Lohnes, 26, d. 26 October 1918, Back Sentry.
18. Olive Naas, 21, d. 28 October 1918, Sentry, housewife.
19. George Langille, 4 months, d. 11 November 1918, Blue Rocks.
20. Mrs. Mary Knickle, 96, d. 13 November 1918, Blue Rocks.
21. Rosavilla Young, 26, d. 8 November 1918, Martin's [*sic*] Brook.
22. Charles Bealer, 35, d. 28? [*October*] 1918, Bridgewater, labourer. [*His father's name was George; he was born in Indian Grant, was Roman Catholic, resided in Bridgewater and was buried there. HVS, Lunenburg County Death Register, Book 43, Page 99, Page 99, Number 336.*]
23. Bernard Robertson, 34, d. 21 October 1918, Bridgewater.
24. Leonard _____ [*no surname on Allan Marble list*], 34, d. 25 October 1918, Bridgewater, master carpenter. [*Original record shows Leonard St. Claire Gelfs/Delfs. Under high magnification, his surname could be either Delfs or Gelfs or even Gelfus. HVS Search Engine identifies him as "Telfer," Book 43, Page 99, Number 339.*]
25. Myrtle Wile, 1, d. 28 October 1918, Bridgewater.
26. Martha Garber, 34, d. 26 October 1918, Bridgewater, housewife.
27. Harry Baker, 31, d. 29 October 1918, Bridgewater, ice dealer.
28. Pearl Himmelman, 18, d. 2 November 1918, Bridgewater.
29. William Smith, 8 months, d. 4 November 1918, Bridgewater.
30. Lucinda Morris, 32, d. 8 November 1918, Bridgewater, secretary.
31. Alfred Dolliver, 19, d. 5 November 1918, Bridgewater, machinist.
32. Medora Whynot, 32, d. 6 November 1918, Bridgewater, housewife.
33. Melburne Lohnes, 29, d. 8 December 1918, Bridgewater, accountant.
34. William Martell, 32, d. 14 December 1918, Bridgewater, clergyman.
35. Bessie Smith, 30, d. 15 October 1918, Barrington.

36. Henry Naugler, 19, d. 18 October 1918, Wynot [*sic*] Settlement, farmer.

37. Irene Franklyn, 6 months, d. 24 October 1918, Dayspring.

38. Carrie Hirtle, 32, d. 27 October 1918, Dayspring, housewife.

39. Grace Brown, 3, d. 25 October 1918, Italy Cross.

40. Bernard Wile, 41, d. 30 October 1918, Wileville, farmer.

41. _____ Conrod, 22, d. 2 November 1918, Upper LaHave, fisherman. [*HVS Database Search Engine gives his surname as M. Conrad, but it is "Conrod, Melassone (Melanson?) in the original record. HVS, Lunenburg County Death Register, Book 43, Page 104, Number 362.*]

42. Ida Wile, 41, d. 22 November 1918, Wileville, housewife.

43. _____ Crouse, male, 4, d. 24 December 1918, LaHave. [*HVS, Lunenburg County Death Register, Book 43, Page 106, Number 372. First name is possibly Garland.*]

44. _____ Crouse [*sic; on Allan Marble list*], female, 8, d. 25 December 1918, West Clifford. [*Evelyn Crouse. She was 8 years and 6 months old. HVS, Lunenburg County Death Register, Book 43, Page 106, Number 373.*]

45. Mary Robar, 5 months, d. 31 December 1918, East Clifford.

46. Agnes Beeler, 67, d. 18 October 1918, Scarsdale, housekeeper.

47. Jane Jefferson, 52, d. 1 November 1918, New Germany, housewife.

48. Ronald Robar, 3, d. 24 November 1918, North River.

49. Grace Westhaver, 20, d. 26 September 1918, Chester, trained nurse. [*Grace was born in Roxbury, Massachusetts; married to William Westhaver of Fox Point, NS. Her early onset date may be the result of a visit home to Massachusetts in September 1918, when the influenza was raging there.*

HVS, Lunenburg County Death Register, Book 43, Page 117, Number 414.]

50. Clarence Croft, 28, d. 20 October 1918, Chester Basin, ship builder.

51. Cecil Croft, 20, d. 9 October 1918, Chester Basin, ship builder.

52. George Pembroke, 18, d. 12 October 1918, Chester, clerk.

53. Pearl Mitchell, 46, d. 19 October 1918, Chester, housewife.

54. Earl Corkum, 26, d. 21 October 1918, Chester, cook.

55. Rhoda Conrod, 22, d. 24 October 1918, Chester, teacher.

56. Eva Katcher, 27, d. 29 October 1918, East River, housewife.

57. Anna Melvin, 25, d. 30 October 1918, East River, housewife.

58. Charles Morris, 61, d. 3 November 1918, Chester, mechanic.

59. James Stanford, 65, d. 11 November, Chester, trader.

60. Evelyn Gates, 2, d. 12 November 1918, Upper Blandford.

61. Henry Gates, 59, d. 28 November 1918, Upper Blandford, fisherman.

62. Effie Turner, 37, d. 19 November 1918, Frauxville [*sic*], housewife.

63. James Hiltz, 49, d. 24 October 1918, Forties Settlement, farmer.

64. Nelson Bezanson, 31, d. 26 October 1918, Fraxville [*sic*], cooper.

65. Maggie Hiltz, 14 d. 29 October 1918, Forties Settlement.

66. Frances Hiltz, 34, d. 30 October 1918, Forties Settlement, housewife.

67. Frances Herget [*Hergot; formerly Herrgott?*], 7 years [*her death record describes her as an "infant," aged "7 mos-9 mos"*], d. 30 October 1918, Forties Settlement [*HVS, Book 43, Page 122, Number 443*].

68. Alice Roach, 19, d. 31 October 1918, Fraxville, housemaid.

69. Crawford Conrad, 21, d. 17 October 1918, Cherry Hill, fisherman.

70. Carl Feener, male, 24, d. 5 November 1918, Italy Cross, nurse in hospital.

71. Charles Falt, 20, d. 9 November 1918, Petite Rivière, labourer.

72. Ray Conrad, 23, d. 24 October 1918, New Dublin, fisherman.

73. Linda Wynacht, 26, d. 17 December 1918, Middle South.

74. Clayton Wentzell, 19, d. 1 January 1918 [sic; 1919], Riverport, fisherman.

75. James Mozeman, 35, d. 16 October 1918, Rose Bay, farmer.

76. Hector Mossman, 29, d. 30 October 1918, Riverport, farmer.

77. George Lohnes, 32, d. 6 December 1918, Riverport.

1919

78. Elizabeth Knickle, 3 weeks, d. 17 February 1919, Lunenburg.

79. William Oxner, 34, d. 1 January 1919, Lunenburg.

80. Annie Demone, 30, d. 19 January 1919, Lunenburg, housewife.

81. Regina Winters, 45, d. 19 February 1919, Bridgewater, housekeeper.

82. Nelson Wile, 72, d. 4 February 1919, Bridgewater, blacksmith.

83. John MacIntosh, 32, d. 23 February 1919, Bridgewater, clergyman.

84. Maurice Hebb, 29, d. 23 February 1919, Bridgewater, electrician.

85. Hilda Montgomery, 30, d. 25 February 1919, Bridgewater, housewife.

86. Uriah Wile, 47, d. 6 January 1919, Wileville, labourer.

87. Edna Wile, 6, d. 21 February 1919, Wileville.

88. Charles Zwicker, 18, d. 5 March 1919, Camperdown, labourer.

89. Everett Zwicker, 6, d. 9 March 1919, Camperdown.

90. Gordon McCarthy, 2, d. 9 March 1919, Conquerall.

91. John Zwicker, 3, d. 9 March 1919, Camperdown.

92. James Frausel, 26, d. 4 March 1919, Poor Farm, Dayspring, pauper.

93. Garfield Fitch, 1 month, d. 11 March 1919, Conquerall Mills.

94. Ethel Veinotte, 17, d. 7 January 1919, Mahone Bay, student.

95. Unnamed male infant, 13 days, d. 14 February 1919, Martin's River.

96. Simeon Carver, 25, d. 26 February 1919, Waldon, farmer.

97. Clifford Levey, 25, 20 March 1919, Little Tancook.

98. Joshua Langill, 55, d. 13 March 1919, Tancook, boatbuilder.

99. Irene Hume, 34, d. 20 February 1919, East Chester, housewife.

100. Ada Bond, 66, d. 6 March 1919, East Chester, housewife.

101. Ellice Hiltz, female, 36, d. 18 February 1918, Fraxville, housewife.

102. Margaret Roach, 59, d. 2 March 1919, Fraxville.

103. Georgiana Himmelman, 32, d. 5 January 1919, LaHave Islands, housewife.

[*The next number in the register is a repeat of the death record for Georgiana Himmelman (as "Georgine"), and is therefore omitted from this list.*]

104. Gladys Levy, 11 d. 22 January 1919, Feltzen South.

1920

105. John Walker, 84, d. 15 January 1920, New Ross.

106. George Veno [*Veinot?*], 30, Northfield, farmer.

107. Emma Spencer, 35, d. 29 February 1920, New Ross, domestic.

108. Jennie Boylon, 27, d. 29 February 1920, New Ross, housewife.

109. Selena Cors____ [Corkum], 29, d. 19 February 1920, East LaHave. [HVS, Book 95, Page 183.]

110. Charles Cor____ [Charles Norman Corkum], d. 19 February 1920, East LaHave, fisherman. [HVS, Book 95, Page 184. He was the son of Josiah and Alice Corkum, and his "racial origin" is given as "German Immigrant."]

111. Phoebe Schnare, 24, d. 6 March 1920, Lunenburg, housewife.

112. Harvey Oxner, 31, d. 11 March 1920, Lunenburg, clerk

113. Laura Anderson, 28, d. 11 March 1920, Lunenburg, housewife.

114. Daniel Zinck, 78, d. 11 March 1920, First South, farmer.

115. St. Clair Greek, 25, d. 22 March 1920, Blue Rocks, fisherman.

116. Lola Feenel, 18, d. 4 March 1920, Bridgewater, schoolteacher.

117. Infant Penny, 7 days, d. 8 March 1920, Bridgewater.

118. Laura Penny, 11 months, d. 11 March 1920, Bridgewater.

119. Elmira Smith, 30, d. 15 March 1920, Dayspring.

120. John Garber, 45, d. 19 March 1920, Newcombville, farmer.

121. Cecil Mader, 20, d. 1 March 1920, Mahone Bay.

122. Mary Emmens, 69, d. 12 March 1920, New Germany, housework.

123. Spurgeon Acker, 23, d. 27 March 1920, Cherryfield.

124. William E. Prisk, 30, d. 4 March 1920, Chester Basin.

125. George Balkes, 31, 2 March 1920, New Ross.

126. George Baker, 32, d. 2 March 1920, New Ross.

127. Abbey Walker, 52, d. 4 March 1920, New Ross.

128. Gladys Walker, 16, d. 5 March 1920, New Ross.

129. Joanna Russell, 76, d. 5 March 1920, New Ross, housewife.

130. Patrick Boylan, 67, d. 6 March 1920, New Ross, farmer.

131. Infant Keddy, 6 months, d. 19 March 1920, New Ross.

132. Leslie Maharney, 10, d. 20 March 1920, New Ross.

133. Lucy Shupe, 87, d. 29 March 1920, Seffernville, housewife.

134. Ella Croft, 32, d. 29 March 1920, West Dublin.

135. Elizabeth Myra, 81, d. 6 March 1920, Feltzen South.

136. Borden Cook, 8 months, d. 1 April 1920, First South.

137. James J. Oickle, 58, d. 20 April 1920, Maitland, farmer.

138. John F. Chesley, 76, d. 7 April 1920, New Germany, farmer.

139. Amy Bezanson, 37, d. 28 April 1920, New Ross, housewife.

Chapter XIV

PICTOU COUNTY

❧⚹⚹❧

IN PICTOU COUNTY, the Great Influenza epidemic killed at least 133 people.

 DR. 'JACK' MACKENZIE IS DEAD
PICTOU, October 12. Doctor John J. MacKenzie, one of the best known physicians in Eastern Nova Scotia, died at two o'clock this morning from bronchial pneumonia following Spanish influenza. As health officer of the town, Dr. MacKenzie on Monday night attended a meeting of the Health Board, at which it was decided to close all theatres, churches and schools to quarantine half a dozen cases of influenza already reported and to take all other precautionary measures to prevent the spread of the disease. On Tuesday Dr. MacKenzie was taken ill and the disease soon turned to pneumonia.

Halifax Evening Mail, 12 October 1918, 1.

✑ Ruth Legge wrote to me about one of her relatives who died, as follows:

✉ Florence Rita Rumley was born 19 Feb 1913, in Stellarton. Little Florence was a daughter of Kenneth Elmer Rumley (1893–1989) and Ethel Grace Ackles (1892–1947). She was 5 years and 9 months when she died of influenza on 20 November 1918. Her parents were living on Bridge Street in Stellarton at the time. When she died, the address is listed as Red Row. I believe that is the miner's row housing in Stellarton, and may be on Bridge St.

Kenneth, her father, was a miner and draegerman (assisted with Moose River rescue and recovery). He was born in Liscomb Mills and was a first cousin once removed of my father. Kenneth's father was Elias Rumley (his mother was Hannah Ferguson of PEI), and Elias was the son of Charles Henry Rumley and Ann "Nancy" Elizabeth Riley, the couple who moved from Halifax to Liscomb Harbour in the 1830s and established the Liscomb area branch of the Rumley family.

Ruth Legge to Ruth Whitehead, email, March 2018.

✑ Florence Rumley wasn't the only child to die in miners' housing in Stellarton. At least one other infant, a boy who lived on Red Row, also died there in the epidemic. His name was James Tolly Jr. He was still a baby.

FORM 6

PROVINCE OF NOVA SCOTIA

CERTIFICATE OF REGISTRATION OF DEATH

198 ✓

1 PLACE OF DEATH
County of *Pictou* Municipality of *New Glasgow* Registered No. _____
(For use of Registrar General only)
City or Town *New Glasgow* Street *Albert St* House No. _____
If in hospital or institution, give name _____

2 NAME OF DECEASED *Miller, Charles Peter*
Residence *Albert St. New Glasgow*
(Usual place of abode)

PERSONAL AND STATISTICAL INFORMATION	MEDICAL CERTIFICATE OF DEATH

3 SEX *Male* **4 RACIAL ORIGIN** *Scotch* **5 Single, Married, Widowed or Divorced (Write the word)** *Single*

6 BIRTHPLACE (Province or Country) *N.S.*

7 DATE OF BIRTH (month, day and year) *Oct 3 1893*

8 AGE Years *27* Months _____ Days _____ If less than one day, _____ hrs. or _____ min.

9 LAST OCCUPATION OF DECEASED
(a) *Auditor* (Trade or occupation or kind of work)
(b) _____ (Kind of industry)
(c) From *about 4 years* (Date from which to so employ’d)

10 FORMER OCCUPATION OF DECEASED
(a) *Clerk in Bank* (Trade or occupation or kind of work)
(b) _____ (Kind of industry)
(c) From *School* to _____ (Date from which to which so employed)

11 LENGTH OF RESIDENCE (In years and months)
(a) At place of death *Life-long*
(b) In province *In Pictou & Here*
(c) In Canada (if an immigrant) _____

12 Name of father *Andrew Miller*
13 Birthplace of father (Province or country) *N.S.*
14 Maiden name of mother *Christena A. Turner*
15 Birthplace of mother (Province or country) _____

16 Informant’s name *Mrs Andrew Miller*
Address *Albert St N.G.*
17 Relationship to deceased *Mother*
18 Place of burial, cremation or removal *Merigomish* Date of burial *Feb 16th 1920*
19 Undertaker *James Ross N.G.* (Name and Address)

20 Date of death *Feby 13* _____ 1920
(Month, day and year)

21 I HEREBY CERTIFY, that I attended deceased from *Feby 6* 19__ to *Feby 13* 19 20 that I last saw him alive on *Feby 13* 19__ and that death occurred, on the date stated above, at *4* P. m.

The CAUSE OF DEATH was as follows:
Pulmonary Tuberculosis
(duration) *1* yrs. *6* mos. _____ dys.
CONTRIBUTORY (Secondary) *Influenza*
(duration) _____ yrs. _____ mos. _____ dys.

22 Where was disease contracted if not at place of death? _____
Did an operation precede death? *No* Date of _____
Was there an autopsy? *No*
(Signed) *J. Ballem* M.D.
Address *New Glasgow*
Date *Feb 14. 1920*

State the Disease causing Death, or in death from Violent Causes, state (1) Means and Nature of Injury, (2) whether Accidental, Suicidal or Homicidal.

23 Registrar’s Record Number _____

24 Filed *Feb 16th 1920* *James Ross*
Division Registrar

(See Instructions on back of Certificate — Statement of OCCUPATION is very important.)

Death record for Charles Miller, an auditor, ill with tuberculosis. He later contracted influenza, and the combination of the two killed him. *(Nova Scotia Archives)*

A SAD STORY

Father Lying At Death's Door—Mother Prepares Their Dead Babe For Burial.

[From the *Eastern Federationist*, New Glasgow]

More than fifty cases of influenza were reported at Stellarton the middle of the week, sixteen in Red Row, north Stellarton, and in that connection The Federationist heard a sad story. It seems some people look upon the disease as a sort of plague, leaving people to prepare their dead for burial [alone]. The case of James Tolly, wife and family was told by a near neighbour and friend.

Mr. Tolly, the man who played the part of a hero at the time of the Allan Shaft explosion, saving several lives, is very ill, seriously ill of influenza and complications. Last Sunday their infant child died, and of course the undertaker was sent for. He is reported to have gone to the house, and handed Mrs. Tolly, through a window, a rule to measure the dead child for its casket. In due course he delivered the coffin, placing it on the doorstep, Mrs. Tolly, taking it in, placed her dead child in it, prepared it for burial, put on the lid, fastened it, and then set the casket containing the remains on the door step, when they were taken away by the nudertaker [*sic*] and buried....Regarding Red Row [miners' housing] and that part of the town, it is said sanitary conditions are bad. Too many open closets [outhouses], not looked after in the most up-to-date way. Many of the dwellings are by no means model work peoples [*sic*] dwellings. The wonder is union labour stands for it.

Pictou Advocate, 6 December 1918, p. 4; reprinted from the Antigonish Casket.
HVS, Pictou County Death Register, Book 45, Page 332, Number 1170.

☞ The HVS record shows him as James Toily [Jr.], father James Toily, "Carcen Row," Stellarton. He was only 3 months old, and died of Influenza after a four-day illness. The HVS Search Engine gives his surname as "Taailey." The undertaker was Herbert MacQuarrie.

WEST RIVER. It is with deep regret that we record the death of Willie Arthur McLean, only son of William McLean of Central West River, which occurred at his home on Sunday 24th, inst. A short time before he had gone to work in Westville and while there contracted Spanish Influenza which rapidly developed into pneumonia.

Eastern Chronicle, 24 November 1918, 1.

WILLIAM A. MCLEAN, WEST RIVER....Died at West River, Nov. 24th, 1918, Willie A. McLean, aged 29 years, only son of Mr. and Mrs. McLean, West River....He had attended celebration of peace in New Glasgow, and contracted influenza, and caught cold, resulting in that dread disease, pneumonia. He had been home one week, came home Saturday night and one week from that day he was called to go.

Pictou Advocate, 13 December 1918, 8.

According to the Town Office register 87 houses in New Glasgow have up to date been placarded for influenza. The reports during the past few days account for the spread with new cases as follows: Thursday 21st, 4 houses; Friday 22nd, 6 houses; Saturday 23rd, 4 houses; Monday 25th, 5 houses.

This would suggest that the citizens would do well to take every individual precaution to stay the epidemic, for the danger point in New Glasgow is by no means over.

We will likely get flayed by the Evening News for making this suggestion, but when one considers that the burden of caring for the sick of necessity falls upon the women of the country, it is deplorable to see a public journal taking the side of relaxed precautions in order to curry favour with advertisers regardless of the sufferings to which innocent people are endangered.

Eastern Chronicle, 26 November 1918, 1.

Miss Floss McKay returned to New Glasgow from Baltimore, bringing the remains of her sister Lillian, which were laid to rest in Riverside Cemetery this afternoon....A young man named Charles Thomas died of influenza on West Side yesterday morning. The remains were sent to St. Peter's C.B. for burial. He had only been a resident of New Glasgow for three weeks....Fourteen additional houses with influenza reported on Monday morning and in some cases there are several victims in a house. The situation is very menacing to say the least. The shire town of Pictou seems to be badly hit at present. Every member of the staff of the Royal Bank there, was down with it on Saturday. Manager Currey included.

Eastern Chronicle, 10 December 1918, 1.

ROBERT F. MCCALLUM, NEW GLASGOW, DIED TUESDAY, DEC. 3
Robert F. McCallum of West Side, New Glasgow, died of pneumonia, following an attack of influenza on Tuesday, Dec. 3. He leaves a widow [Ethel Parker McCallum] and three young sons, Reginald, Seymour and Jack....The deceased came to New Glasgow from Noel, Hants County, and had purchased the Barclay Fraser farm at the held [head] of Willow Avenue. He was an energetic industrious man and well liked by all who knew him. Eastern Chronicle, Dec. 4.

Truro Daily News, 10 December 1918, 7. Courtesy the
Colchester Historeum, Truro.

Mr. McCallum's death is the first recorded for New Glasgow. He was ill nine days, and must have contracted flu on or before October 24.

THE 'FLU' IN WESTVILLE
(Westville Free Lance). In conversation with Mr. J. H. C. Murdoch, druggist, last evening, who is a very busy man nowadays, he informed us—and Mr. R. Fraser, druggist, has the same story to tell—that new cases of influenza are developing in town daily. Mr. Murdoch says that he considers the influenza is slowly but steadily gaining ground and that there are more cases at the present time in Westville than ever before. He further stated that Dr. Bruce has some ten cases of pneumonia, all of them of a critical character, and has a great many cases of influenza to look after as well. These are certainly strenuous days for the doctors....Anything that can be done to save life and to mitigate the suffering should be done and done just as quickly as possible.

Pictou Advocate, 13 December 1918, 8.

PICTOU COUNTY ASYLUM

A meeting of commissioners was held at the Asylum on Thursday last. The superintendent reported the death of one male patient and the admission of one patient since the meeting in October last. The health of the patients was reported to be very good, as the prevailing epidemic of influenza has not yet reached this institution. A strict quarantine against all visitors is maintained.

Pictou Advocate, 17 December 1918, 2.

DEATH ROLL

PERCY ELLIOTT. Percy Elliott, the 17 year old son of Daniel Elliott, of Meadowville, died on Wednesday of influenza.

MRS. ALEX MacKAY. The death occurred at her home at Mount Thom last Saturday of Mrs. Alex MacKay, aged 53 years. Death was due to influenza.

ALBERT RANKIN. Albert Rankin, a young man, 22 years of age, died on Wednesday at his home at Scotch Hill from influenza. The family had moved to Pictou County from the Magadalenes a few years ago.

CLEMENT TURBIDE. Clement Turbide, a young man belonging to the Magdalen Island, while on his way home from Sydney, died in Pictou on Sunday last from the influenza. The young man was 24 years of age. He had only been away from home a few months. His uncle, Father Turbide, was here on his way to the Magdalenes and was with the young man at his death bed. The funeral was held on Tuesday morning to Stella Maris cemetery.

Pictou Advocate, 20 December 1918, 8.

MISS ANNIE JOHNSON. Miss Annie Johnson, Faulkland Street, died on Sunday last, December 22nd, aged 49 years, from pneumonia following an attack of the flu. The funeral was held on Tuesday to Stella Maris Cemetery. Deceased leaves a mother, two brothers, John and Ben, at home, and a third brother, James, in Fall River. Miss Johnson was the home maker for the family, her mother, Mrs. George Johnson, being in poor health, and the two Johnson boys will feel her loss most keenly.

Pictou Advocate, 27 December 1918, 8.

SAD PASSING OF MRS. GEORGE MORAN AND INFANT

Very sad was the death yesterday [1 January] of Mrs. George Moran and her infant child, a few days old. She was only 21 years of age and is survived by her husband and a child one year old. The remains of Mother and infant in the one casket are being taken to Truro this afternoon for interment, accompanied by her mother who was with her when she passed away....

Trenton items in New Glasgow *Evening News*. Mrs. Moran was a daughter of Mrs. M. A. Lear, and granddaughter of Mrs. Timothy Elliott of Lower Onslow. Mrs Lear, who resides with her mother, will care for her little granddaughter, who was one year old the day of her mother's death, and who is at this time recovering from a severe illness of pneumonia following influenza.

Truro Daily News, 2 January 1919, 3.

PICTOU COUNTY, VITAL STATISTICS, DEATH REGISTER, BOOKS 45, 98

1918

1. Robert McCallum, 41, d. 2 December 1918, New Glasgow, miner.

2. Charles Thomas, 24, d. 8 December 1918, New Glasgow, farmer.

3. Charles Mattie, 6, d. 18 December 1918, New Glasgow.

4. John McKenzie, 27, d. 22 November 1918, Piedmont, labourer.

5. Charles Seale, 32, d. 2 December 1918, New Glasgow, labourer.

6. Angus Richard, 29, d. 2 December 1918, New Glasgow.

7. Norman Elms, 18, d. 3 December 1918, New Glasgow, labourer.

8. Hector Penny, 69, d. 22 December 1918, New Glasgow, machinist.

9. Gordon McEachern, 48, d. 28 December 1918, New Glasgow, labourer.

10. Hugh Chisholm, 45, d. 31 December 1918, New Glasgow.

11. Rhoda Penny, 58, d. 12 December 1918, New Glasgow, housekeeper.

12. W. H. Niles, male, 22, d. 13 December 1918, New Glasgow, brakeman.

13. Mrs. David Fraser, 35, d. 19 December 1918, New Glasgow.

14. James Dickie, 38, d. 6 November 1918, New Glasgow, carpenter.

15. Hughena Rankin, 36, d. 10 November 1918, New Glasgow, housekeeper.

16. Michael Hurley, 35, d. 19 November 1918, New Glasgow, fireman.

17. Charles Skinner, 34, d. 28 November 1918, New Glasgow, coal miner.

18. David Douglas, 26, d. 3 November 1918, New Glasgow, operator.

19. Olive De Wolfe, 21, d. 25 November 1918, Stellarton, housewife.

20. Blanche Davidson, 18 months, d. 26 November 1918, Stellarton.

21. Mrs. Mary Martin, 79, d. 3 December 1918, Stellarton, housework.

22. Laurence De Coste, 2, d. 4 December 1918, Stellarton.

23. John Tupper, 18, d. 4 December 1918, Stellarton, railway worker.

24. Arnold Trefery, 3, d. 4 December 1918, Stellarton.

25. Jessie Tupper, 36, d. 5 December 1918, Stellarton, housewife.

26. Vivian Trefery, female, 8 months, d. 7 December 1918, Stellarton.

27. James Carmichael, 29, d. 11 December 1918, Stellarton, railway worker.

28. Evelyn Works, 38, d. 11 December 1918, Stellarton, housewife.

29. Thelema Dean [*Thelma M. Dean*], 11, d. 15 December 1918, Stellarton. [*HVS, Pictou County Death Register, 1918, Book 45, Page 329, Number 1159.*]

30. John McDonald, 8 months, d. 31 December 1918, Stellarton.

31. James Toiley, 8 months, d. 1 November 1918, Stellarton.

32. Rosey Maniah, female, 15 [*16 and 6 months*], d. 3 November 1918, Stellarton, housewife. [*HVS, Pictou County Death Register, Book 45, Page 332, 1171, has her name as "Marish." She was living on Red Row, Stellarton.*]

33. Joseph Waitaitas, 10 months, d. 10 November 1918, Stellarton. [*HVS, Pictou County Death Register, 1918, Book 45, Page 333, Number 1170; living at Cricket Row, Stellarton. HVS Search Engine has his name as "Waitaetos."*]

34. George Hood, 28, d. 15 November 1918, Stellarton, machinist.

35. Walter Curry, 42, d. 12 November 1918, Stellarton, miner.

36. Annie Johnson, 24, d. 13 November 1918, Stellarton, housewife.

37. Sarah Faulds, 42, d. 16 November 1918, Stellarton, housewife.

38. Florence Rumley, 5, d. 20 November 1918, Stellarton.

39. Harold Morgan, 4 months, d. 21 November 1918, Stellarton.

40. David Carrol, 21, d. 22 November 1918, brakeman on railway.

41. Joseph Welsh, 28, d. 2 December 1918, Thorburn, miner.

42. Mrs. Herbert Canning, 20, d. 4 December 1918, Thorburn, housewife.

43. Isabell MacDougal, 4, d. 10 December 1918, Thorburn.

44. Audrie Dwyer, 7 months, d. 26 December 1918, Thorburn.

45. Edgar Foote, 19, d. 27 November 1918, Barney's [sic] River Station, farmer.

46. Margaret Hoggart, 10 months, d. 25 November 1918, Marshy Hope.

47. John McKenzie, 26, d. 22 November 1918, Piedmont, labourer.

48. Ernest Grant, 22, d. 22 October 1918, Sunny Brae.

49. John McQuarrie, 38, d. 8 December 1918, Hopewell, labourer.

50. William Hughes, 13, d. 26 October 1918, Westville, student.

51. Paul Le Blanc, 45, d. 16 November 1918, Westville, labourer.

52. Jessie Robertson, 22, d. 17 November 1918, Westville.

53. George Livingstone, 3, d. 17 November 1918, Westville.

54. Ruth Wood, 3, d. 20 November 1918, Westville.

55. John Dooley, 53, d. 20 November 1918, Westville.

56. Melville Thompson, 13 months, d. 25 November 1918, Westville.

57. Christine Langille, 24, d. 25 November 1918, Westville, housewife.

58. John Matheson, 75, d. 26 November 1918, Westville, labourer.

59. Isabelle MacLeod, 31, d. 29 November 1918, Westville, housewife.

60. Robert Russell, 31, d. 30 November 1918, Westville, miner.

61. Murray Sutherland, 32, d. 1 December 1918, Westville, brakeman, railway.

62. Clarence Rector, 27, d. 7 December 1918, Westville, machinist.

63. Jennie Muir, 26, d. 20 December 1918, Westville, schoolteacher.

64. Alex Thomson, 36, d. 26 December 1918, Westville, miner.

65. John Emery, 64, d. 29 December 1918, Westville, miner.

66. Jane MacLeod, 71, d. 4 November 1918, Burnside, housewife.

67. John J. McKenzie, 45, d. 12 October 1918, Pictou, physician.

68. Victoria Banks, 18, d. 20 October 1918, Pictou.

69. Albert Arseneau, 26, d. 28 November 1918, Pictou, labourer.

70. John McInnis, 33, d. 5 December 1918, Pictou, schoolteacher.

71. Francis Heighton, 4, d. 9 December 1918, Pictou.

72. Clement Turbide, 24, d. 15 December 1918, Pictou, labourer.

73. Annie Johnson, 52, d. 22 December 1918, Pictou.

74. Mrs. Robert Tanner, 66, d. 2 November 1918, Central Cariboo.

75. Albert Rankin, 23, d. 18 December 1918, Scotch Hill, farmer.

76. Hugh McDonald, 23, d. 21 October, Loganville, farmer.

77. Joseph Dorrington, 27, d. 15 December 1918, Trenton, fireman.

78. Myrtle Moran, 21, d. 18 December 1918, Trenton, housewife.

79. Fred Arsenault, d. 16 October 1918, Trenton, steel worker.

80. Frederick Bernard, 19, d. 17 October 1918, Trenton, steel worker.

81. Joseph McEachern, 23, d. 15 November 1918, Trenton, steel worker.

82. Laurence Munroe, 6, d. 25 November 1918, Trenton.

83. Daniel McDonald, 16, d. 29 November 1918, Trenton, steel worker.

84. Mrs. Burton Langille, 21, d. 2 December 1918, Trenton.

85. Leola Thomson, 20, d. 5 December 1918, Trenton, stenograph [*sic*].

1919

86. James McKay, 84, d. 24 March 1919, Abercrombie.

87. Laura Currie, 2, d. 31 March 1919, New Glasgow.

88. Annie McDonald, 4, d. 1 January 1919, Evansville (near Stellarton).

89. Gordon Clark, 27, d. 8 January 1919, Stellarton, miner.

90. Angus McKenzie, 35, d. 10 January 1919, Stellarton, miner.

91. Mrs. Marcella Fraser, 38, d. 23 January 1919, Stellarton, housewife.

92. Joseph Lohez [*Lohey*], 5 months, d. 17 February 1919, Stellarton. [*HVS, Pictou County Death Register, 1919, Book 45, Page 381, Number 13.*]

93. Julia Dyer, 10 months, d. 24 February 1919, Stellarton.

94. George Cummings, 20 months, d. 4 March 1919, Stellarton.

95. Howard McEachern, 17 d. 5 March 1919, Stellarton, miner.

96. Mrs. Leah Cummings, 30, d. 5 March 1919, Stellarton, housewife.

97. John Pearson, 33, d. 18 March 1919, Stellarton, stationary engineer.

98. Mrs. Mary Whyte, 45, d. 23 March 1919, Stellarton, housewife.

99. Jean McKenzie, 18 months, d. 25 March 1919, Stellarton.

100. Elma McKenzie, 2, d. 31 March 1920, Stellarton.

101. Charles Arbuckle, 28, d. 8 January 1919, Ponds, farmer.

102. Thomas McKay, 18, d. 9 January 1919, St. Paul's [*sic*], farmer.

103. Ressie Gray, female, 24, d. 29 March 1919, Westville.

104. Colin Bull, 36, d. 2 January 1919, Pictou, labourer.

105. Mary Rudolph, 19 months, d. 11 February 1919, Pictou.

106. Annie Cameron, 17, d. 26 February 1919, Mulgrave.

107. Michael Andrews, 6 months, d. 17 March 1919, Trenton.

108. David Cameron, 11 months, d. 26 March 1919, Trenton.

109. Earl Dunn, 5, d. 1 January 1919, Trenton.

1920

110. Charles Miller, 27, d. 13 February 1920, New Glasgow, auditor.

111. John H. Bonvie, 44, d. 25 February 1920, New Glasgow, labourer.

[*Dr. Marble's list shows Number 112 as Donald B. MacVicar, 22, d. 22 February 1920, from Merigomish, died in Boston, fireman. Since he did not die in Pictou County, his name has been removed from the present list, so that death counts may be accurate for the county.*]

112. Mrs. Annie E. Mitchell, 34, d. 19 February 1920, Pictou.

113. John P. Bentley, 61, d. 3 March 1920, New Glasgow, labourer.

[*Dr. Marble's list show Number 114 as Rosella MacCallum, 26, d. 5 March 1920, housewife. No place of residence is listed by Dr. Marble, and no Nova Scotian death register carries her name. As with Donald McVicar, above, she almost certainly died elsewhere. Since she did not die in Pictou*]

County, her name has been removed from the present list, so that death counts may be accurate for the county.]

114. John D. McKay, 4, d. 12 March 1920, New Glasgow.

115. Cassie Newbury, 31, d. 13 March 1920, New Glasgow, housekeeper.

116. Mary Jane McKay, 74, d. 13 March 1920, New Glasgow, housekeeper.

117. William G. Arthrelt [*Arthrell*], 1 month, d. 7 March 1920, Thorburn. [*HVS, Death Register, 1920, Book 98, Page 276, shows him the son of Harry and Clara M. Vachuisse Arthrell. He was born in Thorburn, died there, but was buried in Stellarton.*]

118. Mrs. James McKay, 89, d. 17 March 1920, Stellarton.

119. William H. E. Murray, 50, d. 21 March 1920 at the Asylum in Riverton.

120. Abraham Langille, 42, d. 21 March 1920 at the Asylum in Riverton. [*HVS, Book 98, Page 299 shows "Occupation: patient," and that he had lived at the asylum for the last seven years, and had never had a previous occupation of any sort.*]

121. Isabel Sutherland, 40, d. 21 March 1920 at the Asylum in Riverton.

122. Thomas Donohue, 75, d. 24 March 1920 at the Asylum in Riverton.

123. Andrew Hood, 35, d. 28 March 1920 at the Asylum in Riverton.

124. John McIntosh, 60, d. 31 March 1920 at the Asylum in Riverton.

125. Elizabeth Broderick, 62, d. 8 March 1920, Pictou.

126. Mrs. Annie MacLeod, 56, d. 15 March 1920, Salt Springs.

127. Chester McMullen, 4 months, d. 15 March 1920, Trenton.

128. Mary Bennoit, 29, d. 14 April 1920, Vale Road.

129. Eva McGregor, 2 months, d. 25 April 1920, Big Island. [*HVS search engine gives her name as "MacGregor, Eva Donella"; the actual death record, Book 98, Page 348, clearly shows her name was Eva Donelda McGregor.*]

130. John J. MacLellan, 62, d. 26 April 1920, East River.

131. Andrew Davidson, 58, d. 9 April 1920 at the Asylum at Stellarton [*sic*].

132. Hugh Rogers, 64, d. 13 April 1920 at the Asylum in Riverton.

133. Mrs. Daniel MacGregor, 80, d. 6 May 1920, Big Island.

Chapter XV

QUEENS COUNTY

꙳ꙨꙨ꙳

IN QUEENS COUNTY, there were only twenty-five deaths from the Great Influenza: twenty-three dead between 4 August 1918 and 27 April 1919, and two deaths between April 18 and May 5, 1920. Perhaps because of the low number of flu victims in the county, there is almost no newspaper coverage on what was happening vis-à-vis influenza here in 1918–20. People got most of this minimalist reportage on the epidemic from newspapers elsewhere.

☞ The majority of the deaths from influenza in Queens County clustered around Liverpool and the surrounding area. The death register is a bit odd: the first death recorded by Dr. Marble for Queens County is that of Burnard Hemeon, 39, a fisherman of West Berlin, NS, who died in Gloucester, Massachusetts, on 19 September 1918, after a four-day illness of "Spanish influenza." He shouldn't be in this register at all because he didn't die in this county, but there he is. Nevertheless, his name is not included on the amended list of county dead, at the end of this chapter.

HVS, Lunenburg County Death Register, 1918, Book 46, Page 309, Number 710.
The search engine for HVS database gives his name as "Bernard Hemeon."

☞ The next two deaths that Dr. Marble recorded from the register were even earlier: they were those of elderly ladies, beginning with Mrs. Hugh Bradley, 83, a widow of Whiteburn, Queens County. An Irish Roman Catholic, she was buried in West Caledonia. She began to fail in July, and on August 4 died of "Old Age/ La Grippe." This is either an early onset for the Second Wave of Influenza in Nova Scotia, or else a final gasp from the First Wave, (as was the death of Margaret Cole, below, another person who did not die in Queens County.)

HVS, Lunenburg County Death Register, 1918, Book 46, Page 319, Number 738.

☞ Margaret Cole, 79, died on August 31 in Maitland [Bridge], Annapolis County, according to Dr. Allan Marble's list by counties. She had been ill for three weeks, the cause being "LaGrippe and pneumonia." Because she died outside of the county, she is not on the Queens County amended list, but has been transferred to Annapolis County. Her name is on Dr. Marble's list of Queens County dead because it appears in the Queens County death register, which he was transcribing. So even though the register clearly says she was born in Caledonia, but resided, died, and was buried in "Maitland, Annapolis County," there she is anyway.

HVS, Queens County Death Register, 1918, Book 46, Page 320, Number 743.

☞ Two further deaths are recorded for the month, one person dying on the October 20, and the other on the October 31, but it is in November that the influenza really started to take off. Influenza deaths continued into 1919, from January until April 1919, when Mr. Ingram Gardner of Brooklyn lost his daughters Evelyn, aged 9, on April 23; and Olethia Harriet, aged 2, on the April 27. They were the last recorded deaths from the Second Wave of influenza. There occurred only two deaths in 1920, from the Third Wave. The first was Sadie Smith, 47, a Liverpool housewife, who died on April 18, 1920, followed by Violet Crouse, aged 8, who died on May 5, 1920, in West Berlin, Queens County.

The death of Bernard Hemeon, West Berlin, occurred in a hospital in Gloucester [Massachusetts], September 20th. He was only ill a short time with Spanish Influenza and his death came as a shock to his family and the community. The remains were brought home for burial, interment taking place in St. John's cemetery on Wednesday last....Besides a wife and two small sons he leaves an aged father, five sisters and two brothers to mourn their loss.

Liverpool Advance, 2 October 1918, 2.

OBITUARY. A very wide circle of friends will receive with sincere regret, news of the death on Sunday, September 24th, following a short illness from Spanish Influenza, of Eliza, wife of H. Freeman Conrad. Her husband, who was with her at the time of her death, accompanied the remains to East Berlin, the funeral taking place Saturday from the home of her mother, Mrs. Eva Wolfe. The deceased, who was but 25 years of age, was a devoted member of the Church of England, and deeply interested in any work connected with the church. She leaves to mourn their loss, a husband and infant son, also a mother, two sisters and three brothers.

Liverpool Advance, 2 October 1918, 2.
HVS, Queens County Death Register, 1920, Book 46, Page 332, Page 776.

☞ The register states that Eliza Hilda Conrad died of "pneumonia/child bearing," after an illness of four days. This is why Dr. Marble left her off the list, but the newspaper says she had Spanish Influenza, to which pregnant or post-partum women were the most vulnerable of all its victims.

OBITUARY. Mrs. Maude Feener, wife of Levi Feener of this town, died Thursday, Oct. 31st, of pneumonia, following influenza. Deceased was 65 years of age, and besides her husband is survived by two sons and three daughters— James, of Liverpool, and Leonard, of Calgary; Mrs. Gaston Ledrun, Mrs. Arthur Lebman, in the United States, and Mrs. George VanNorden, Liverpool. Also two brothers, Reuben and Leonard Clattenburg, East Port Medway.

Liverpool Advance, 6 November 1918, 2.

Her name was Matilda Maude Clattenburg Feener. A possible relation, Frank Clattenburg, 47, of Port Medway, also died of influenza, on 23 March 1919.

HVS, Queens County Death Register, 1918, Book 46, Page 328, Number 763.

The death occurred on Friday [November 1], at the residence of Levi Feener, after a brief illness of influenza and pneumonia, of Miss Lillian Black, daughter of the late James G. and Martha Black, in the 37th year of her age. Miss Black is survived by two brothers, Oscar J. and John, residing in Boston, and one sister, Mrs. J.L. Boynton, Lynn, Mass. A. H. Boucher, of this town, is a half-brother of the deceased.

Liverpool Advance, 6 November 1918, 2.

Perhaps Lillian Black was at the Feener home to help nurse Matilda Maude, Levi's wife, who had died the day before.

Much sympathy is expressed for Mr. and Mrs. William Fraelic, Western Head, in the loss of their only son, William, whose death took place from pneumonia, on Friday, Nov. 1st. Deceased was 24 years of age, and a very promising and popular young man, and leaves a host of friends who regret his demise.

Liverpool Advance, 6 November 1918, 2. HVS, Queens County Death Register, 1918, Book 46, Page 325, Number 751.

The HVS register gives his name as William Stanley Frellick, a fisherman who died of "Influenza/Pneumonia" after an illness of five days.

DEATHS. At Milton, Nov. 17th, William Boutilier, aged 18 years.

Liverpool Advance, 20 November 1918, 3.

 His death record says he died of influenza and pneumonia; a single man, a labourer, Anglican, and the son of "Daniel Boutlier." His name appears as "William Boutlier," and the HVS search engine has him in as "William Bouthier."

HVS, Queens County Death Register, 1918, Book 46, Page 330, Number 770.

In this town [Liverpool], Nov. 17th, Evily [Evelyn], wife of James Roy, aged 45 years.

Liverpool Advance, 20 November 1918, 3. HVS, Queens County Death Register, 1918, Book 46, Page 346, Number 831. Cause of death is influenza and pneumonia.

 In this town, Nov. 18th, of pneumonia following Spanish influenza, Hattie May [Whynot], wife of Freeman Whynot, aged 28 years, leaving a husband and four children to mourn their loss.

Liverpool Advance, 20 November 1918, 3.

DEATHS. At Eagle Head, Nov. 28th, of Spanish influenza, Willard Colp, son of Erlin and Cora May Colp, aged 18 years 2 mos. Leaving a wife.

At Eagle Head, Dec. 1st, of Spanish influenza, Cora May, wife of Erlin Colp, aged 46 years, 7 months.

Liverpool Advance, 4 December 1918, 3.

Willard was a fisherman. He became ill on November 17, and died after eleven days. His mother, Cora May, was ill only seven days. Both were "Episcopalians" and were buried at Eagle Head.

HVS, Death Register, Queens County, 1918, Book 46, Page 332, Number 779 (Willard), and Number 781 (Cora).

The death of Dianah E. Phalen, occurred at her home at East Port Medway on the 12th of January after an illness of only one week of influenza and heart trouble, at the age of 85 years. Deceased was the wife of the late James Phalen, and leaves to mourn their loss three daughters, Mrs. Henry Tarr, Western Head; Mrs. Donald Smith, Portland, Me.; and Mrs. Reuben Smith, East Port Medway; and two sons, Capt. Leander and Adelbert Phalen, at East Port Medway – also sixteen grandchildren and four greatgrandchildren.

Liverpool Advance, 22 January 1919, 2.

DEATHS. In this town, Feb. 11th, of pneumonia, following influenza, Margaret Kathryn, daughter of Robie and Alice Eleanor Millard, aged 15 years, 6 mos. Funeral Thursday, Feb. 13th, at 3 p.m.

Liverpool Advance, 12 February 1919, 3.

Dr. Marble and other researchers found no newspaper references to the two victims who died in 1920. This county had one of the lowest death totals for mainland Nova Scotia during the Great Influenza.

QUEENS COUNTY, VITAL STATISTICS, DEATH REGISTER, BOOKS 46, 101

1918

[Burnard Hemeon, 39, d. 19 September 1918, died in Gloucester, Massachusetts; resided in West Berlin, Queens County, NS; a fisherman. His name has been removed from Dr. Marble's list as his death did not take place in this county, although he is in the register as dying in West Berlin. See the newspaper story above.]

[Margaret Cole, 79, d. 31 August 1918 in Maitland, Annapolis County. Although in the Queens County records, she did not die in the county and has also been removed, in order to give an accurate death count.]

1. Mrs. Hugh Bradley, 83, d. 4 August 1918, Whiteburn, Queens County.
2. William Frellish [Frellick], 24, d. 1 November 1918, Western Head, fisherman.
3. Hattie Whynot, 28, d. 18 November 1918, Liverpool, housework.
4. Winnie Farmer, female, 6, d. 7 November 1918, Liverpool.
5. Herbert Farmer, 8, d. 9 November 1918, Liverpool.
6. Alice Conrad, 17, d. 20 October 1918, Liverpool, house work.
7. Matilda Feener, 65, d. 31 October 1918, Liverpool, housewife.
8. Lillian Black, 36, d. 1 November 1918, Liverpool, housework.
9. Evelyn Roy, 45, d. 17 November 1918, Liverpool, housework.
10. Lois Hemeon, 48, d. 15 November 1918, West Berlin, housewife.
11. John MacEwan, 18, d. 23 November 1918 in Liverpool. *[Dr. Marble's lists show that Mr. McEwan was erroneously recorded in the Yarmouth County Register. His name in this amended list has been moved here from the Yarmouth County list to give an accurate death total for Queen's County, but his home was in Yarmouth County.]*
12. Willard Colp, 19, d. 28 November 1918, Eagle Head, fisherman.
13. Cora Colp, 46, d. 1 December 1918, Eagle Head, housewife.
14. Martha McGowan, 58, d. 16 March 1919, Hunts Point, housewife.
15. Margaret Millard, 15, d. 13 February 1919, Liverpool, student.
16. Laurie Smith, 28, d. 27 January 1919, Port Mouton, engineer.
17. Joseph Francis, 1, d. 6 November 1918, Milton.
18. William Boutelier, 18, d. 17 November 1918, Milton, labourer.

1919

19. Diana Phalen, 85, d. 12 January 1919, East Port Medway, housewife.
20. Etta Holland, 26, d. 2 January 1919, Greenfield, housekeeper.
21. Frank Clattenburg, 47, d. 23 March 1919, Port Medway, cook.
22. Evelyn Gardner, 9, d. 23 April 1919, Brooklyn. *[Evelyn Constantina Gardner was sister to Olethia Harriet Gardner (below); Ingram Gardner was their father. Book 46, Page 361, Number 867.]*
23. Olethia Gardner, female, 2 years and 8 months, d. 27 April 1919, Brooklyn. *[HVS database gives Olethier Harriet Gardner, Queens County Death Register, 1919, Book 346, Page 361, Number 868.]*

1920

24. Sadie Smith, 47, d. 18 April 1920, Liverpool, housewife.
25. Violet Crouse, 8, d. 5 May 1920, West Berlin. *[HVS, Book 101, Page 72, gives her name as Violet Barbara Crouse.]*

Chapter XVI

RICHMOND COUNTY

THE SEVERITY OF the Great Influenza that laid waste to Richmond County took at least eighty-one lives, and probably more.

Every chapter of this book has turned out differently, due to the situation in each county, and its surviving data. Richmond County has only four newspaper stories preserved, and but a single newspaper obituary, all of which were published in papers of other counties. Isle Madame's small fishing villages in Richmond County were hit so hard, and so early, that it is almost as if there was no time even to let the outside world know what was going on, or to ask for help—only to survive or die. Yet it is from Isle Madame that the folk memory of the Great Influenza is the strongest, and from which we were given the most amazing oral histories of the entire book.

 INFLUENZA IN RICHMOND COUNTY
Nine Funerals in One Day at Little Village of Petit de Grat [sic]
(Arichat Record). Seven deaths on Sunday and two on Monday from Spanish influenza in Petit de Grat is the appalling record of mortality since the Record's last report and there may be more to announce before we go to press. The poor victims had not even the comfort of religious consolation to accompany them into the other world. Nine burials on Monday were held at Petit de Grat [sic], four of the victims being taken out of one house.

Sydney Daily Post, 29 October 1918, 7.

☞ The *Post* originally picked up this story from the *Arichat Record*. There are no copies of this newspaper in the Nova Scotia Archives, and one wonders if the staff all came down with influenza, and it ceased publication. There is currently no website for it, past or present.

 TWENTY-FIVE DEAD IN ONE HUNDRED FAMILIES. RAVAGES OF INFLUENZA AT PETIT DE GRAT [*sic*]
ARICHAT, November 1. Spanish influenza of a most virulent type has broken out at Petit de Grat [*sic*]. In this small community of about one hundred families, twenty-five persons have passed away and many are seriously ill. Whole families

Death record for Lena Samson (Mrs. Andrew) and Minnie Samson Landry (Mrs. Albert), Petit-de-Grat, Richmond County. Both women were pregnant, but influenza killed them before their babies could be born. *(Nova Scotia Archives)*

are stricken with the disease. In one case the mother and three children have died. One particularly sad case reported is the deaths of Mrs. Felix Sampson [Samson] and her eldest son. She leaves a husband who has been a cripple for some years and six small children. Dr. Cyr, of Arichat, who was in attendance, was taken ill and Dr. A. D. LeBlanc was summoned from Sydney to attend the stricken people.

Halifax Evening Mail, 4 November 1918, 14.

☞ This influenza made its first Richmond County appearance in Petit-de-Grat, brought in by the sick crew of the schooner *Athlete,* out of Gloucester, Massachusetts. By the end of September, the Great Influenza had spread throughout Massachusetts; in one week there were seventy-five thousand people ill with it.

WHOLE CREW HAD DISEASE
Gloucester Schooner Made Cape Breton Port with Difficulty— One Man Died

Special to the Morning Chronicle

A Cape Breton Port, September 28: The Gloucester schooner *Athlete*, Capt. Berhan [Bonham], arrived here last Tuesday [Petit-de-Grat, September 24] to load fish for the Gordon Pew [Gorton-Pew] Fish Co., of Gloucester, the cargo having been bought by them from our Bay fishermen. Shortly after leaving Gloucester sickness developed among the crew, and when the vessel arrived it was with difficulty she was sailed into port, as all the members of the crew were afflicted with the disease, which the doctors have pronounced Spanish influenza. Frank Pools [Poole], one of the crew, died of the disease today and was buried at Petit de Grat [*sic*] this afternoon. He was a native of Newfoundland and twenty-four years of age. The other members of the crew have recovered or are recovering from the disease.

Halifax Morning Chronicle, 2 October 1918, 1.

Reports from St. Peters tell us that the influenza situation there is not very severe, there being only one or two cases. There is no epidemic of the disease generally throughout the county; the only places where there is an epidemic are Petit de Grat [*sic*] and Louisdale, is doubtless due to the fact that those who became infected did not obey instructions, and when a death occurred rushed from the house panic stricken and mingled with the people, thus spreading the disease and inviting an epidemic.

Sydney Daily Post, 29 October 1918, 7.

☞ How the people reacted, which the newspaper had no real way of knowing, had nothing to do with the spread of influenza. The minute that infected schooner crew sailed into Petit-de-Grat, the result was a foregone conclusion.

☞ Here are the influenza deaths that resulted from that initial infection, deaths from all the little communities on Isle Madame and a few close neighbouring areas, extracted from "Vital Statistics for Richmond County, Book 47," the list of Richmond County deaths transcribed from the Death Register of 1918–1920 by Dr. Allan Marble.

You will notice a few persons, dying of influenza, who are listed as sick for months; those were people with pre-existing conditions such as tuberculosis, which contributed to the severity of the flu. Usually death came quickly with this flu, but these death records added any time sick with a contributing condition, thus recording a *total* combined time ill and not the time ill of influenza.

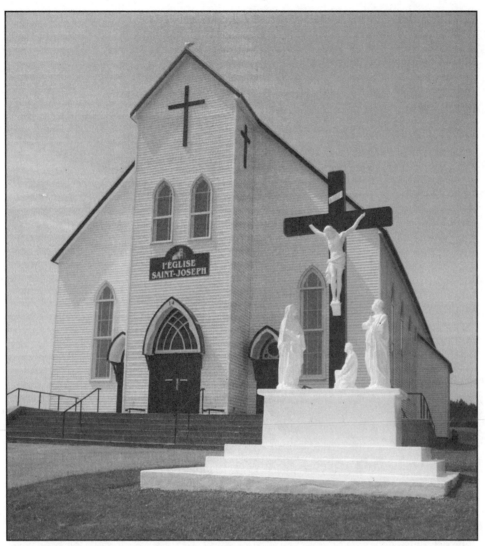

L'Eglise Saint-Joseph, Petit-de-Grat, Richmond County. Many victims of the Great Influenza lie in unmarked graves behind this church, including Frank Poole, crew member of the *Italy*, a fishing schooner out of Gloucester, Massachusetts. Its infected crew brought the epidemic to Richmond County. *(Gordon Hammond)*

Alderney Point
No deaths recorded

Arichat

Hureau, John	19	Arichat	26 December 1918	05 days ill

[This young fisherman died "on board a vessel" in Cape Breton County waters, hence he has an entry in that county's death register, Book 30, Page 99, Number 549. Apparently, after his body was sent home to Arichat for burial, he was erroneously given an entry in that county's register as well: Book 47, Page 460, Number 985.]

Goyetch, Irene	30	Arichat	03 January 1919	04 days
Boudreau, Romeo	11m	Arichat	04 February 1919	08 days
Doyle, Florence	35	Arichat	15 February 1919	05 days
Doyle, Mary	13m	Arichat	18 February 1919	04 days
Malzard, Jean	5d	Arichat	28 February 1919	04 days
Phelan, James	81	Arichat	16 March 1919	14 days
Burke, Mary	8m	Arichat	31 April 1919	14 days
Burke, Mrs. John	21	Arichat	03 May 1919	9 months

Boudreauville

Boudreau, Godfrey	21	Boudreauville	21 October 1918	09 days
Boudreau, Francis	22	Boudreauville	27 October 1918	08 days

Cabbage Cove

[The hamlet was renamed legally after the war, and is now Samsons Cove. This tiny community sent men to help unload the Athlete, and quickly lost a large proportion of people from flu, as shown below: ten people from three families.]

Martell, Mary	07	Cabbage Cove	21 October 1918	06 days
Martell, Willie	---	Cabbage Cove	21 October 1918	not given
Samson, Gorgie	01	Cabbage Cove	21 October 1918	not given
Samson, Lucy	53	Cabbage Cove	21 October 1918	08 days
Samson, Wilfred	25	Cabbage Cove	23 October 1918	02 days
Martell, Albert	---	Cabbage Cove	24 October 1918	not given
Boudreau, Catherine	16	Cabbage Cove	26 October 1918	05 days
Martell, Sabeth	---	Cabbage Cove	03 November 1918	not given
Boudreau, Mary	18d	Cabbage Cove	22 February 1919	08 days

Cape Auguet

Boudreau, Charles	10m	Cape Auget [sic]	19 November 1918	07 days
Boudreau, Anita	02	Cape Auget [sic]	07 December 1918	04 days

D'Escousse

Samson, Georgina	25	Descousse	07 December 1918	11 days
Poirier, Casimer	28	Descousse	23 January 1919	12 days
Harding, Alexander	14	Descousse	09 February 1919	14 days

Lennox: No deaths recorded.

Little Anse: No deaths recorded.

Lochside: No deaths recorded.

Louisdale

Hill, Rose	13m	Louisdale	8 October 1918	04 days
McRae, James	03m	Louisdale	8 October 1918	02 days
Marchand, Barbara	29	Louisdale	27 January 1919	10 months, flu & TB

Martinique

Boudreau, Leo	18m	Martinique	11 December 1918	14 days
Lowry, Emma	7m	Martinique	01 January 1919	21 days

Petit de Grat [*sic*]

This village had the earliest occurrence of the disease, and the greatest number of its victims.

Benoit, James	37	Petit de Grat	17 October 1918	8 days
Bouchie, Jervos	15m	Petit de Grat	17 October 1918	03 days
Boudreau, Joseph	25	Petit de Grat	19 October 1918	02 days
Samson, Albany	23	Petit de Grat	21 October 1918	08 days
Samson, Martha	29	Petit de Grat	21 October 1918	15 days
Bouchie, Marah	02	Petit de Grat	21 October 1918	not given
Bouchie, Jentie	3 wks	Petit de Grat	21 October 1918	not given
Landry, Minnie	30	Petit de Grat	25 October 1918	22 days
Samson, Lena	24	Petit de Grat	25 October 1918	06 days
Boudreau, Sabine	26	Petit de Grat	26 October 1918	15 days
Poole, Frank	24	Petit de Grat	28 October 1918	04 days
Samson, Mary	33	Petit de Grat	31 October 1918	12 days
Samson, Leon	18	Petit de Grat	01 November 1918	06 days
Boudreau, Clarence	17	Petit de Grat	03 November 1918	not given
Samson, Cecelia	22	Petit de Grat	05 November 1918	04 days
Landry, Joseph	2m	Petit de Grat	03 January 1919	2 months

Poirierville

Petitpas, Rebecca	48	Poirierville	09 May 1919	09 days

Pondville: No deaths recorded.

Pondville South: No deaths recorded.

Port Royal

Marchand, Marie	62	Port Royal, C.B.	28 October 1918	? days

Poulamon

Boudreau, Joseph	6m	Poulamond [*sic*]	25 April 1919	05 days
Fougere, Francis	6m	Poulamond [*sic*]	06 April 1919	04 days

Rocky Bay: No deaths recorded.

Samsons Cove: (see Cabbage Cove, above)

West Arichat

Mury, Louis	14	West Arichat	08 February 1919	07 days
Boyer, Emma	23	West Arichat	06 March 1919	21 days
Boyer, Joseph	35	West Arichat	07 March 1919	14 days

☞ Harriet McCready, Parrsborough Shore Historical Society, knew that this project hoped to find more about the cluster of deaths in Isle Madame, especially around the tiny community of Cabbage Cove. This community was renamed Samsons Cove, and it is an example of communities on the master list which are no longer identifiable by that name. Such changes are important to know about so that those Cabbage Cove deaths could appear in the right spot on the map of Nova Scotia, for a video piece on the flowage of the disease through the province. This can be seen on the Nova Scotia Museum of Natural History website.

Having connections to West Arichat, Harriet McCready set to work to help us. She had a former son-in-law from West Arichat, Stephen Poirier, and thought he might help. When she couldn't get in touch with him, she called his daughter (her granddaughter), Caitlin. Here is what Harriet turned up, beginning through Caitlin, and the stages through which her research went as she examined the 1918 influenza epidemic in Isle Madame. It makes for a fascinating story. She went from informant to informant, as suggested by those she interviewed: Caitlin McCready-Carswell (daughter of Stephen Poirier of West Arichat), to Lori Poirier Forgeron (Stephen's sister), to Viola Samson (Lori's friend), to Lena Samson (Viola Samson's sister-in-law), and finally to Lena Samson's old history teacher, Gabriel LeBlanc, author (in 2017) of *Mon Isle Madame*.

To demonstrate how research proceeds, and how helpful was the detailed information offered by various people in Isle Madame's communities, the data is presented here just as it came in—pieces of the jigsaw puzzle from oral histories.

☞ Info transcribed from four text messages from Lori Poirier Forgeron on Isle Madame to Harriet McCready:

✉ I contacted a Nicholas Boudreau from Petit de Grat [*sic*], he is about mid-80s. He told me he did hear about Cabbage Cove, most of what he knows was from what his father told him. He remembered his father said that a ship had thrown a mattress overboard and it was thought that this brought the flu to the area. He said a lot of them starved to death as well because no one would want to go near them to bring food etc., because they did not want to get sick; he said his father had said many were buried together, but did not know of any cemetery.

Just got some more information, Viola Samson, a friend, said she remembered her mother talking about the big flu, some called it the plague, she remembered it started in at the Pointe in Petit de Grat [*sic*], more people died there than in Cabbage Cove. She said it started when a man came from one of the ships; he left the ship because of the number of people that were sick on board. It is said that anyone who went to visit the sick people would get sick as well.

They gave me another name to contact, her sister-in-law Lena, I tried to call but no answer, try later.

✑ Harriet McCready's text to Ruth Whitehead:

✉ Lena Samson...very interesting person. Here is what I got from her: Cabbage Cove was renamed Samson's [sic] Cove. It was renamed by Lena's grandfather Sylvaire Samson, who was high in government. It was said that it was called Cabbage Cove because they grew cabbages and ate the middle of the cabbage and gave the rest to the animals.

Lena said her mother told her a ship docked in Petit de Grat [sic] and a gentleman was very sick and had died. They burnt his clothes on land and it is said the germs escaped into the air and people got sick. Including Lena's uncle, who lived in Samson's [sic] Cove, his wife, and their little boy. "My grandmother [her uncle's mother] went to visit them from La Pointe in Petit de Grat [sic] and all 3 got sick and died. She said most of them were buried behind the Petit de Grat [sic] church [St. Joseph's]; most were buried 5 in the same tomb (no coffins); you will not find their graves as the cemetery area was bulldozed since then."

Lena said this sickness was not only here it was called the Spanish Flu, she said you can call her "but a really good person to talk to would be Gabriel LeBlanc, he wrote many books on Isle Madame and its history, he was also a schoolteacher of mine."

✑ Harriet later clarified: the uncle's wife did not die, but the grandmother did, as well as (elsewhere) one of the grandmother's daughters.

✑ Lena Samson to Harriet McCready:

✉ Forgot to tell you the guy from the ship was a Spanish person and the epidemic caused many people to die between Oct and Nov of that year.

✑ The crewman who died was named Frank Poole. He was born in Newfoundland, and lived in Gloucester, Massachusetts. Perhaps the 'Spanish' memory came from the name of the influenza.

✑ Harriet McCready re: her calls to Lena Samson:

✉ Notes transcribed from my own shorthand: Her [Lena's] uncle, Wilfred Samson, got sick and died. His wife Evangeline did not die [ill, but survived]. They lived in Sampson [Samsons, formerly Cabbage,] Cove. Her grandmother Lucy Samson (from La Pointe in Petit de Grat [*sic*]) went to visit them and got sick and died there. She [Lena] thought most people were sick about one day. I found them on Dr. Marble's list:

Samson, Lucy, 53, Cabbage Cove, d. 21 October 1918, [days ill] 08

(Lena's grandmother, who was from La Pointe, Petitde Grat [*sic*], died in Cabbage Cove visiting Wilfred Samson, her son; the death record assumed she lived there.)

Samson, Wilfred, 25, Cabbage Cove, d. 23 October 1918, [days ill] 02

Samson, Gorgie, 01, Cabbage Cove, d. 21 October 1918, days ill not given

(His child died, Lena did not remember name, but I found this and called her [Lena] again, she confirmed.

Landry, Minnie, 30, Petit de Grat [*sic*], 25 October 1918, [days ill] 22.

Wilfrid's sister, (Lena Samson's aunt Minnie), lived in Petit de Grat [*sic*]; she died from this flu, but *her* husband, Albert L. Landry, survived.

↝ Harriet McCready, interviews with Gabriel LeBlanc:

✉ Hello M. Gabriel. Thanks so much for speaking with me this evening. As promised, I am sending you the list of deaths on Isle Madame from the Spanish Flu. As I mentioned, Ruth Whitehead compiled this list from the master list of those known to have died from this devastating illness. I have highlighted the four people Lena Samson told me about; her grandmother, her uncle, his child, and his sister, Lena's aunt.

I am hoping you can find out something about some of the rest. You mentioned that Lockeport and Petit de Grat [*sic*] were among the hardest hit, and so it would be good to have information about these people.

Your own connections are very interesting, and I do hope you can make time to write down what you told me: (your grandfather bringing ashore the body of Frank Poole, who died on board the ship bringing salt to the Comeau Brothers fish plant, your great-grandfather who picked up bodies each morning with his horse and wagon, the order from Halifax to bury bodies immediately without a church service, and the rest!)

I confess I added these snippets of the stories for Ruth's benefit, whom I have copied. She initiated this search and I would encourage you to contact her directly as I am sure she would be most appreciative.

Harriet McCready to Gabriel LeBlanc, email, 18 March 2018.

☞ Gabriel LeBlanc replied, and has been extraordinarily helpful. He actually had two eyewitness accounts to share. Everything he told us had come to him via people uniquely placed to know exactly what they were reporting on, and he has added enormously to the history of this sad time.

Gabriel LeBlanc, on Cabbage Cove location:

✉ Cabbage Cove is located on the Island of Petit de Petit (Aldernay Island); it is located between Little Anse and Petit de Grat [*sic*]. It is now called Samson's [*sic*] Cove.

Gabriel LeBlanc to Harriet McCready, email, 18 March 2018.

☞ Gabriel LeBlanc to Harriet McCready, 18 March 2018, email on the coming of influenza to Petit-de-Grat:

✉ The schooner (Italy) arrived in Petit de Grat [*sic*] to the Comeau Brothers' fish plant with a full load of salt. She came from the Caribbean. A crew member named Frank Poole had died during the voyage. That was the first victim of the flu in Petit de Grat [*sic*]. The [local] people unloaded the schooner; shortly after, the flu spread through the village and neighbouring parishes like wild fire. Petit de Grat [*sic*] lost over ten per cent of its population in four months. According to statistics Petit de Grat [*sic*] and Lockport [Shelburne County] were the hardest hit coastal communities.

My grandfather (James/Jacques Desire LeBlanc), was harbour master, and had to remove M. Poole's body from the schooner. He never became a victim of the flu. My great grandfather collected the cadavers with his horse and wagon. He also escaped the flu. He credits the Black Rum for saving him from the flu. His name was Jeffrey Marchand. Remi Boudreau, the casket maker of the parish, could not keep up. Therefore, many bodies were just wrapped in cloth and buried; several bodies were buried in the same graves. Wooden crosses were used as markers but have long disappeared.

The people of Petit De Grat [*sic*] thought that it was the revenge of the Germans. That German spies had poisoned the wells. The symptoms were very high fever and the spitting of blood—some people died in the snow banks trying to lower their temperature. The houses were quarantined, the afflicted were fed through houses' windows and isolated. The health authorities from Halifax ordered all bodies to be buried immediately without church services. My great aunt with tears in her eyes said, "They threw them in a hole just like animals." She had lost several members of her immediate family. It was a time of high anxiety, fear, and hard times.

Gabriel LeBlanc to Harriet McCready, email, 18 March 2018; slightly edited for
clarity. His oral history, with few exceptions, has proved accurate to the
last degree, and we thank him.

Frank Poole's Death Record:

Name of Deceased: Frank Poole
Sex: Male
Date of Death: Sept 28/18
Age: 24 yrs.
Residence: Gloucester, Mass.
Occupation: Fisherman
Single, Married, or Widowed: Single
If Single, give name of Father: William
Where Born: Beleorme [Belleorme] Fortune Bay (Nfland)
Cause of Death: Spanish Influenza
Length of Illness: Eight days
Religion: Roman Catholic [his family in NL was Anglican]
Race: White
Name of Physician Attending: LeBlanc, Dr. R.A.
Name of Undertaker: Merchand [Marchand], Alex
Place of Burial: St. Joseph's [Roman Catholic] / Petit de Grat [*sic*]
Name of Person Making Return: Bonham, Thomas, Capt. [of the schooner *Athlete*]
Date of Return: Sept. 28/18

Nova Scotia Archives: HVS (Historical Vital Statistics) database, Death Register, Richmond County, Year 1918, Book 47, Page 438, Number 941.

☞ Frank Poole became ill on September 20, if the length of illness (eight days) and the date of death, September 28, shown in the death record are correct. He had been ill for four days when the schooner made port, and was obviously quarantined aboard his vessel until he died aboard her. Then the body was brought on shore and buried.

Salt Trade

☞ Gabriel LeBlanc stated that the schooner coming in with sick crew aboard was bringing salt from the Caribbean. The salt trade from the Caribbean came mainly from Turks Island. It was essential to the fishing industry, and vessels were continuously loading cargos of salt for transport to wherever the fisheries were. These Lunenburg newspaper notices are but a few of a thousand examples:

The schooner *Eugene Creaser* has discharged a cargo of salt at Riverport. The vessel took lumber from Halifax to to Demarara, and brought salt in return from Turks Island.

The schooners *Bertha L. Walters*, *Lillian B. Corkum*, and *Mary Ruth*, will bring cargoes of salt to Lunenburg from Turk's Island. Their outward cargoes were dry fish to Porto Rico.

Lunenburg Progress Enterprise, 17 March 1920, 1.

Gorton-Pew, the Massachusetts fisheries company which sent their schooner *Athlete* into Petit-de-Grat, advertised that they were providers of salt in bulk. They owned a fleet of fifty-four other schooners and kept them on the go continuously—fishing, loading salt, and transporting orders of equipment to fishermen.

For more on this salt trade, see smithsonianmag.com/history/white-gold-how-salt-made-and-unmade-the-turks-and-caicos-islands-161576195/.

Gorton-Pew Fisheries, Massachusetts, Purveyors of Salt and Buyers of Fish Catches

By the mid-nineteenth century Gloucester's fishing industry was the largest of any port in America and the second largest in the world. During the heyday of the fishing schooner in the 1880s, Gloucester had a fleet of 400-500 sailing vessels....

The glory days of Gloucester fishing came in the second half of the nineteenth century. The key figure in the city's success was a man who became a fisherman only accidentally. Slade Gorton started his work life as a mill worker in a Rhode Island textile factory; by the time he was in his twenties, he had been made an overseer. He moved to Rockport, took a job as overseer of the Annisquam Cotton Mill, married and raised a family. He might have spent his entire career there, had a tragic fire and an energetic wife not intervened.

In 1883 the Annisquam Cotton Mill burned to the ground. At 51, the unemployed Gorton tried to help out his wife, who ran a boarding house for mill workers, by catching and packaging fish for her to salt, smoke, and serve. According to Gorton legend, his wife took the next step. With the money she had saved from running the boarding house, she bought a fishing boat, rented Rockport's now famous *Motif #1* for a shop, and announced to her husband, "We are now in the fish business."

On March 31, 1906...Gorton's would merge with three other Gloucester fish companies. Formally known as Gorton-Pew, but generally called "Gorton's," the new company would become the largest fishing business on the Atlantic Coast. Over 1,000 fishermen manned 55 vessels; another 1,000 men and women worked on shore salting, drying, boning, cutting, grinding, smoking, and packaging millions of pounds of fish.

From massmoments.org/moment-details/gloucester-fish-companies-merge.html

☞ The Halifax newspaper states that the schooner that arrived in Petit-de-Grat in late September 1918 was named *Athlete*. She was delivering fish to Gorton-Pew. This vessel was there, says modern historian Gabriel LeBlanc, to do business with the Comeau Brothers Fish Plant—to deliver a load of salt, and pick up a load of fish. He had been told this schooner was named *Italy*.

Roger Marsters, at the Maritime Museum of the Atlantic, has searched the register of ships for Massachusetts in 1918, which shows that there were none called *Italy* on the books, let alone any of that name owned by Gorton-Pew. Gorton-Pew Fisheries were, however, the owners of a schooner *Athlete* and they were the sellers of the salt cargo, and the buyers of the fish cargo in Petit-de-Grat. They were based in Gloucester, Massachusetts, as the newspaper account states. It would seem likely that the contemporary newspaper account, however, has the more likely version of the name.

Perhaps a Francophone such as LeBlanc's grandfather would be accustomed to pronounce a *th* in *Athlete* as a hard *t*—as "Atlete"—which then comes very close to "Italy," as he remembered hearing it from his grandfather all those years before, and one hundred years ago now since his grandfather first heard it. Apart from this very natural blurring, every single thing we were told by Gabriel LeBlanc was correct.

Halifax Morning Chronicle, 2 October 1918, 1.
Roger Marsters to Ruth Whitehead, personal communication, May 2018.

Elsewhere in Richmond County

☞ It should be noted that the small Mi'kmaw population living in Barra Head, Richmond County, was also affected by this influenza, beginning in late September 1918 and peaking in October of that year. There were five deaths, but none appear in the HVS database maintained by the Nova Scotia Archives, Halifax. These names, however, do occur in the original death registration ledgers for Richmond County, 1918, and were extracted by Dr. Allan Marble, in his rough-draft list of deaths by counties, Vital Statistics for Richmond County, Book 47. Information extracted from this list appears below.

- [Mrs.] Stephen Michael, aged 50, widow, lived Barra Head; died 1 October 1918, Influenza, ill one week. Fell ill around 24 September 24, 1918; another very early onset date for Richmond County, and also, coincidently, the date the *Athlete* came into Petit le Grat, her entire crew down with "Spanish Influenza." Given as "Indian" in Allan Marble's draft list, she has no record in the HVS database for Richmond County Death Register. She appears in the original ledgers, Nova Scotia Archives.

- Mrs. Paul Nicholas, aged 35, married, lived Barra Head; died October 8, 1918, Influenza, ill one week. Fell ill October 1,1918. Given as "Indian" in Allan Marble's draft list, but no HVS record.

- Alice Johnston, aged 50, married, lived Barra Head; died October 10, 1918, Influenza, ill one week. Fell ill October 3, 1918. Given as "Indian" in Allan Marble's draft list, but no HVS record.

- Michael Nicholas, aged 1 year, lived Barra Head; died October 15, 1918, Influenza, length of illness not recorded. Given as "Indian" in Allan Marble's draft list, but no HVS record.

- Joe Nicholas, aged 8 years, lived Barra Head; died October 11, 1918, Influenza, ill three days. Fell ill October 8, 1918. Given as "Indian" in Allan Marble's draft list, but no HVS record.

☞ The Indian Agency Report for 1918 makes no mention of this Mi'kmaw community falling ill, or of the deaths which occurred there. There was no newspaper coverage of this localized outbreak. There were no newspaper obituaries, postings, or memorials of any kind to the Mi'kmaw dead. It is difficult to say with any certainty, therefore, how this pathogen was introduced into the group, nor have we any way of knowing how many people became ill and survived, or the dates when they fell sick. The length of time the first three victims on this list were ill is given as "one week." No "days-ill" were recorded for the fourth victim at all. One might speculate that the doctor did not arrive until after these first four people listed had died, and in filling out the returns for the deaths, one week was a guesstimate, either by local folk or by the doctor himself. The final listed victim, who died on October 11, shows a more specific length of time ill, in days, on his returned record, and he may have been the only one actually attended by a doctor.

How was influenza introduced to this small community? All we know for sure is that the Mi'kmaq of Barra Head had become infected at around the same time as Frank Poole (taken ill September 20, made port on September 24, and died there, in Petit-de-Grat, on September 28). The disease spread out from there, and parts of Richmond County would shortly reach epidemic status. It is plausible that someone either from Barra Head, or passing through the community, had been in Petit-de-Grat when the Athlete arrived. They became infected and then infected in turn the Barra Head Mi'kmaq. If so, the carrier was possibly travelling by sea, and certainly could have done it in under a day.

Conclusion

⟶ And the influenza roared on. In just three months, by the end of 1918, at least forty-nine people had died. We hope that someone will come up with more oral histories for Richmond County as a whole, during the entirety of the epidemic. Newspaper accounts are almost non-existent. One such comes from an Antigonish newspaper:

At Arichat, February 15, 1919, of influenza followed by pneumonia, Florence, beloved wife of E.C. Doyle, in the 35th year of her age. The deceased was the possessor of those rare charms of mind and heart that won her the esteem and love of all who knew her. She was the youngest daughter of Capt. Alex Boutin of West Arichat, and was married at the Cathedral, Antigonish, by Father McAdam on February 8, 1917. Two children were born of the union, one of which, little daughter Mary, subsequently succumbed to the same dread disease and followed her dear mother to that land where sorrow is unknown. There remains the one child, Edward Boutin, and her sorrowful husband to mourn the loss of a true and devoted wife and mother. Eternal rest give her, oh Lord, and let perpetual light shine upon her.

Antigonish Casket, 15 February 1919. Courtesy the Antigonish Heritage Museum.

⟶ Almost three years after it struck, with the last death in 1920—that of Jane Malcolm, 25, of Bear Island, who died on May 10—influenza finally loosened its grip on Richmond County, and silently departed the wreckage.

Additional Research

⊂▷ Because I have found no further information published during the years 1919–20, I have prepared two further lists for descendants, or friends of the dead, and for the use of researchers:

⊂▷ List A: to make a complete roster of the Richmond County people dead in this epidemic, Dr. Alan Marble transcribed the names of those killed by "Spanish Flu," from the Richmond County Death Registers, 1918–1920. The list beginning on the next page has been edited, and was generated from the data he recorded (each county chapter has this information at the end of the chapter).

Additional information [in brackets] has been provided to this list. I have further edited it for errors in transcription, as it is often quite difficult to read the original handwritten entries. This was done using the high-magnification feature of the camera app on my cellphone, to clarify a number of entries. (I recommend this technique; it solved almost all my questions.)

⊂▷ List B: I have generated a table, set out chronologically from earliest to latest onset dates for the disease across the county, beginning with the actual date each person became ill, their dates and places of death, and then their individual entries from the unpublished Dr. Marble list for Richmond County. This will allow readers to track the spread of the sickness over three years. Keep in mind that only the *deaths* from flu are recorded, not the total number of people taken ill. There is, to date, no reliable information on that, for anywhere in the province. List B begins immediately after List A.

LIST A

RICHMOND COUNTY, VITAL STATISTICS, DEATH REGISTER, BOOKS 47, 102

1918

1. Mrs. Stephen Michael, 50, d. 1 October 1918, Barra Head, widow.

2. Charles Boudreau, 10 months, d. 19 November 1918, Cape Auget [*sic*].

3. Anita Boudreau, 2, d. 7 December 1918, Cape Auget [*sic*].

4. Albany Samson, 23, d. 21 October 1918, Petit de Grat [*sic*], fisherman.

5. Martha Samson, 29, d. 21 October 1918, Petit de Grat [*sic*], housewife.

6. Godfrey Boudreau, 21, d. 21 October 1918, Boudreauville, fisherman.

7. Lucy Samson, 53, d. 21 October 1918, Cabbage Cove [*now Samsons Cove*], housewife.

8. Mary Martell, 7, d. 21 October 1918, Cabbage Cove [*now Samsons Cove*], schoolgirl.

9. Willis Martell, d. 21 October 1918, Cabbage Cove [*now Samsons Cove*].

10. Gorgie Samson [*Georgie?*], 1, male, d. 21 October 1918, Cabbage Cove [*now Samsons Cove*],

11. Wilfred Samson, 25, d. 23 October 1918, Cabbage Cove [*now Samsons Cove*], fisherman.

12. Albert Martell, d. 24 October 1918, Cabbage Cove [*now Samsons Cove*], fisherman.

13. Lena Samson, 24, d. 25 October 1918, Petit de Grat [*sic*], housewife.

14. Minnie Landry, 30, d. 25 October 1918, Petit de Grat [*sic*], housewife.

15. Sabine Boudreau, 26, d. 26 October 1918, Petit de Grat [*sic*], housewife.

16. Cathrine Boudreau [*sic*], 16, d. 26 October 1918, Cabbage Cove [*now Samsons Cove*], servant.

17. Francis Boudreau, 22, d. 27 October 1918, Cabbage Cove [*now Samsons Cove*], fisherman.

18. Mary Samson, 33, d. 31 October 1918, Petit de Grat [*sic*], housewife.

19. Leon Samson, 18, d. 1 November 1918, Petit de Grat [*sic*], fisherman.

20. Clarence Boudreau, 17, d. 03 November 1918, Petit de Grat [*sic*], labourer.

21. Sabeth Martell, d. 3 November 1918, Cabbage Cove [*now Samsons Cove*], student.

22. James Benoit, 37, d. 17 October 1918, Petit de Grat [*sic*], fisherman.

23. Joseph Boudreau, 25, d. 19 October 1918, Petit de Grat [*sic*], labourer.

24. Jervos Bouchie, 15 months, d. 17 October 1918, Petit de Grat [*sic*].

25. Jentie Bouchie, male, 3 weeks, d. 21 October 1918, Petit de Grat [*sic*].

26. Marah Bouchie, male, 2, d. 21 October 1918, Petit de Grat [*sic*].

[*James Boudreau, 21, d. 5 November 1918 in Cogswell Military Hospital, Halifax, soldier; formerly Number 27 on Dr. Marble's list. Since he did not die in Richmond County, his name has been removed from the present list. He is instead listed under Halifax County.*]

27. Mary Boudreau, 17, d. 6 November 1918, Little Ance [*sic*], housemaid.

28. Cecelia Samson, 22, d. 5 November 1918, Petit de Grat [*sic*], tailor.

29. Sophie Boudreau, 12, d. 27 October 1918, Poulamond [*sic*].

30. Theresa Landry, 5, d. 7 November 1918, Poulamond [*sic*].

31. Charles Gouthro, 39, d. 5 December 1918, Tracadie, labourer.

32. Georgina Samson, 25, d. 7 December 1918, Descousse [sic], housewife.

33. Emanuel McNamara, 13 months, d. 7 October 1918, Lower River Inhabitants.

34. Wallace White, 36, d. 30 November 1918, Whiteside, fisherman.

35. Mrs. Paul Nicholas, 35, d. 8 October, Barra Head.

36. Alice Johnston, 50, d. 10 October, Barra Head.

37. Michael Nicholas, 1, d. 15 October, Barra Head.

38. Joe Nicholas, 8, d. 11 October 1918, Barra Head.

39. Deline Martell, 47, d. 3 November 1918, L'Ardoise, housemaid, "epidemic influenza."

40. Marie Marchand, 62, d. 28 October 1918, Port Royal C.B., housework.

41. Peter Bonin, 3 months, d. 2 December 1918, Jordin's [Jourdain's] Harbour. [HVS, 1918, Book 47, Page 487, Number 1064.]

42. Leo Boudreau, 18 months, d. 11 December 1918, Martinique.

43. Angus McDonald, 35, d. 23 November 1918, Stirling C.B., farmer.

44. Katie McDonald, 30, d. 23 November 1918, Stirling C.B.

45. Roderick McDonald, 29, d. 18 October 1918, Point Tupper, engineman.

46. Elizabeth Walsh, 40, d. 21 October 1918, Point Tupper, housemaid.

47. Rose Ann Hill, 13 months, d. 8 October 1918, Louisdale.

48. James McRae, 3 months, d. 8 October 1918, Louisdale.

1919

49. Mary Doyle, 13 months, d. 18 February 1919, Arichat.

50. Jean Malyard [Malzard], female, 5 days old, d. 28 February 1919, [Arichat. Death record says her family was English, Episcopalian, her father was Charles Malzard. She was buried at St. John's Arichat. Book 47, Page 497, 1088.]

51. James Phelan, 81, d. 16 March 1919, Arichat, merchant.

52. Roméo Boudreau, 11 months, d. 4 February 1919, Arichat.

53. Irene Goyetch, 30, d. 3 January 1919, Arichat, matron.

54. Florence Doyle, 34, d. 15 February 1919, Arichat, matron.

55. Joseph Landry, 2 months, d. 3 January 1919, Petit de Grat [sic].

56. Mary Boudreau, 18 days, d. 22 February 1919, Cabbage Cove [now Samsons Cove].

57. Casimir Poirier, 28, d. 23 January 1919, Descousse [sic], mariner.

58. Alexander Harding, 14, d. 9 February 1919, Descousse [sic].

59. Lucy Roche, 23, d. 15 November 1918, Rockdale, housemaid.

60. Emma Lowry, 7 months, d. 1 January 1919, Martinique.

61. Louis Mury, 14 months, d. 8 February 1919, West Arichat.

62. Emma Boyer, 23, d. 6 March 1919, West Arichat, housework.

63. Joseph Boyer, 35, d. 7 March 1919, West Arichat, fisherman.

64. Barbara Marchand, 29, d. 27 January 1919, Louisdale.

65. Mrs. John Burk, 21, d. 3 May 1919, Arichat, housewife. [HVS, 1918, Book 47. Page 522, Number 1157, shows Mrs. John W. Burke, no first name of her own. Mother of Mary, below.]

66. Mary Burk, 8 months, d. 31 April 1919, Arichat. [HVS, 1918, Book 47. Page 522, Number 1158, shows "Mary Ann Burk, daughter of John Burk, Burk Shore, Arichat." The woman immediately above was her mother.]

67. Francis Fougère, 6 months, d. 6 April 1919, Poulamond [*sic*].

68. Joseph Boudreau, 6 months, d. 25 April 1919, Poulamond [*sic*].

69. Rebecca Petitpas, 48, d. 9 May 1919, Poirierville, housewife.

70. Clarence McDonald, 5 months, d. 5 April 1919, Grantville.

71. Mrs. Sarah Shanahan, 28, d. 27 February 1919, St. Peters, housewife.

72. Louise Mary Martell, 2 months, d. 27 March 1919, West L'Ardoise.

73. Philomèn [*Philomène*] Angeline Martell, 2 months, 31 March 1919, West L'Ardoise.

1920

74. Mrs. Bella MacIntosh, "about" 80, d. 6 March 1920, Black River.

75. Mrs. Peter Nelson, 85, d. 11 March 1920, Black River, housework.

76. Susie Fougère, 10, d. 4 April 1920, River Bourgeois, student.

77. Matthew Dugas, 80, d. 7 April 1920, River Bourgeois, farmer.

78. Ida Samson, 18, d. 10 April 1920, River Bourgeois. [*HVS Search Engine names her "Ida May Sampson," but the death record (Book 102, Page 110), gives "Samson" as the correct surname. She died of "Tuberculosis," following an attack of "LaGrippe."*]

79. John McNeil, 26, d. 3 April 1920, Johnstown.

80. Jane Malcolm, 25, d. 10 May 1920, Bear Island, housewife.

[*Dr. Marble suspects that there may be more victims, whose information was never recorded.*]

LIST B

RICHMOND COUNTY, VITAL STATISTICS, BOOKS 47, 102

Onset on:	Death on:	Name, Age, Location, Occupation, Length of Illness
1918		
1918 09 24	1918 10 01	Mrs. Stephen Michael, 50, Barra Head, widow, ill 7 days.
1918 10 01	1918 10 08	Mrs. Paul Nicholas, 35, Barra Head, ill 7 days.
1918 10 03	1918 10 10	Alice Johnston, 50, d. Barra Head, ill 7 days.
1918 10 03	1918 10 25	Minnie Landry, 30, Petit de Grat [*sic*], housewife, ill 22 days.
1918 10 04	1918 10 08	Rose Hill, 13 months, Louisdale, ill 4 days.
1918 10 04	1918 10 07	Emanuel McNamara, 13 months, Lower River Inhabitants, ill 3 days.
1918 10 06	1918 10 21	Martha Samson, 29, Petit de Grat [*sic*], housewife, ill 15 days.
1918 10 06	1918 10 08	James McRae, 3 months, Louisdale, ill 2 days.
1918 10 08	1918 10 11	Joe Nicholas, 8, Barra Head, ill 3 days.
1918 10 08	1918 10 18	Roderick McDonald, 29, Point Tupper, engineman, ill 10 days.
1918 10 09	1918 10 17	James Benoit, 37, Petit de Grat [*sic*], fisherman, ill 8 days.
1918 10 11	1018 10 26	Sabine Boudreau, 26, Petit de Grat [*sic*], housewife, ill 15 days.
1918 10 12	1918 19 21	Godfrey Boudreau, 21, Boudreauville, fisherman, ill 9 days.
1918 10 13	1918 10 21	Albany Samson, 23, Petit de Grat [*sic*], fisherman, ill 8 days.
1918 10 13	1918 10 21	Lucy Samson, 53, Cabbage Cove [*Samsons Cove*], housewife, ill 8 days.
1918 10 14	1918 10 17	Jervos Bouchie, 15 months, Petit de Grat [*sic*], ill 3 days.
1918 10 15	1918 10 27	Sophie Boudreau, 12, Poulamond [*sic*], ill 12 days.
1918 10 16	1918 10 21	Elizabeth Walsh, 40, Point Tupper, housemaid, ill 5 days.
1918 10 17	1918 10 19	Joseph Boudreau, 25, Petit de Grat [*sic*], labourer, ill 2 days.
1918 10 17	1918 10 21	Mary Martell, 7, Cabbage Cove [*Samsons Cove*], schoolgirl, ill 6 days.
1918 10 19	1918 1025	Lena Samson, 24, Petit de Grat [*sic*], housewife, ill 6 days.
1918 10 19	1918 10 27	Francis Boudreau, 22, Cabbage Cove [*Samsons Cove*], fisherman, ill 8 days.
1918 10 19	1918 10 31	Mary Samson, 33, Petit de Grat [*sic*], housewife, ill 12 days.
1918 10 19	1918 10 31	Mary Boudreau, 17, Little Ance [*sic*], housemaid, ill 13 days.
1918 10 21	1918 10 26	Cathrine Boudreau 16, Cabbage Cove [*Samsons Cove*], servant, ill 5 days.
1918 10 21	1918 10 23	Wilfred Samson, 25, Cabbage Cove [*Samsons Cove*], fisherman, ill 2 days.
1918 10 24	1918 10 06	Mary Boudreau, 17, Little Ance [*sic*], housemaid, ill 13 days.
1918 10 25	1918 11 01	Leon Samson, 18, Petit de Grat [*sic*], fisherman, ill 6 days.
1918 10 26	1918 10 28	Marie Marchand, 62, Port Royal C.B., housework, ill 2 days.
1918 10 27	1918 11 03	Deline Martell, 47, L'Ardoise, maid, "epidemic influenza," ill 7 days.
1918 10 31	1918 11 07	Theresa Landry, 5, Poulamond [*sic*], ill 8 days.
No data	1919 01 03	Joseph Landry, 2 mos, Petit de Grat [*sic*], ill since birth; cause of death influenza.
No data	1918 10 15	Michael Nicholas, 1, Barra Head, no time ill given.
No data	1918 10 21	Gorgie Samson, 1, Cabbage Cove [*Samsons Cove*], time ill not given.
No data	1918 10 21	Willis Martell, Cabbage Cove [*Samsons Cove*], time ill not given.
No data	1918 10 21	Jentie Bouchie, male, 3 weeks, Petit de Grat [*sic*], time ill not given.
No data	1918 10 21	Marah Bouchie, male, 2, Petit de Grat [*sic*], time ill not given.

No data   1918 10 24   Albert Martell, Cabbage Cove [*Samsons Cove*], fisherman, time ill not given.

No data   1918 11 03   Clarence Boudreau, 17, Petit de Grat [*sic*], labourer, time ill not given.

No data   1918 11 03   Sabeth Martell, Cabbage Cove [*Samsons Cove*], time ill not given.

1918 11 01   1918 11 05   Cecelia Samson, 22, Petit de Grat [*sic*], tailor, ill 4 days.

1918 11 01   1918 11 15   Lucy Roche, 23, Rockdale, housemaid, ill 7 days.

1918 11 02   1918 11 05   James Boudreau, 21, d. in Cogswell Military Camp, Halifax, soldier, ill 3 days. [*Richmond County Death Register, 1918, Book 47, Page 465, Number 1010: later crossed out, as he didn't die in Richmond county.*]

1918 11 12   1918 11 19   Charles Boudreau, 10 months, Cape Auget [*sic*], ill 7 days.

1918 11 16   1918 11 23   Angus McDonald, 35, Stirling C.B., farmer, ill 7 days.

1918 11 16   1918 11 23   Katie McDonald, 30, Stirling C.B., ill 7 days.

1918 11 20   1918 11 30   Wallace White, 36, Whiteside, fisherman, ill 10 days.

1918 11 25   1918 12 02   Peter Bonin, 3 months, Jordin's [*sic*] Harbour, ill 7 days.

1918 11 27   1918 12 11   Leo Boudreau, 18 months, Martinique, ill 14 days.

1918 11 27   1918 12 05   Charles Gouthro, 39, Tracadie, labourer, ill 9 days.

1918 11 27   1918 12 07   Georgina Samson, 25, Descousse [*sic*], housewife, ill 11 days.

1918 12 03   1918 12 07   Anita Boudreau, 2, Cape Auget [*sic*], ill 4 days.

1918 12 11   1919 01 01   Emma Lowry, 7 months, Martinique, ill 21 days.

1918 12 31   1919 01 03   Irene Goyetch, 30, Arichat, matron, ill 4 days.

1919

1919 01 11   1919 01 23   Casimir Poirier, 28, Descousse [*sic*], mariner, ill 12 days.

1919 01 26   1919 02 09   Alexander Harding, 14, Descousse [*sic*], ill 14 days.

1919 01 31   1919 02 04   Romeo Boudreau, 11 months, Arichat, ill 4 days.

No data   1919 01 27   Barbara Marchand, 29, Louisdale, ill 10 months, flu & TB.

1919 02 01   1919 02 08   Louis Mury, 14 months, West Arichat, ill 7 days.

1919 02 10   1919 02 18   Mary Doyle, 13 months, Arichat, ill 8 days.

1919 02 10   1919 02 15   Florence Doyle, 34, Arichat, matron, ill 5 days.

1919 02 13   1919 03 06   Emma Boyer, 23, West Arichat, housework, ill 21 days.

1919 02 14   1919 02 22   Mary Boudreau, 18 days, Cabbage Cove [*Samsons Cove*], ill 8 days.

1919 02 20   1919 02 27   Mrs. Sarah Shanahan, 28, St. Peters, housewife, ill 7 days.

1919 02 21   1919 03 07   Joseph Boyer, 35, West Arichat, fisherman, ill 14 days.

1919 02 24   1919 02 28   Jean Malyard [*Malzard*], female, 5 days old, [*Arichat*], ill 4 days.

1919 03 02   1919 03 16   James Phelan, 81, Arichat, merchant, ill 14 days.

1919 03 23   1919 03 27   Louise Martell, 2 months, West L'Ardoise, ill 4 days.

1919 03 23   1919 03 31   Philomèn Martell, 2 months, West L'Ardoise, ill 8 days.

1919 03 29   1919 04 05   Clarence McDonald, 5 months, d. 5 April 1919, Grantville, ill 7 days.

1919 04 02   1919 04 06   Francis Fougère, 6 months, Poulemond [*sic*], ill 4 days.

1919 04 16   1919 04 30   MaryAnn Burk, 8 months, Arichat, ill 14 days.

1919 04 20   1919 04 25   Joseph Boudreau, 6 months, d. 25 April 1919, Poulamond [*sic*], ill 5 days.

1919 04 30   1919 05 09   Rebecca Petitpas, 48, d. 9 May 1919, Poirierville, housewife, ill 9 days.

No data   1919 05 03   Mrs. John Burk, 21, Arichat, housewife, time ill not given.

1920

1920 02 27	1920 03 06	Mrs. Bella MacIntosh, 80, Black River, ill 23 days.
1920 03 01	1920 03 11	Mrs. Peter Nelson, 85, Black River, housework, ill 10 days.
1920 03 04	1920 04 04	Susie Fougère, 10, River Bourgeois, student, ill 1 month.
1920 03 18	1920 04 07	Matthew Dugas, 80, River Bourgeois, farmer, ill 20 days.
1920 03 24	1920 04 03	John McNeil, 26, Johnstown, ill 10 days.
No data	1920 04 10	Ida Samson, 18, River Bourgeois, time ill not given; flu, TB.
No data	1920 05 10	Jane Malcolm, 25, Bear Island, housewife, ill 3 months, flu, TB.

Chapter XVII

SHELBURNE COUNTY

꙳ᘉ⥢ᘓ⥤ꙻ

SHELBURNE COUNTY HAD at least sixty-four confirmed deaths from the Great Influenza. Most of these deaths took place during the most vicious Second Wave of this influenza. It typically made its appearance in mid-September to early October 1918, in the majority of Nova Scotian counties. Dr. Marble recorded one death, however, that does not fit this pattern. Annie Heckman, 14, of Central Woods Harbour, died of "LaGrippe" on July 14, after a two-month illness. Either she died in the First Wave of this flu, which began in the early spring of 1918, or the Second Wave in Shelburne County began earlier than expected.

Shelburne County Death Register, 1918, Book 49.

⊂▷ Annie does not appear in the HVS database, but Dr. Allan Marble found her death record while transcribing the originals in the 1918 Shelburne County Death Register, Book 49. He does not, however, give a page or number reference.

⊂▷ Lockeport, a fishing community, apparently was the first point of entry into Shelburne County for the more common Second Wave time period. The earliest person to die first showed symptoms on October 2; more followed on October 4, 5, 7, and 9. After that, so many people, including the local doctor, became ill that some names reported in the newspaper don't even *have* death certificates, and there are only a few newspaper accounts, all from other counties. No one reported the situation to Provincial Health Officer Dr. Hattie until October 14. Dr. Hattie immediately accorded Lockeport epidemic status, in a report published on October 16.

Halifax Morning Chronicle, 16 October, 2.

⊂▷ How was the virus introduced? The obvious first guess is that it arrived on fishing vessels, either from Massachusetts, or in those having had contact with Massachusetts.

Fishermen as Disease Vectors

⊂⊃ George McIntosh, the first person to die, was a fisherman. He brought his infection home (from wherever he picked it up) and passed it to his daughter Minnie, who died of it on October 18. This was a particularly virulent influenza, perhaps fresh out of Gloucester, Massachusetts. It attacked Lockeport in late September or early October, however introduced, and began spreading outward to the rest of the county and beyond—in a number of cases, via infected fishermen.

The Sutherland Grocery, a Hot Spot

⊂⊃ The 1911 Canadian Federal Census has Fred Sutherland as a retail grocer in Lockeport. His son William was a grocery salesman, and his son Frank, a bank teller. In 1918, at the time of their deaths, sons John and Max are described as "clerks," perhaps working for their father, as Max was still in his teens. Wherever they all worked, they had multiple contacts with the public all day long. However they picked it up, they took it home to dinner, and then influenza consumed them. The whole Sutherland family—Frederick Sr., wife Louisa, and six of nine children: Frederick Jr., John, Rupert, Max, Robert, and Grace—fell ill. John and Max died. Murray and William were away, serving as soldiers. Victoria, called Queenie, was in Toronto training as a nurse at Toronto General Hospital; she came home to assist the family, after losing two brothers. I mention the Sutherland Grocery just as one possibile point of contact. Anywhere there were people coming and going—and especially a grocery store where visiting infected fishermen or others might come in to resupply—that is, anywhere there were crowded situations, influenza could flourish.

RG 31 –C-1, Nova Scotia Shelburne & Queens Cos. ED 52-22, Lockeport, page 7. Nova Scotia Archives, HVS, Shelburne County Death Register, 1918, Book 49, Page 318, Numbers 768 (John) and 769 (Max).

⊂⊃ This venue or others like it, however, merely facilitated the spread of influenza. How it first came into the community is still unclear. Still less clear to the community was *what* it was, or how seriously it should be taken. Notice in the excerpt on the next page, Spanish influenza is not mentioned—even influenza is not mentioned.

NORTH EAST POINT NOTES (From a Correspondent.) Mr. Clarence Penny is quite ill, and almost the entire family of Mrs. Gilbert Atkinson and several members of the family of Mr. Bradford Smith are on the sick list. Matthias Krafve, Mrs. Benjamin Gladwin, and Sidney Krafve, who have been quite ill, are slightly improved....Mr. Angus Goodwin is quite ill.

HAWK POINT NOTES (From a Correspondent.) We regret to report Mrs. Coleman Smith very ill at time of writing.

Yarmouth Telegram, 11 October 1918, 2.

The first newspaper account of Lockeport's influenza came from information received on October 14, by a Liverpool newspaper, another county over. The day George McIntosh, Mary Lavinia Lewis, and Max Sutherland died in Lockeport, October 16, this Queens County newspaper, the *Liverpool Advance*, ran the story about the influenza then raging in Lockeport:

There have been upwards of one hundred and fifty cases of Influenza at Lockeport during the last week. In some houses every member of the family has been down with the disease. There were two deaths on Friday last. Mr. Henry Bangay, foreman of the smoking department of the cold storage, was sick but a day or two, and died on Friday morning. Mr. Bangay was a widower and leaves two children. On Friday afternoon Mrs. Roache of West Head, who was sick but a few hours, passed suddenly away, leaving a husband and several small children. A great many are still very sick. The schools, churches and all public gatherings have been closed for two weeks.

Since writing the above, there passed away at Lockeport on Sunday at noon, one of the brightest of our young men, Avery Lewis, aged 19 years and 6 months. Avery was the son of Mr. and Mrs. David H. Lewis, formerly of Port L'Herbert [*sic*]. The family moved to Lockeport the first of June last. Avery started some weeks ago to learn the blacksmith trade, and worked with Mr. John Day. Last week he was stricken down with influenza, which quickly developed into pneumonia, and he died on Sunday, leaving a sorrow-stricken family to mourn the loss of one who was greatly beloved by all who knew him. Lockeport, Oct. 14th, 1918.

Liverpool Advance, 16 October 1918, 2. HVS, Shelburne County Death Register, 1918, Book 49, Page 318, Number 767 shows "John Henry Bangay," occupation: "Fish Curer." Book 49, Page 319, shows Ardella Roache (773), her mother-in-law Mary Roache (774), and her daughter Louise Roache (778) as flu victims.

NURSES NEEDED IN LOCKEPORT

HALIFAX, October 16....Dr. sends out an urgent call for help for Lockeport, particularly for nurses. Extra medical help has been secured, BUT NURSES ARE REQUIRED. Dr. Ford, of Liverpool, is there; Miss [Florence] Murray a third year medical student, has gone down and Mrs. Anderson, a fourth year medical, goes today. Nurses are urgently needed.

Dr. Hattie states that any strong girls—from four to six of them anyway— who will volunteer, even if they are without nursing training, will be welcomed in the service to work under the direction of trained nurses attending the sick at Lockeport.

Halifax Evening Mail, 16 October 1918, 10.

LOCKEPORT WANTS EXPERIENCED NURSES

Spanish influenza and pneumonia has caused a number of deaths in Lockeport during the past week, and advices from that town this morning state the situation is steadily growing worse. In some cases whole families are down with the disease.

John Sutherland, twenty-two years of age, son of Frederick Sutherland and brother of Frederick Sutherland, jr., commercial traveller, of this town, succumbed to the disease yesterday, and a younger brother is not expected to recover.

The resident doctor has been in poor health for some time, and in response to a call from the inhabitants for medical aid, Dr. T. R. Ford left here on Friday and has been rendering all the assistance possible to the sufferers. He reports there is great need of nurses and has asked Mayor Hendry to secure all the experienced nurses available in this county.

One trained nurse, Miss Fannie Hunt, of Greenfield, went to Lockeport last week, and is reported to be rendering valuable assistance. Our readers will confer a favour by sending Mayor Hendry the names of any experienced nurses who are willing to offer their services.

Liverpool Advance, 16 October 1918, 2.

SITUATION AT LOCKEPORT IS SERIOUS

Three Hundred Cases of Influenza in the Town, and Appeal is Made for Nurses.

Dr. Hattie, Provincial Health Officer, has received an urgent appeal for nurses, or if they cannot be obtained, for anyone who can care for those suffering from Spanish influenza at Lockeport. The situation in this town is more serious than anywhere else in Nova Scotia. There are three hundred cases of influenza, the majority of them critical, and last night some twenty-eight pneumonia cases had developed, several of them apparently fatal. A large part of the population is stricken, and the few who have escaped have worked day and night caring for the sick. Now they are exhausted and can do no more. Because of their depleted strength, they are themselves menaced by the disease. It has been impossible to obtain nurses from neighbouring points. Although he spent the greater part of yesterday trying to obtain nurses or help of any kind, Dr. Hattie was unsuccessful, because of the increase of the epidemic in this city....If there is anyone who can answer the call, they should communicate with Dr. Hattie, and he will arrange their transportation.

Halifax Morning Chronicle, 16 October 1918, 5.

MISS IRENE SMITH. The death took place at the home of her parents, West Head, Cape Sable Island, on Friday, of Miss Irene, second daughter of Mr. and Mrs. J. Grant Smith, after a brief illness of pneumonia, following Spanish Influenza....Miss Smith had just reached her 23d birthday.

Yarmouth Telegram, 18 October 1918, 1.

MRS. BENJAMIN L. GOODWIN. Spanish influenza followed by pneumonia claimed another victim on Monday when Mrs. Benjamin L. Goodwin, of North East Point, Shelburne Co., passed away after only a few days illness....She leaves her husband and several children.

Yarmouth Telegram, 18 October 1918, 1.

LOCKEPORT NOTES (FROM A CORRESPONDENT)
The influenza is still a serious matter here and in neighboring villages. Recent deaths are Henry Bangay; Lavania Lewis, Little Harbor; Mrs. Leander Roache [Ardella], West Head; Avery Lewis, Mrs. James Symonds, George MacIntosh, John Sutherland and Max Sutherland, sons of F. W. Sutherland. Three trained nurses and a lady doctor are already here and several nurses are expected to-day. Dr. Ford, of Liverpool, is assisting Dr. Lockwood.

Mr. George Stephens and Mrs. James Roach [Mary], two aged residents of Western Head, died to-day. Timothy [Tilley] Chivers, of Lockeport, died in Shelburne on Wednesday.

There have been upwards of one hundred and fifty cases of influenza here during the last week. In some homes every member of the family has been down with the disease. There were two deaths on Friday last. Mr. Henry Bangay, foreman of the smoking department of the cold storage, was sick but a day or two and died on Friday morning. Mr. Bangay was a widower and leaves two children. On Friday afternoon Mrs. [Leander] Roach [Ardella Roach], of West Head, who was sick but a few hours, passed away suddenly, leaving a husband and several small children. [Her daughter Louise had died of flu as well.] A great many are still very sick. The schools, churches and all public gatherings have been closed for two weeks...."

Yarmouth Telegram, 18 October 1918, 2.

☞ Mary Roach, mother of Leander Roach, died of influenza, probably caught in the same vector of infection as killed her daughter-in-law Ardella, and her granddaughter Louise.

Tilley James Chivers was born to Sarah A. Prince Chivers and her husband, Tilley Richardson Chivers. She had been born in Newfoundland in 1882. Tilley Richardson Chivers was a Nova Scotian, born in in 1865 in Sable River, Shelburne County. They married in Boston in 1902. Their son Tilley James was born on 16 November 1903; by then the family had returned to Sable River. His father died a year later. Tilley Jr. died of influenza on 15 October 1918 in Shelburne, and is buried there, in the Pine Grove Cemetery.

From Leslie Richardson's Genealogy website.

☞ A subsequent report, from the Liverpool paper published October 23, shows *some* victims' names and death dates (see below). Actual death certificates are still the best source of information, however; this account is just a list of names, there are errors and omissions, and it is eight days late in publishing a death that occurred October 16, of someone who fell ill on October 2.

 ### FIFTEEN DEATHS IN NINE DAYS AT LOCKEPORT OF INFLUENZA AND PNEUMONIA

Lockeport, October 21. Influenza is still quite serious in Lockeport. The majority, however, who have been sick with the disease, have improved so they are able to help others. There are still some who are very sick. The upper room of the Temperance Hall has been fitted up for an emergency hospital. Four patients were moved in there on Sunday afternoon, and nurses are in attendance all the time. There are several nurses here from Halifax and Liverpool. A lady doctor and an assistant are doing all they can and are as busy as they can be in attending to the sick, not only in the town, but in the outlying districts. Committees are at work in every possible way to relieve the sick and suffering. A kitchen is kept going day and night supplying gruel, broths, etc., which is hurriedly despatched to the sick and needy. The clergymen are on the go day and night, doing their best in visiting the sick, burying the dead, and helping in every possible way. There were five burials on Saturday and three on Sunday. Rev. Mr. Phalen attended at the burial of eight persons in six days, and Rev. Mr. Meadows attended nine burials in nine days....The following are the deaths in the town and neighboring communities from influenza since Oct. 11th:

Oct. 11,   Henry Bangay, aged 39 years.
"   11,   Mrs. Leander Roach [Ardella], 34 years.
"   13,   Avery Lewis, 19 years, 6 mos.
"   14,   Catherine Townsend, 17 years.

" 15,   John Sutherland, 22 years.
" 16,   Max Sutherland, 16 years, 6 mos.
" 16,   Mary Lavinia Lewis, 18 years, 10 mos.
" 16,   George McIntosh, 50 years.
" 17,   Annie L. Farrington, 16 years.
" 18,   Minnie McIntosh, 19 years.
" 18,   Pearl Goodick, 17 years.
" 18,   Lulu Young, 17 years.
" 18,   A Stanley child, 3 years [Stella]
" 19,   Mrs. Frank Townsend, 35 years.
" 19,   A Roache child, 11 years. [Louise Roach, daughter of Leander and Ardella]

Besides these, Sidney, son of Captain Enos Page, died in Montreal and was brought home for burial....Up to the hour of writing, we have heard of no deaths either on Sunday or this morning. There are now quite a number of serious cases at East and West Green Harbor.

Liverpool Advance, 23 October 1918, 2.

⊂▷ Here are names of additional victims, and further information for some of the listed dead:

- Goodick, Pearl, is Annie Pearl Goodick, Lockeport, aged 17. No death record found; no female Goodicks except a much older woman, Eleanor. Identified as "Annie Pearl Goodick," via website *findagrave*. Yet even searching for Annie Pearl Goodick (or variants thereof) produced no Death or Birth Record for Shelburne County.

  See website, Annie Pearl Goodick (1901-1918)—Find A Grave Memorial
findagrave.com › ... › Shelburne County › Lydgate › Lockeport Cemetery."
In Cemetery Records of Shelburne County, Volume VIII (2002) Shelburne
County Genealogical Society.

- "Robertson, R.B.H., d. Lockeport, aged 34." No death record found, either under Robertson or Robinson, for this person. The *Lunenburg Outlook*, 25 October 1918, page 1, reads "R.B.H. Robertson, barrister of Bridgewater, died of influenza and pneumonia." A search of death records for Lunenburg reveals that he was born in Shelburne, but died in Bridgewater, where he resided and practised law. He was Presbyterian, and had been ill one week. In the HVS search engine, his name is given as Robertson, R. Bernardo, but that is possibly incorrect.

- "A Stanley child, d. Lockeport, aged 3." 'A (SURNAME) Child' —this is the newspaper format: they use 'A Roach child' for Louise Roach, for example. Dr. Marble's list interpreted this as "Stanley, A." Death Record shows she was Stanley, Stella.

- "Townsend, Roy, d. Lockeport, aged 4." Death Record not found. This is an error for Townsend, Gordon Earle, a child who has a death record for the proper period, but isn't mentioned in this list. (There is a 1918 record for a child surnamed Townsend, in Book 49, but this child, Harold, died of spinal meningitis.)

- "Williams, William Earl, d. Lockeport, aged 2." This is an error for William Earle Stephens, son of James Stephens.

- "Simmonds, Mrs. James, d. Lockeport, aged 33." This is an error for Mrs. James Symonds.

- "Died in Shelburne. (Shelburne Gazette). Mrs. Thomas Buchanan [Margaret Firth Buchanan], of Jordan Branch, fell a victim to pneumonia, following Spanish Influenza, and passed away on Monday night. The deceased was 62 years of age and leaves a husband and seven children."

Bridgetown Monitor, 23 October 1918, 4.

 INFLUENZA AT LOCKEPORT

The influenza situation in Lockeport, N.S. continues to be very serious. A large proportion of the citizens are ill and there are one to four deaths daily. Doctors and nurses from outside have been called to assist and the Temperance Hall has been converted into a temporary hospital.

Liverpool Outlook, 25 October 1918, 1.

☞ All throughout this epidemic, one man was working night and day to fashion the caskets and do the burials. His name was Lewis Huskilson. His family business has survived into the present, and they have a website, which notes "The H.M. Hulskilson's Funeral Homes and Crematorium Limitied had its modest beginning in 1878 near Lockeport, Shelburne County, when Elendur Huskilson, an Icelandic immigrant and a carpenter by trade, began making caskets for deceased community members. His son, Lewis Huskilson, followed in his father's footsteps, and opened a funeral home in Lockeport in 1909."

huskilson.net

TWENTY-THREE DEATHS AT LOCKEPORT IN FOURTEEN DAYS FROM SPANISH INFLUENZA

Situation Now Improved

Lockeport, Oct. 28. The influenza conditions are a little more favourable than a week ago. There have been no new cases developed during the last two days. A few cases are still quite serious, but for the most part many are gradually improving.

There are now six patients in the emergency hospital who are being cared for by trained nurses. Altogether twenty-three have died from influenza and pneumonia within fourteen days in the town and near neighbourhoods. The following have died since the report in last week's ADVANCE:

Oct. 20,   Erma Thompson, aged 17 years [death record has Thompson, Irma Pearl]
"   21,   Mrs. James Simmonds, 33 years [death record has Symonds, Gertrude; husband James Symonds]
"   21,   Mrs. Jos. F. Williams, 32 years [Gertrude; husband Joseph]
"   22,   Mrs. Walter Chemist, 23 [Gertrude; death record has Gertrude Chymist; husband Walter Chymist]
"   22,   Roy Townsend, 4 [Gordon Earle Townsend]
"   24,   Wm. Earle Williams, 1 yr., 9 mos. [William Earle Stephens , with father given as James Stephens]
"   26,   Victor Huskins, 17 years

At time of writing, the patients in hospital and elsewhere are resting quite comfortably, and hopes are entertained for their recovery. Quite a few are down with the disease at Allendale, Sable River and Green Harbour.

Owing to the prevalence of influenza, business is very dull. The stores, barber shops, and all public places are being closed at 6 p. m. Fishing vessels are tied up at the wharves or anchored in the stream with no men to man them. There is very little doing in and around the town.

Miss Victoria (Queenie) Sutherland, who has been in training at the General Hospital at Toronto, is visiting at her home. She started for home when she heard of the serious illness, but before she arrived her two brothers, John and Max, had passed away. It was a sad home-coming....

Mr. J.C. McLeod, a theological student, who has been supplying the Presbyterian Church here for the summer months, is a victim to influenza. He is much better this morning, and it is to be hoped he will soon be around again at his work.

Liverpool Advance, 30 October 1918, 2.

 At Sable River, Nov. 1, of influenza, Mrs. Lewis Harlow [Ida], aged 49 years, leaving her husband, five daughters, and one son.

Yarmouth Telegram, 8 November 1918, 8.

Health Officer Fuller [for Yarmouth] reported that a vessel had arrived from the fishing grounds on Tuesday with several cases aboard; three were taken to the Hospital on arrival], and on Wednesday the other afflicted [on the schooner] had so far recovered as not to deem it necessary for them to go to that institution. He had a suspicion that the men had contracted the disease while the vessel was at Lockeport for bait.

Yarmouth Telegram, 8 November 1918, 1.

👉 A further account, from the same source, said that this vessel was the *Francis A.*, and that one of her crew had died that night. (See the Yarmouth County chapter.)

OBITUARY. Two or three weeks ago the Gazette published the marriage of Captain Jonathan Locke Johnston, son of Mr. and Mrs. Wynne Johnston, of Lockeport, the event taking placing in England. To-day it is our duty to report the death of this young soldier, which occurred in Horton County of London War Hospital [*sic*] on Nov 1st, after an illness of influenza. The deceased was familiarly known as 'Jock' and was universally popular. He enlisted in the 64th battalion as a private and rapidly rose in the service. The following despatch to his father from the Records office, tells of his death: 'Deeply regret to inform you that captain and adjutant Quartermaster Jonathan Locke Johnston, medical services, seriously ill in Horton County of London War Hospital, Epson, Oct. 31st, with influenza, died Nov. 1st.' It is unnecessary to say that the sympathy of their many friends will be extended to the grief-stricken parents and the bride-widow. (Shelburne Gazette).

Liverpool Advance, 13 November 1918, 2.

👉 Horton County of London War Hospital should be read as Horton (County of London) War Hospital. It was located in Epsom, Surrey, and had been an asylum previously.

At Christie's Point, Dec. 12. Blanche, wife of Roscoe Smith, and on the same day—15 minutes later—their son, Fernwood, both victims of influenza. Mr. Smith and a young son are yet ill of the same disease. Mrs. Smith was a daughter of Mr. Burns Madden, and leaves five sisters.

Yarmouth Telegram, 20 December 1918, 3. Thanks to Deborah Trask for placename identification.

Conclusion

⊂⊃ So, Lockeport, Cape Sable Island, and the rest of Shelburne County—how did the disease first take hold here? We just don't know. Did it come in with George McIntosh, a fisherman? Did it arrive on a schooner from Massachusetts? Or could it have been brought somehow from Yarmouth, Halifax, Sydney, or from Arichat by more local fishermen?

Gertrude Williams fell ill the same day that Mr. MacIntosh became ill, namely, October 2; her husband was almost certainly a fisherman. See her death record, where Occupation is listed as "fisherman" by the husband, who then realized it wanted *her* occupation, and scratched a line through the word.

Leander Roache, another fisherman, lost his daughter Louise, who fell ill on October 9; his mother, Mary, sickened on October 12, and his wife, Ardella, on October 14. All three died. There is no way to know if Leander was ill as well, even earlier than they, but recovered. He certainly lived long enough to sign and return their death records. All that was left of his house, however, were himself and his young son.

A number of other fishermen fell victim to the flu, including a large cluster on Cape Sable Island, in the villages or hamlets of Cape Island and of South Side, Cape Island, as well as at Clarks Harbour, Newellton, The Hawk, North East Point, West Head, and Stoney Island. At Cape Island, Edward Quinton, 18, died October 15, 1918; he showed symptoms first on October 4. Percy Nickerson, 35, fell ill on October 24, and died on October 28. Judah Nickerson, a fisherman at South Side, Cape Island, died on November 2, aged 31. At Clarks Harbor, the dead included Russell Nickerson, aged 30, who became ill October 11 and died on October 17.

Others in these communities, in many cases related to fishermen, were dying as well. Irene Smith, 23, West Head, died October 17, 1918. Deborah (Mrs. Benjamin L.) Goodwin, born at Newellton, resided and died at North East Point, cause "pneumonia," according to the death record, but the newspaper account of her death states it had developed out of influenza. Perhaps the deaths of other Cape Sable Island neighbours at this time, listed as "pneumonia," should also be re-evaluated, such as that of L. Freda [Elfrida?] Swain, 24, wife of Joseph Swain of Stoney Island, who died of pneumonia after an illness of five days.

Minard Nickerson of Clarks Harbor, aged 19, died on 12 November 1918 of "Spanish influenza," after a week's illness. Rayford Crowell, 24, described as "yacht man," died on November 9 at Clarks Harbor (no death certificate under that name in HVS search engine). He had been ill since November 3. The earliest death, however, was that of Goldie A. Smith, aged 4, of Cape Island, who died on September 17, 1918, of "La Grippe," after a week's illness. Douglas Nickerson, aged 9 months, South Side, Cape Island, died on November 2. Doane Atwood, 66, a blacksmith at Newellton, died on November 8, of influenza, after fighting it for a month.

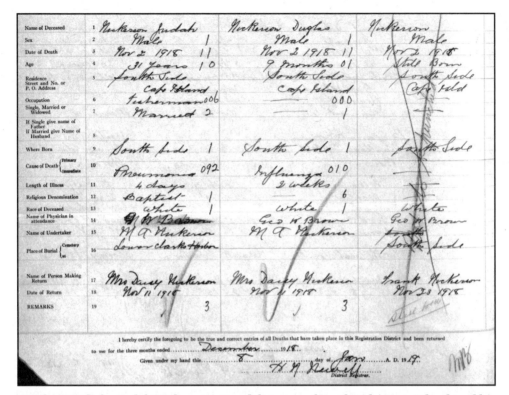

Name of Deceased	1	Nickerson Judah	Nickerson Duglas	Nickerson
Sex	2	Male	Male	Male
Date of Death	3	Nov 2 1918	Nov 2 1918	Nov 2 1918
Age	4	31 Years	9 months	Still Born
Residence Street and No. or P. O. Address	5	South Side Cape Island	South Side Cape Island	South Side Cape Island
Occupation	6	fisherman		
Single, Married or Widowed	7	Married		
If Single give name of Father If Married give Name of Husband	8			
Where Born	9	South Side	South Side	South Side
Cause of Death	10	Pneumonia	Influenza	
Length of Illness	11	4 days	2 weeks	
Religious Denomination	12	Baptist		
Race of Deceased	13	White	White	White
Name of Physician in attendance	14	G W Baker	Geo W Brown	Geo W Brown
Name of Undertaker	15	M C Nickerson	M C Nickerson	
Place of Burial	16	Lower Clark Harbor		South Side
Name of Person Making Return	17	Mrs Daisy Nickerson	Mrs Daisy Nickerson	Frank Nickerson
Date of Return	18	Nov 11 1918	Nov 11 1918	Nov 23 1918
REMARKS	19			

I hereby certify the foregoing to be the true and correct entries of all Deaths that have taken place in this Registration District and been returned to me for the three months ended............December............1918.

Given under my hand this............8............day of............Jany............A. D. 19.9.

............H. M. Newell............
District Registrar.

Death records for Judah Nickerson, 31, a fisherman of South Side, Cape Island, and his nine-month-old son, Douglas. Both died on 2 November, 1918—Douglas of influenza, his father of pneumonia (almost certainly as a result of influenza). Influenza had taken neighbour Percy Nickerson five days earlier. *(Nova Scotia Archives)*

Influenza went through Cape Sable Island, a conflagration, an almost instant killer. The island seems to have been in just as bad a shape as Lockeport, but it didn't get the newspaper coverage. Just as an example, the same page, 334, in the online death register for Shelburne County, Book 49, has two people who died of influenza (Percy Nickerson, Douglas Nickerson), two who died of pneumonia (Margaret Nickerson, wife of Everett Nickerson, and Judah Nickerson), plus one (Muriel L. Duncan, Number 810), for whom the cause of death is illegible—it looks like "Immediate," then states she was ill for four days. One cannot help but wonder if these pneumonia deaths arose out of influenza. All of the victims lived on the island. All of them were Baptists. They died between October 19 and November 2, less than two weeks apart. Two were fishermen. They had ample opportunity to spread this disease around amongst themselves. But where did it come from initially?

Judah Nickerson, 31, died after four days of pneumonia, on November 2, 1918 at South Side, Cape Island. His return (Book 49, Page 334, Numbers 811 and 812) was sent in by Mrs. Daisy Nickerson on November 11. She also sent in the return for Douglas Nickerson, 9 months old, who died on the same day, November 2, at South Side Cape Island. One assumes that she was Judah's wife and Douglas's mother.

Other fishermen dying elsewhere in the county of the flu included Mitchell Enslow, 19, of West Green Harbor, who got sick in late December 1918, and died on January 12, 1919. Oliver Thomas, 33, of Cape Negro, died on January 20, 1919, after falling ill in December 1918. David Perry, 38, died on January 21, 1919 at Roseway, of influenza and pneumonia, after a week's illness.

Were Sable Island or Lockeport infected by fishermen, or by a visitor from elsewhere in Nova Scotia? Possibly a returning family member, friend, or customer? Were there multiple vectors? To date, there is no discernible smoking gun. This influenza does, however, seem very like the virulent form of extremely contagious influenza that hit Petit-de-Grat, in Cape Breton, and, at the other end of the province, western Nova Scotia, beginning in Yarmouth, about the same time. Both those epidemics were kicked off by one or two symptomatic fishermen from Gloucester, Massachusetts.

At any rate, this flu spread all over the county. Deaths were reported from Central Woods Harbor, Cape Island, Shelburne, Jordan River, Enslows Point, Sandy Point, Birchtown, East Jordan, Western Head, Lydgate, Sable River, West Green Harbour, West Middle Sable, Upper Middle Sable, Clarks Harbour, Newelltown, Baccaro, Port LaTour, East Sable River, Upper Ohio, Roseway, Charleville, Jordan Ferry, East Ragged Island, Louis Head, Cape Negro, Malden, West Baccaro, and Woods Harbour. It raged from September 1918 through March 1919. Sixty-two people died. Then in 1920, it popped up again, killing three people: Susan Nickerson, February 2, 1920; Mary Whiteway, May 4, 1920; and Leonard Smith, June 16, 1920.

☞ It is perhaps just a coincidence that the last person to die was another fisherman.

SHELBURNE COUNTY, VITAL STATISTICS, DEATH REGISTER, BOOKS 49, 103

1918

1. Annie Heckman, 14, d. 14 July 1918, Central Woods Harbour.
2. Goldie Smith, 4, d..17 September 1918, Cape Island.
3. Leith Clow [*Luther Bertram Clow*], d. 11 November 1918, Shelburne. [*HVS, 1918, Book 49, Page 309, Number 733*].
4. Sarah McCarthy, 27, d. 21 November 1918, Shelburne, housewife.
5. Tilly Chivers, 15, d. 15 October 1918, Shelburne.
6. Dudley Matthews, 3, d. 25 October 1918, Shelburne.
7. George Jacklin, 16, d. 31 October 1918, Shelburne, blacksmith's helper.
8. Anthony Acker, 1, d. 28 October 1918, Shelburne.
9. James Matthew, 5 months, d. 9 October 1918, Jordan River.
10. Margaret Buchanan, 62, d. 14 October 1918, Enslows Point, housewife.
11. Francis Goulden, 1, d. 17 October 1918, Sandy Point.
12. Lucinda Acker, 2, d. 5 November 1918, Birchtown.
13. Aesop Lohnes, 25, d. 24 November 1918, Jordan River, lumberman.
14. Edwin Corkum, 26, d. 24 November 1918, Jordan River, lumberman.
15. Harold Wolfe, 2, d. 29 November 1918, East Jordan.
16. Gertrude Chymist, 23, d. 22 October, Lockeport, housewife.
17. John Sutherland, 22, d. 15 October 1918, Lockeport, clerk.
18. Max Sutherland, 16, d. 16 October 1918, Lockeport, clerk.
19. George McIntosh, 53, d. 16 October 1918, Lockeport, fisherman.
20. Minnie McIntosh, 18, d. 18 October 1918, Lockeport, schoolteacher.
21. Mrs. James Symonds, 34, d. 21 October 1918, Lockeport, housewife.
22. Ardella Roach, 37, d. 11 October 1918, Western Head, housewife.
23. Mary Roach, 84, d. 16 October 1918, Western Head, housekeeper.
24. Stella Stanley, 2, d. 17 October 1918, Lydgate.
25. Luke Young, 17, d. 18 October 1918, West Green Harbour.
26. Louise Roache, 13, d. 18 October 1918, Western Head.
27. William Stephens, 1, d. 23 October 1918, Lydgate.
28. Victor Huskins, 18, 28 October 1918, West Green Harbour, labourer.
29. Kathleen Townsend, 17, d. 14 October 1918, Lydgate.
30. Irma Thompson, 17, d. 20 October 1918, West Middle Sable.
31. Ida Harlow, 47, d. 1 November 1918, Sable River, housewife.
32. Winnifred Nickerson, 30, d. 7 October 1918, Upper Woods Harbour, domestic.

[*The next entry in Dr. Marble's list, taken from the death register, is for Robert Abbott, 63, Yarmouth, "hotel keeper," ill a "few days." He died 18 October 1918; his death return was mistakenly entered in Shelburne County and later crossed out. Since it is not a death happening in this county, it has been transferred to Yarmouth County, the place of his death.*]

33. Edward Quinton, 18, d. 15 October 1918, Cape Island, fisherman.
34. Russel Nickerson, 30, d. 17 October 1918, Clark's [*sic*] Harbour, fisherman.

35. Percy Nickerson, 35, d. 28 October 1918, Cape Island, fisherman.

36. Douglas Nickerson, 9 months, d. 2 November 1918, Cape Island.

37. Doane Atwood, 66, d. 8 November 1918, Newellton, blacksmith.

38. Minard Nickerson, 19, d. 12 November 1918, Clark's [sic] Harbour, sailor.

39. Rayford Crowell, 24, d. 9 November 1918, Clark's [sic] Harbour, yacht man.

40. Blanche Smith, 21, d. 12 December 1918, Baccaro, housewife.

41. Clinton Smith, 3, d. 12 December 1918, Baccaro.

42. Augustus Morgan, 32, d. 22 October 1918, Port Latour, clergyman.

43. Hilda Smith, 26, d. 27 October 1918, Port Latour, housewife.

44. Albert Nickerson, 1, d. 28 October 1918, Baccaro.

1919

45. *Infant* Ringer, female, 9 days, d. 21 January 1919, Shelburne.

46. Dorothy Miles, 6 weeks, d. 29 January 1919, Shelburne.

47. Nellie Oickle, 10 months, d. 4 March 1919, Shelburne.

48. Selena Legrayley, 8 months, d.18 March 1919, Shelburne.

49. Victor Gower, 10 weeks, d. 10 January 1919, Upper Ohio.

50. David Perry, 38, d. 21 January 1919, Roseway, fisherman.

51. George Crowe, 23, d. 31 January 1919, Sandy Point, servant.

52. Julia McKenzie, 52, d. 15 February 1919, Jordan Ferry, housewife.

53. Mitchell Enslow, 19, d. 12 January 1919, West Green Harbour, fisherman.

54. Alice Matthews, 54, d. 17 March 1919, East Ragged Island, housewife.

55. Alice Arey, 1, d. 27 February 1919, East Sable River.

56. Ida Kraft, 52, d. 28 December 1918, Louis Head. [*A belated 1918 entry, in the 1919 Death Register for Shelburne County. HVS Search Engine says she died in 1919, because she's in that register. Book 49, Page 353, Number 873.*]

57. Robert Chetwynd, 3 months, d. 8 April 1919, Charlesville.

58. Alford Nickerson, 16, d. 1 January 1919, Malden, landsman.

59. Mertis Madden, 27, d. 5 January 1919, West Baccaro, housewife.

60. Oliver Thomas, 33, d. 20 January 1919, Cape Negro, fisherman.

61. Alice Matthews, 54, d. 17 March 1919, East Ragged Island, housewife.

1920

62. Susan Nickerson, 78, d. 2 February 1920, Woods Harbour, housewife.

63. Mary Whiteway, 37, d. 4 May 1920, housekeeper.

64. Leonard Smith, 18, d. 16 June 1920, Baccaro, fisherman. [*This young man, son of John and Mary Smith, had been fishing for several years before he died. He apparently had caught influenza "a year ago," which is given as a contributory cause of death, along with the "Pulmonary Tuberculosis" he also developed "a year ago." The influenza developed into his fatal lung condition. (There have been others found, whose cause of death was a "tuberculosis" developing out of this influenza. As an example, see Colchester County, above.) HVS, Book 103, Page 164.*]

SHELBURNE COUNTY, VITAL STATISTICS, BOOKS 49, 10

Onset on:	Death on:	Name, Age, Location, Occupation, Religion, Length of illness

1918

No data	1918 07 14	Annie Heckman, 14, Central Woods Harbour, ill "2 months."
1918 09 10	1918 09 18	Goldie Smith, 4, Cape Island, ill 7 days.
1918 10 01	1918 10 15	Tilly Chivers, 15, Shelburne, ill 14 days.
1918 10 02	1918 10 16	George McIntosh, 53, Lockeport, fisherman, ill 14 days.
1918 10 02	1918 10 09	James Matthews, 5 months, Jordan River, ill 7 days.
1918 10 02	1918 10 23	William Stephens, 1, Lydgate. ill 21 days.
1918 10 03	1918 10 17	Francis Goulden, 1, Sandy Point, ill 14 days.
1918 10 04	1918 10 16	Max Sutherland, 16, Lockeport, clerk, ill 12 days.
1918 10 04	1918 10 15	Edward Quinton, 18, Cape Island, fisherman, ill 11 days.
1918 10 05	1918 10 15	John Sutherland, 22, Lockeport, clerk, ill 10 days.
1918 10 07	1918 10 14	Margaret Buchanan, 62, Enslows Point, housewife, ill 7 days.
1918 10 07	1918 10 21	Mrs. James Symonds, 34, Lockeport, housewife, ill 14 days.
1918 10 08	1918 10 22	Gertrude Chymist, 23, Lockeport, housewife, ill 14 days.
1918 10 09	1918 10 11	Ardella Roach, 37, Western Head, housewife, ill 2 days.
1918 10 09	1918 10 18	Louise Roache, 13, Western Head, ill 9 days.
1918 10 09	1918 10 18	Luke Young, 17, West Green Harbour, ill 9 days.
1918 10 10	1918 10 17	Stella Stanley, 2, Lydgate, ill 7 days.
1918 10 11	1918 11 08	Doane Atwood, 66, Newellton, blacksmith, ill 28 days.
1918 10 11	1918 10 18	Minnie McIntosh, 18, Lockeport, schoolteacher, ill 7 days.
1918 10 11	1918 10 17	Russel Nickerson, 30, Clark's [sic] Harbour, fisherman, ill 6 days.
1918 10 12	1918 10 16	Mary Roach, 84, Western Head, housekeeper, ill 4 days.
1918 10 13	1918 10 20	Irma Thompson, 17, West Middle Sable, ill 7 days.
1918 10 17	1918 10 22	Augustus Morgan, 32, Port Latour, clergyman, ill 5 days.
1918 10 18	1918 10 28	Albert Nickerson, 1, Baccaro, ill 10 days.
1918 10 19	1918 11 02	Douglas Nickerson, 9 months, Cape Island, ill 14 days.
1918 10 20	1918 10 27	Hilda Smith, 26, Port Latour, housewife, ill 7 days.
1918 10 21	1918 10 28	Anthony Acker, 1, Shelburne, ill 7 days.
1918 10 21	1918 10 28	Victor Huskins, 18, West Green Harbour, labourer, ill 7 days.
1918 10 24	1918 10 28	Percy Nickerson, 35, Cape Island, fisherman, ill 4 days.
1918 10 24	1918 10 31	George Jacklin, 16, Shelburne, blacksmith's helper, ill 7 days.
1918 10 25	1918 11 01	Ida Harlow, 47, Sable River, housewife, ill 7 days.
1918 10 30	1918 11 05	Lucinda Acker, 2, Birchtown, ill 7 days.
No data	1918 10 14	Kathleen Townsend, 17, Lydgate, ill 14 months, flu and TB?
Eliminated	1918 10 18	Robert Abbott, 63, Yarmouth, hotel keeper, ill a few days.
		In Richmond County Register, later crossed out. Not kept in this list.
No data	1918 10 07	Winnifred Nickerson, 30, Upper Woods Harbour, ill a "few days."
No data	1918 10 25	Dudley Matthews, 3, d. 25 October 1918, Shelburne, ill "few days."
1918 11 03	1918 11 09	Rayford Crowell, 24, Clark's [sic] Harbour, yacht man, ill 6 days.
1918 11 05	1918 11 12	Minard Nickerson, 19, Clark's [sic] Harbour, sailor, ill 7 days.
1918 11 17	1918 11 24	Aesop Lohnes, 25, d. 24 November 1918, Jordan River, lumberman.
1918 11 17	1918 11 24	Edwin Corkum, 26, Jordan River, lumberman, ill 7 days.
No data	1918 11 11	Luther Bertram Clow, age not given, Shelburne, time ill not given.
No data	1918 11 21	Sarah McCarthy, 27, Shelburne, housewife, ill "two months."
No data	1918 11 29	Harold Wolfe, 2, East Jordan, time ill not given.
1918 12 05	1918 12 12	Blanche Smith, 21, Baccaro, housewife, ill 7 days.

1918 12 06	1918 12 12	Clinton Smith, 3, Baccaro, ill 6 days.
1918 12 22	1918 12 28	Ida Kraft, 52, d. 28 December 1918, Louis Head, ill 6 days.
1918 12 22	1919 01 12	Mitchell Enslow, 19, West Green Harbour, fisherman, ill 14 days.
1918 12 25	1918 01 01	Alford Nickerson, 16, Malden, landsman.
1918 12 26	1919 01 20	Oliver Thomas, 33, Cape Negro, fisherman, ill 25 days.
1918 12 30	1918 01 05	Mertis Madden, 27, West Baccaro, housewife.

1919

1919 01 03	1919 01 10	Victor Gower, 10 weeks, Upper Ohio, ill 7 days.
1919 01 15	1919 01 21	David Perry, 38, Roseway, fisherman, ill 7 days.
1919 01 16	1919 01 21	*Infant* Ringer, female, 9 days, Shelburne, ill 5 days.
1919 01 17	1919 01 31	George Crowe, 23, Sandy Point, servant, ill 14 days.
1919 01 25	1919 01 29	Dorothy Miles, 6 weeks, Shelburne, ill 4 days.
1919 01 25	1919 02 15	Julia McKenzie, 52, Jordan Ferry, housewife, ill 21 days.
1919 02 06	1919 02 27	Alice Arey, 1, East Sable River, ill 21 days.
1919 02 28	1919 03 04	Nellie Oickle, 10 months, Shelburne, ill 7 days.
1919 03 11	1919 03 18	Selena Legrayley, 8 months, d.18 March 1919, Shelburne, ill 7 days.
No data	1919 03 17	Alice Matthews, 54, East Ragged Island, housewife.
No data	1919 04 08	Robert Chetwynd, 3 months, Charlesville, ill "a few days."

1920

No data	1920 02 02	Susan Nickerson, 78, Woods Harbour, housewife, time ill not given.
No data	1920 05 04	Mary Whiteway, 37, d. 4 May 1920, housekeeper, time ill not given. [*HVS, 1920, Book 103, page 127: Mary M. (Burrage) Whiteway, born at Lower Pelican, Newfoundland, living Shelburne, Shelburne County. Cause of death: TB and Influenza. No time-ill given for onset of influenza. HVS search engine calls her Mary Whitman.*]
No data	1920 06 16	Leonard Smith, 18, Baccaro, fisherman, time ill, one year. Cause of death: TB, resulting from Influenza; both arising "a year ago."

Chapter XVIII

VICTORIA COUNTY

VICTORIA COUNTY SUFFERED through "several" cases of influenza, with only a few confirmed deaths from the Great Influenza: three in November–December 1918, and five between April 19 and May 20, 1919. There were no cases at all in 1920, according to Dr. Marble, who so noted at the end of his lists of the deaths in Victoria County: "1920: nil." Victoria County's death rate was by far the lowest of any Nova Scotia county.

Influenza was furiously spreading through the rest of the province. Victoria County, by contrast, had only eight recorded flu deaths in three years. There are no newspaper reports from the county itself, only a smattering of news from other counties.

Death record for Patrick J. Williams, a fisherman from South Bay, and his son George, aged two. (*Nova Scotia Archives*)

Oral histories might give us more information about how many got sick, what happened when they did, and how many died. As yet this has not been done.

 One case of the disease at Cape North is understood to have been traced directly to Spain in its origin, having been contracted from a Newfoundland man who had returned from a voyage to Spanish ports.

Sydney Record, 24 September 1918, 2.

☞ This is the first reference to influenza in Victoria County. The county's first death also occurred in Cape North, that of Henry Christie, who became ill on October 31.

☞ Statistics were being published almost daily by the provincial medical officer, based in Halifax, and on October 18, 1918, Dr. Hattie included Cape North in his list.

 Reports of the influenza epidemic for the 24 hours up to noon yesterday, as compiled by the Nova Scotia health department, are as follows:

Halifax	28	Little Bass River	01
Dartmouth	01	Tusket	01
Hopewell	01	Bells Rock	06
Foxbrook, Pictou	01	Wallbrook Mountain	06
Eureka Mills	16	Clare District	10
Stellarton	50	Glace Bay	05
Cape Sable Island	06	Windsor	17
Woods Harbor	25	Hantsport	04
Shaw Harbor	05	Mount Denison	02
Barrington Passage	08	Avonport	02
North West Harbor	05	Lockeport and vicinity	25
Port Saxony	03	Canning	04
Grosvenor	02	Blomidon	01
Morin	01	Kingsport	03
Tracadie	01	Canard	04
Fairmont	11	Vernon Mines	05
Pictou	02	Victoria Harbor	08
Salmon River	08	Cambridge	08
Upper Brookfield	15	Aylesford	10
Fairview	02	Black Rock	02
Great Village	01	South Berwick	10

Sommerset	01
South Wentworth	04
New Waterford	04
Main a Dieu	10
Cariboo Marsh	06
Truro	07
Digby	04
Lunenburg	07
Cape North	several
Stewiacke	06
Gay's River	13
Miller's Siding	15

Halifax Evening Mail, 18 October 1918, 10. "Several" is not very informative.

☞ "Christie, Henry, aged 15, Cape North, died 06 November 1918, ill 07 days." This child's death was the first in the county. Henry Christie's father's name was John Christie, and they resided at Bay Valley Road, Cape North, the place where Henry had been born. John Christie buried his son at "St. Margaret's Village" cemetery. The family were Roman Catholics. The death register says Henry Christie died of "Influenza (supposed to be)."

HVS, Victoria County Death Register, 1918, Book 48, Page 295, Number 58.

☞ Henry Christie's death notice is also the end of any newspaper coverage that Dr. Allan Marble, Sam Howard, or I have been able to find for Victoria County. The shadow of death that was the Great Influenza had almost entirely passed over this county.

The next death came on December 20, when Leo Moran, a South Ingonish fisherman, passed away. Leo Moran was followed on December 30, by Mrs. Mary Duggan, a Dingwall housewife, aged 42. Hers was the last death of 1918.

There was a lull, and then in April of 1919, there occurred a fourth death, that of "Mrs. Neil A. McKay." She died after a six-day struggle with influenza. She had been born in Englishtown, and was taken back there for burial. Hers is an interesting death record in that Mrs. McKay is described as a farmer at Cape Dauphin, although this word is blurred and might also be read as "tanner" or even something stranger.

HVS, Death Register, Victoria County, 1919, Book 48, Page 321, Number 624.

☞ During this research, I have found that when a woman was identified only as Mrs. 'Husband's Name', not by her own name, the husband was still living. That was the case for Mrs. McKay. She was identified as married, not as widowed, and her own first name was not used. I have also found that persons making out the return of death sometimes got confused when asked for "occupation," and put in the husband's occupation. See Cumberland and Shelburne County examples. Sometimes it was corrected, other times not. Perhaps that is what happened here.

Angus D. McDonald, 52, died on May 11, 1919. He had lived in a place recorded as "Plaster North Shore" which is not easily identifiable today, where he farmed.

The final two deaths both occurred in the Williams family of South Bay. The first was that of 2-year-old George Williams, who died on May 14. This child's father was Patrick J. Williams. He was born in Sydney Mines. George's father, Patrick Williams, died two days later. He had been born in South Ingonish. The family was Roman Catholic, and father and son were both buried in South Bay.

HVS, Victoria County Death Register, 1919, Book 48, Page 325, Numbers 635, 636.

VICTORIA COUNTY VITAL STATISTICS, DEATH REGISTER, BOOK 48

1918

1. Leo Moran, age not given, d. 20 December 1918, South Ingonish, fisherman.
2. Henry Christie, 15, d. 6 November 1918, Bay Road Valley, Cape North.
3. Mary Duggan, 47, d. 30 December 1918, Dingwall, housewife.

1919

4. Mrs. Neil McKay, 45, d. 8 April 1919, Cape Dauphin, farmer.
5. Neil McAskill, 35, d. 20 May 1919, Englishtown, farmer.
6. Angus McDonald, 52, died 11 May 1919, Plaster North Shore, farmer.
7. George Williams, 2, died 14 May 1919, South Bay.
8. Patrick J. Williams, 32, died 16 May 1919, South Bay, fisherman.

</>

Chapter XIX

YARMOUTH COUNTY

※〜ﾚⱭﾚ〜※

IN YARMOUTH COUNTY, there were at least seventy-two confirmed deaths from the Great Influenza. It all began with one fishing schooner out of Gloucester, Massachusetts. On Tuesday, September 24, disease and death sailed into Yarmouth. They came aboard a schooner, the *Natalie Hammond*, whose story is told below. Dr. Allan Marble feels that it was this schooner, and perhaps others like it, that infected not only Yarmouth, but the whole of western Nova Scotia (see his unpublished manuscript, *Medical History of Nova Scotia, Vol. III*).

September 24 was also the day a fisherman named Frank Poole took ill aboard another Massachusetts schooner, the *Athlete*, all of whose crew were down with the Great Influenza when they made port at Petit-de-Grat, Richmond County, a few days later. Frank Poole died. The disease, thus introduced, rapidly infected that county.

The situation in Massachusetts itself was dire. The *Halifax Evening Mail* reported:

Boston, September 30—Governor McCall to-night received from Lieutenant-Governor McCallum Grant of Nova Scotia, the following telegram: "This province cannot fail to recall with gratitude the magnificent and immediate resource Massachusetts made in the time of our urgent need at Halifax [in 1917]. Some nurses have already gone to help you and more both of doctors and nurses will follow as you may require them."...State Health Commissioner E. R. Kelly, in a telegram to Surgeon-General Blue, of the United States public health service, covering the situation up to one o'clock today says: "Reports from 55 cities and towns outside Boston total 5,500 new cases of influenza. There are at least 75,000 cases of influenza in Massachusetts today, excluding the number in Cantonments [army training barracks, all very overcrowded]. Nurses and doctors most urgently needed."

Halifax Evening Mail, 1 October 1918, 7.

☞ It's easy to see, with the strong connection between Massachusetts and Nova Scotia, how the disease could have been imported here. The fisheries alone would have seen to it. Fishing vessels were back and forth all the time between Nova Scotia and Massachusetts.

 SOREN BJURUN. The death of Mr. Soren Bjurun [Søren Bjerrum: a good Danish name] took place at Yarmouth Hospital this morning. The deceased was one of the crew of the Gloucester sch. *Nathalie J. Hammond* [*Natalie Hammond*], which landed him in Yarmouth. He was then in a very precarious condition suffering, apparently, from Spanish Influenza. The deceased was born in Denmark 24 years ago but for many years past had been a resident of Gloucester, Mass., where his widow resides. Instructions are awaited regarding the disposition of the remains.

Yarmouth Telegram, 27 September 1918, 1.

FISHERMAN DIES OF INFLUENZA
Member of Crew of Gloucester Schooner Passes Away at Yarmouth Hospital.
Special to the Morning Chronicle. YARMOUTH, N.S. September 27.
Sorun B. Jurun [Søren Bjerrum], of Gloucester, Mass., died at Yarmouth Hospital this morning [Friday, September 27] from what is known as Spanish Influenza. The deceased was one of the crew of the Gloucester schooner Nathalie Hammond and was taken ill whilst his vessel was on the Banks. His condition grew steadily worse and the Hammond's captain put into Yarmouth on Tuesday [September 24] and Jurun was taken to the hospital. The deceased was a native of Denmark, and was twenty-four years of age. Some years ago he came to America and settled in Gloucester, Mass., where his widow resides.

Halifax Morning Chronicle, Saturday, 28 September, 1918.

☞ There were *two* fishermen offloaded in Yarmouth from the *Natalie Hammond*. Both of them died. The crewman who died first was called "Soren Bjurun" and "Sorun B. Jurun," in the above newspaper accounts. Here is his record from the Death Register for Yarmouth, 1918, under *almost* his real name, which was (note the slashed ø) Søren Bjerrum.

Name of Deceased: Bjerrum, Soren [Søren]

Sex: Male

Date of Death: Sept. 27, 1918

Age: 28 years

Residence: 10 Pearl St. / Gloucester, Mass.

Occupation: Fisherman

Single, Married or Widowed: Married

Place of Birth: Denmark

Cause of Death: Spanish Influenza /Pneumonia

Length of Illness: about 10 days

Religion: Lutheran

Race: White

Name of Physician Attending: Farish, J. W. S.

Undertaker: Van Stone, A. L.

Place of Burial: Gloucester, Mass. U.S.A.

Name of Person Making Return: Watson, Mary A.

Date of Return: September 28, 1918

> Søren Bjerrum, Death Registration, Yarmouth County, Year 1918, Book 51, Page 75, Number: 253. Died Yarmouth Hospital, Yarmouth, Yarmouth County, NS.

The second crewman to die was Augustus Thompson, also of Gloucester, Massachusetts.

DEATH IN YARMOUTH FROM INFLUENZA
Gloucester Man Succumbs to the Disease After a Couple of Weeks Illness

YARMOUTH, October 1

The death took place at Yarmouth hospital today of Augustus Thompson, of Gloucester, Mass. The deceased was one of the two members of the crew of the Gloucester fishing schooner *Nathalie Hammond* [*Natalie Hammond*] which that vessel left in Yarmouth two weeks ago today seriously ill with Spanish Influenza. The disease at the time of their arrival had become very deeply seated and the physicians feared for their recovery. They continued to fail, pneumonia having developed and the other [Søren Bjerrum] passed away on Friday last [September 27], whilst Thompson lingered until this morning. He is survived by a widow and five children in Gloucester, where he settled after coming to North America from Norway, his native country.

Halifax Morning Chronicle, 2 October 1918, 13.

Name of Deceased: Augustus Thompson
Sex: Male
Date of Death: Oct. 1st, 1918
Age: 49 years
Residence: 123 Rogers St. / Gloucester, Mass.
Occupation: Fisherman
Single, Married or Widowed: Married
Place of Birth: Norway
Cause of Death: Spanish Influenza /Pneumonia
Length of Illness: 12 days
Religion: Lutheran
Race: White
Name of Physician Attending: Farish, C. W. T.
Undertaker: Sweeny, V.S. [Vernon S.]
Place of Burial: Gloucester, Mass. U.S.A.
Name of Person Making Return: Watson, Mary A.
Date of Return: October 2, 1918

> Augustus Thompson, Yarmouth County, Death Register, 1918, Book 51, Page 107, Number 321.

☞ Yarmouth undertaker Sweeny's "Ledger 9 (2 Feb 1918 to 23 Mar 1920)" shows that the American Consulate had asked that the body of Augustus Thompson be shipped to Boston; shipping was to be charged to a "Miss Thompson." Deceased had been a Lutheran.

> Information courtesy of Deborah Trask, Curator Emeritus, Nova Scotia Museum, whose mother, Gwen Trask, CG-C (Certified Genealogist, Canada), had a copy of a transcript of the ledger.

☞ The schooner *Natalie Hammond* made it safely back to Gloucester, arriving September 27. But she had had other cases of influenza on board, and had offloaded ailing men in a Massachusetts port even before coming into Yarmouth.

CAPTAIN COLSON'S CREW HARD STRICKEN

Capt. Charles Colson, of the schr. Natalie Hammond, which arrived here last Friday [September 27], reports six of the Hammond's crew taken ill during the last trip, two [and it would be at least three] of whom have died of the Spanish influenza and pneumonia. After the first day out of port, three weeks ago last Friday, Wallace Doucette, of Lynn, was taken ill and three others, Peter Doucette, William Tarnun and David White, were stricken with the disease and landed by Capt. Colson in Provincetown. Doucette died in Provincetown.

A week ago last Tuesday Capt. Coulson landed two more of his crew, Augustus Thompson and Soren Bjerm [Søren Bjerrum], at Yarmouth, N.S., the latter [and shortly thereafter, the former] passing away at the hospital there. Both dead men [all three of them] were married. Doucette is [was] about 38 years of age and lives in Lynn. He registered in his home city the day the Hammond left and he jumped on board just before the craft left port. Bjerm was 28 years old [24 years old] and leaves a widow and little daughter in this city. Sixteen of the Hammond's crew with her captain arrived home well.

Yarmouth Telegram, 4 October 1918, 2, from the *Gloucester Times*, September 30.

☞ Augustus Thompson, the second crewman unloaded in Yarmouth from the *Natalie Hammond*, died on October 1, 1918.

☞ Deborah Trask sent further information gleaned from Vernon Sweeny's Ledger 9, of burials performed for victims of Influenza in Yarmouth:

✉ I went to Yarmouth this weekend to visit my mother and yesterday we went over to Port Maitland to the cemetery called the Island cemetery—here is a general photo of the site (you can see Port Maitland in the distance) and another of the stone for Lyndon Porter, died 4 Jan. 1919 [not shown].

Afterward I got into mum's genealogical library—she has a copy of the Sweeny Funeral home records, which were computerized and indexed by some folks in Tusket area a long time ago. There I found a couple of interesting things.

The Ledger for 1918/19 is #9, and the first reference to "spanish influenza" in Ledger 9 is for Elizabeth L. Cann who died 23 Sept 1918, and the last was for Mary Owen Hurley who died Lower Argyle 8 Feb 1919, age 26. There's a couple of influenza deaths after that [to the end of Feb./19], but not called 'spanish'. Selda Atkinson (you have indexed as Atkins), died 29 Nov 1918, age 6, buried in Mountain Cemetery.

Also interesting to see that quite a number of Yarmouth people died in Massachusetts but were brought home for burial. For example, Harold Churchill, age 26 died 28 Sept 1918, place died: Lynn of Essex, funeral 16 Oct, burial Darling's Lake.

Deborah Trask, Curator Emeritus, Nova Scotia Museum, whose mother, Gwen Trask, CG-C (Certified Genealogist, Canada), had a copy of a transcript of the ledger, to Ruth Whitehead, 19 March 2018, email.

SAYS U-BOATS SPREAD INFECTION
Washington, D.C., Sept. 18.

Atrocities by German submarine commanders have reached their apex in the spreading of Spanish Influenza germs in America, according to Lieutenant Colonel Philip S. Doane, head of the Health and Sanitation Section of the Shipping Board. German submarines, he reports, have traversed the ocean, loaded with these germs, which have been released in this country, with especially baneful effects upon the intellectual [*sic*] population of Boston.

Yarmouth Telegram, 27 September 1918, 4.

Doctor G. G. Melvin, chief medical officer for New Brunswick, was interviewed on the subject of "Spanish Flu":

Without a doubt it is caused by minute vegetable growths known as germs, which find access to the breathing organs by way of the mouth and nose.... The affected person is most likely to spread the disease to those near him by coughing or sneezing. These actions expel very small—almost invisible particles of moisture from the air passage. These particles are known as droplets and are likely to carry the germ within or upon them.

Yarmouth Telegram, 27 September 1918, 2.

This was the state of knowledge of influenza in 1918. The cause, a virus, had not yet been identified—indeed, even the term 'virus' was poorly understood as to its nature, even its existence, or worse yet, no one knew that there were a gazillion viruses, or that they continually mutated.

The death took place at the Yarmouth Hospital yesterday morning, of Bernard Crowell, son of Mr. and Mrs. John Crowell of Argyle, after an illness of twelve days of Pneumonia. The deceased was a fisherman living at Yarmouth Bar when he was taken ill, and remained there for several days or until the disease became deeply seated. When a physician was finally summoned, he was found to be in a very precarious condition. He was at once taken to the hospital, where it was soon found that there was little or no hope for his recovery, and he gradually failed until yesterday morning, when he passed away. He was a bright and promising young man of 19 years.

Yarmouth Telegram, 4 October 1918, 2. Note that he was taken ill on September 22, and was a fisherman.

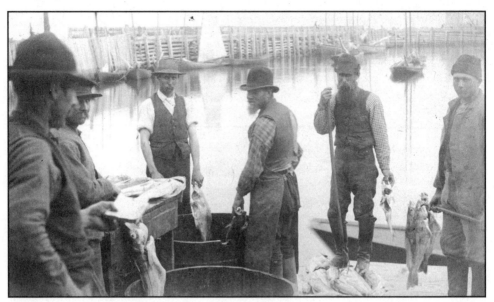

Fishermen at Port Maitland, Yarmouth County, with the south wharf in the background. *(Courtesy of the Yarmouth County Museum Archives)*

HAROLD CHURCHILL. The sad news was received by relatives in Darling's Lake and Plymouth, Yarmouth Co., on Wednesday, of the death of Mr. Harold Churchill in Lynn, Mass. A previous telegram a day or so before told of his serious illness, which, to a degree, prepared his relatives for the depressing news that came on Wednesday....The remains will be brought home for burial as soon as Mrs. Churchill, who is also ill, has recovered sufficiently to allow her to travel.

Yarmouth Telegram, 4 October 1918, 2.

The Spanish Influenza in Yarmouth is being kept well within bounds and what does exist is only of a very mild type, in many cases being little more than an ordinary fall cold. Yesterday three houses were quarantined and three to-day and in each instance it was done only as a precautionary measure, and not, as reported, owing to the seriousness of the cases. There are two in the hospital and both are in a ward by themselves. One of these, Gunner Guennox Y. Vos, of a French patrol ship, who was recently landed at a Nova Scotia Atlantic port; the other, Adolphus Fitzgerald, of H.A. Amiro's schooner Dawn, which arrived yesterday. But these patients have very mild cases and to-day are much improved.

Yarmouth Telegram, 11 October 1918, 1.

☞ The authorities were still calling this a "very mild type." They would quickly be disabused.

BOARD OF HEALTH
The Council then met as the Board of Health and at the request of the Deputy Solicitor, passed the following resolution:
Resolved, that Spanish Influenza be, and is hereby declared to be, an infectious and contagious disease, dangerous to the public health, and that all by-laws of this Board relating to the prevention of epidemic disease shall apply thereto. Hiram Goudry, Secretary Board of Health, Yarmouth, NS, Octr. 9, 1918.

Yarmouth Telegram, 11 October 1918, 2, 4.

PUBLIC NOTICE
The Health Board of the Municipality of Yarmouth, in order to prevent the spread of the epidemic disease commonly known as Spanish Influenza, has determined, under the authority conferred upon it by the Public Health Act, that all churches, theatres, moving picture shows and schools both public and private and other places where people assemble or congregate shall be closed from this date until further order, and persons having control of such places are hereby notified to comply with such directions, and for failing so to do will incur the penalties provided by law in that behalf. J. ARCH. BLACKADAR, Sec'y. Yarmouth, N.S., Oct. 9, 1918.

Yarmouth Telegram, 11 October 1918, 4.

REGINALD B. CHURCHILL. The death took place at Port Maitland early on Wednesday morning, of Mr. Reginald B. Churchill, after an illness of only a few days of pneumonia. The deceased was one of the County's most progressive and energetic young farmers and fishermen....Mr. Churchill was the son of Mr. and Mrs. Ernest Churchill, of Port Maitland, and was 27 years and 5 months old. He leaves, besides his parents, his widow and infant.

Yarmouth Telegram, 18 October 1918, 1.

A meeting of the Board of Health was held in the Council Chamber last evening....The question of shipping arrivals was also discussed, and the Health Officer was instructed to work in conjunction with the Chief of Police, in watching the waterfronts and to enforce the act that masters of all incoming vessels must show a clean bill of health before any of the crew is allowed to land.

Yarmouth Telegram, 18 October 1918, 1.

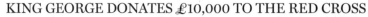
KING GEORGE DONATES £10,000 TO THE RED CROSS

King George, in a most appreciative and congratulatory letter to the Red Cross Society of Canada, says: "Impressed as I am by the vast obligations which must still fall on the joint societies, I have much pleasure in contributing the sum of £10,000."

Yarmouth Telegram, 18 October 1918, 1.

Yarmouth District Registrar

In 1918, the Municipal Clerk and District Registrar for Yarmouth was Hiram Goudey. He was to die a year later. Perhaps Mr. Goudey was not in the best of health in 1918, as there are mistakes in the 1918 Death Register. He died of nephritis on November 12, 1919; his brother sent in the return of death, and it was filed in the 1919 Death Register, and the name of the District Registrar who did sign this page, is "Hiram Goudey / Dist. Registrar, Yarmouth N.S."—his own name! He must have signed off on a number of blank pages in the register before his final illness.

Other mistakes made by Mr. Goudey show up in the case of Robert Abbott, a Yarmouth hotel proprietor on Hawthorne Street, aged 63, born in Forbes Point, Shelburne County. He died October 16, 1918, in the Yarmouth Infirmary. Mr. Abbott ended up with two death records, one of which, in the Shelburne County Register, was later crossed out, but had been sent in by the district registrar for *Yarmouth* County, who signed off on Mr. Abbot's Yarmouth County register entry, as well as sending a return of Abbott's death to Shelburne County, his birthplace.

Yarmouth County, 1918, Book 51, Page 108, Number 332:
Abbott, Robert James, male, 63, d. October 18, 1918. He was a "hotel keeper," residing on Hawthorne Street, Yarmouth. His death is given here as caused by bronchial pneumonia, after an illness of six days. His doctor was A. M. Perrier. Mr. Abbott was married, a Baptist, born in Forbes Point, Shelburne County, and buried there in the "Public Cemetery." The undertaker's name was A. X. Van Horne. Return of Death was sent in by "Abbott, Nellie" on 19 October 1918, the day after his death; she was likely his wife.

At the bottom of this very page (108) in the death register, we find: "I hereby certify the foregoing to be the true and correct entries of all Deaths that have taken place in this Registration District and have been returned to me for the three months ended Dec. 31 1918. Given under my hand this 15th day of Feb'y A.D. 1919. Hiram Goudey."

☞ Shelburne County, 1918, Book 49, Page 329, Number 796½:

Abbott, Robert James, Male, 63, d. October 18, 1918. In the register's line for Occupation appears "Prop. & Keeper of a store." Written above in a blank space is, "Hawthorne Hotel, Yarmouth." *This* record says he died from influenza, after an illness of "a few days." Mr. Abbott, as above, was married, a Baptist, born in Forbes Point, and buried there in the "Public Cemetery." In the section labeled "Return sent in by:" appears the name of "Goudey, Hiram / Dist. Registrar / Yarmouth County." There is no date on the return, so it makes it impossible to say which record came first, but Hiram Goudey had a hand in both.

Nellie Abbott's prompt return of death, on October 19, is probably the earlier record. She says he died in Yarmouth.

Mr. Abbot's Shelburne County record was entered in the Register of Deaths for the year 1918, in "District No. 5, Woods Harbour, Barrington, Shelburne County." Therein, Number 796½ is entered *between* Numbers 796 (Nickerson, Winnifred), and 797 (Murphy, Gladys), in the original ledger, a very strange way of recording, not seen elsewhere in research for this book. The whole record was later crossed out. To further complicate matters, Nova Scotia Archives' HVS Search Engine results for this name are headlined, "Robert James Abbott, died 1918 in Yarmouth, Shelburne County"! Their HVS heading gives the record number as 796, but below this title, one can see, on their photograph of the original ledger, that it is 796½, indicating that it had been shoehorned in at a later date.

☞ There were so many Yarmouth and Shelburne County deaths during this period of October 16 through December 31, 1918, it is no wonder that doctors, nurses, families, and even registrars were overwhelmed.

MRS. GEORGE FORBES. The death of Martha, wife of Mr. George Forbes, who at one time was a landscape gardener about town, occurred at their home, Pleasant Lake, on Wednesday after only a few days illness of pneumonia. The deceased was 65 years of age.

Yarmouth Telegram, 25 October 1918, 1.

Passengers arriving in Yarmouth by steamers are of the impression that they are being discriminated against by the recent ruling of the Board of Health, which compels them to remain aboard the steamer until the arrival of Health Officer Fuller. They claim that dozens of passengers arrive daily by the D.A.R. and H.&S.W. express, and that they come from points infected quite as serious[ly] as those at which the steamers call, yet no doctor or health officer molests them, and they land from the trains and go their way as before any epidemic prevailed.

Yarmouth Telegram, 25 October 1918, 1.

CAPT. GEORGE FARISH DIES OF INFLUENZA
Was Taken Ill on Wednesday Last, Pneumonia Quickly Developing. Was Paymaster of the First Depot Battalion

Halifax, October 27. Very wide is the circle in which the sorrowful news of the death at an early hour this morning of Captain George Farish, of the widely-prevalent Spanish influenza, death being due to pneumonia which developed with incredible swiftness, will be received with a sense of shock and of loss. His father, H.C. Farish, and his cousin, Dr. Farish and Mrs. Farish, of Yarmouth, came to the city by motor, having been summoned by the news of the gravity of his condition. To Mrs. Farish [the widow] his death, as will be readily understood, is an overwhelming blow. She is at present with Mr. and Mrs. George E. Nicholls, Coburg Cottage, with her little daughter, an infant of two months, and on all sides are heard expressions of deep sympathy for her in her bereavement.

Halifax Evening Mail, 28 October 1918, 1.

THE CLOSURE WILL CONTINUE. AND THE RULING IS TO BE MOST RIGIDLY ENFORCED

A meeting of the Board of Health was held yesterday morning, Mayor Grant presiding, all Councillors present, together with Health Officer Fuller. Mayor Grant informed the Board that seventy-four houses had been placed under surveillance. Health Officer Fuller spoke as to condition of affairs and said that the thirty-two houses did not limit the epidemic to that many cases, as there were in some instances more than one case to a dwelling....The Health Officer reported concerning the disease amongst the fishing vessels and stated that a very careful watch had been kept on all arrivals and he felt there had been no spread from that source. He thought that a considerable fear of the disease had emanated amongst the public, and that the precautions taken by the people generally had gone a long way towards keeping the disease well in hand. Some had complained about the coastal steamers being held up, while trains and autos were allowed to come unmolested from many of the affected sections. He said such inconveniences were experienced in any Maritime port on which a quarantine was placed.

In his opinion the handling of the trains was a matter for the Provincial Board of Health to look after, by issuing an order to forbid the sale of a railroad ticket to any person who could not produce a clean bill of health.

Coun. Lonergan asked the Health Officer if there was not some complaint caused by his delay in visiting the incoming steamers.

Dr. Fuller replied that he made a point to visit those steamers just as soon after arrival as he possibly could. The delay in Yarmouth is not greater than in other parts where a quarantine exists, for no matter how large the port may be or how extensive the number of arrivals, a quarantine officer never sleeps on the docks, but is summoned on arrival.

Yarmouth Telegram, 1 November 1918, 4.

 At East Pubnico, Nov. 1, of influenza and pneumonia, Mr. Adelbert Nickerson, aged 37 years, leaving his mother and three sisters.

Yarmouth Telegram, 8 November 1918, 8.

 THE BAN LIFTED THIS MORNING
A meeting of the Board of Health was held yesterday morning, Mayor Grant presiding, all Councillors present, together with Health Officer Fuller.

Health Officer Fuller reported that a vessel had arrived from the fishing grounds on Tuesday with several cases aboard; three were taken to the Hospital on arrival [see Alfred Pothier, below], and on Wednesday the other afflicted [crew members on the schooner] had so far recovered as not to deem it necessary for them to go to that institution. He had a suspicion that the men had contracted the disease while the vessel was at Lockeport for bait....He also referred to the great deal of extra work he had been put to in attending the incoming steamers and vessels in connection with his duties. He asked the Board considered that that work should come within the duties which his stipend of $100 per annum covers.

Yarmouth Telegram, 8 November 1918, 1.

 ALFRED POTHIER. Mr. Alfred Pothier, son of Mr. and Mrs. Daniel Pothier, died at the Yarmouth hospital last evening, aged 22 years. The deceased had for some time past been a member of the crew of the schooner Francis A., which arrived from the fishing grounds on Tuesday. Mr. Pothier, with two others of the crew, was seriously ill at that time with influenza and pneumonia and was immediately taken to the hospital, where the precariousness of his condition was at once realized and his relatives were given little or no encouragement for his recovery.

Yarmouth Telegram, 8 November 1918, 1.

 MRS. JOHN JACQUARD. The death of Olive, beloved wife of Mr. John Jacquard, took place at her home, Wedgeport, on Thursday morning. The deceased had been in poor health for some time past and a few days ago contracted a severe cold which developed into influenza and pneumonia. Owing to her impaired health she was unable to withstand the inroads of that dread disease and failed rapidly.

Yarmouth Telegram, 8 November 1918, 1.

MRS. MICHAEL BOUDREAU. Another death which cast much gloom over Wedgeport also occurred yesterday morning when Mary, wife of Mr. Michael Boudreau, passed away. The deceased had for months past been suffering from tubercular trouble but the direct cause of her death was pneumonia which developed from a cold, and her final illness was very brief.

Yarmouth Telegram, 8 November 1918, 1.

HAROLD RAY. A very distressing death took place yesterday at his home on Water Street, when Mr. Harold Ray, formerly of Port Mouton, passed away. The deceased was 25 years of age and leaves his widow, who at present is dangerously ill, and two young children, one 10 months old and the other 10 days.

Yarmouth Telegram, 8 November 1918, 1.

Health Officer Fuller...addressed the Council in regard to the influenza situation. There had been 45 new cases since the last meeting—6 so far this week. They were largely among the poorer class and a number of the cases had been so serious that he had deemed it necessary to send them to the hospital. There were 13 cases there at that time, and the hospital could not accommodate any more owing to the lack of beds, which at present could not be bought in Yarmouth. The hospital charged nothing less the $2 per day for the cases and he would like to get the view of the Council in the matter. Some of these cases, he was sure, could never pull through, as they were not in a position to receive any care whatever.

Yarmouth Telegram, 13 December 1918, 2.

The death took place in Yarmouth yesterday of Miss Rosie, the 17-year-old daughter of Mr. Frank Frauten, of Springhaven. The deceased had been ill of influenza and had practically recovered, when she suffered a relapse which developed into pneumonia and it was soon apparent that little or nothing could be done for her.

Yarmouth Telegram, 20 December 1918, 1.

YARMOUTH COUNTY, VITAL STATISTICS, DEATH REGISTER, BOOKS 51, 110

1918

1. Elizabeth Cann, 38, d. 23 September 1918, Yarmouth.

2. Søren Bjerrum, 24, d. 27 September 1918 in Yarmouth, [*Danish*] fisherman from Gloucester, MA.

3. Volucien Doucet, 36, d. 16 September 1918, Tusket, fisherman.

4. Alfred Muise, 24, d. 25 September 1918, Belleville, soldier.

5. Augustus Thompson, 49, d. 1 October 1918 in Yarmouth, fisherman from Gloucester, MA.

6. Bernard Crowell, 19, d. 3 October 1918, Argyle, labourer.

7. Robert Abbott, 63, d. 18 October 1918, Yarmouth, hotel keeper. [*Entered in Shelburne County Death Register and later crossed out; not listed in Yarmouth County Death Register, due to a registrar's error. His name has been transferred here to give a corrected total of Yarmouth deaths.*]

8. George Robard, 68, d. 23 October 1918, Yarmouth, labourer.

9. Mary Koritem, 45, d. 27 October 1918, Yarmouth.

10. Alfred Pothier, 22, d. 7 November 1918, Yarmouth, fisherman.

11. Harold Ray, 25, d. 8 November 1918, Yarmouth, fisherman.

12. Kenneth Sweeny, 28, d. 9 November 1918, Yarmouth, merchant.

13. Joshua Doucette, 28, d. 9 November 1918, Wedgeport, fisherman.

14. Harriet Muise, 16, d. 9 November 1918, Yarmouth, mill hand.

15. Mary Nelson, 2, d. 12 November 1918, Yarmouth.

[*Next on Dr. Marble's list from the Yarmouth Death Register was John MacEwan, 18, d. 23 November 1918 in Liverpool. Eliminated here, and moved to Queens County death registration list.*]

16. Nora Grannon, 33, d. 27 November 1918, Yarmouth, housewife.

17. Monde Surette, 36, d. 10 December 1918, Yarmoth [*sic*], labourer.

18. Percy Surette, 5 months, d. 11 December 1918, Yarmouth.

19. Lottie Whitten, 17, d. 13 December 1918, Yarmouth, housekeeper.

20. Florence Kinney, 28, d. 15 December 1918, Yarmouth.

21. Edith Van Emburg, 3 months, d. 18 December 1918, Yarmouth.

22. Annie Morton, 31, d. 21 December 1918, Yarmouth.

23. Edward Smith, 26, d. 23 December 1918, Yarmouth, moulder.

24. Laurence Pothier, 17, d. 29 December 1918, Yarmouth, fisherman.

25. Sarah Watkins, 17 months, d. 21 October 1918, Yarmouth.

26. Nathan Moses, 36, d. 27 December 1918, Ohio, NS, farmer.

27. Adelbert Jenkins, 38, d. 28 December 1918, Hebron, labourer.

28. Reginald Churchill, 27, d. 16 October 1918, Port Maitland, fisherman.

29. Seldon [Selda M., female] Atkinson, 6, d. 29 November 1918, Darlings Lake.

30. George Ellis, 9, d. 2 December 1918, Port Maitland.

31. Celenie Surette, 27, d. 23 October 1918, Wedgeport.

32. Charles Surette, 23, d. 24 October 1918, Wedgeport, fisherman.

33. Emilie Cotreau, female, 30, d. 27 November 1918, Wedgeport.

34. Lloyd LeBlanc, 12, d. 4 November 1918, Wedgeport

35. Mary Boudreau, 27, d. 7 November 1918, Wedgeport.

36. Olive Jacquard, 72, d. 7 November 1918, Wedgeport

37. Judith Muise, 36, d. 9 November 1918, Belleneck, Argyle.

38. Jeremie LeBlanc, 39, d. 11 November 1918, Abrams River, fisherman.

39. Laura Muise, 2, d. 14 November 1918, Belleneck.

40. Marie Bourque, 21, d. 20 December 1918, Eel Brook, housework.

41. Clemente Surette, 17, d. 5 October 1918, Middle West Pubnico, housework. [*HVS Search Engine gives her a male name, Clement, but she is female, thus 'Clemente', which can be seen on her record.*]

42. Adelbert Nickerson, 37, d. 11 October 1918 at East Pubnico, farmer.

43. Stephen Surette, 52, d. 18 October 1918, West Pubnico, farmer.

44. Dorothy D'Eon, 4, d. 30 October 1918, West Pubnico.

45. Augustine Moulaison, male, 3 months old, d. 18 December 1918, Surette Island. [*He was born and lived on Morris Island, but died on nearby Surettes Island. No father's name given, and no family noted. Roman Catholic, buried on Surettes Island. The undertaker sent in the return.*]

46. George Moulaison, 9, d. 7 December 1918, Sluice Point.

47. Rose Moulaison, 9, d. 21 December 1918, Sluice Point.

48. Mary Frotten, 17, d. 19 December 1918, Argyle, housemaid.

49. Raymond Cann, 3, d. 5 November 1918, Comeau's [*sic*] Hill.

1919-20

50. Maud Roach, 49, d. 25 March 1919, Yarmouth, housekeeper.

51. Mabel Higley, 28, d. 4 January 1920, Yarmouth, factory worker.

52. James Crowell, 77, d. 7 January 1919, Yarmouth, expressman.

53. Harry Fox, 32, d. 9 January 1919, Yarmouth, boiler maker.

54. William Morton, 2, d. 1 January 1919, Yarmouth.

55. George Bain, 36, d. 19 January 1919, Yarmouth, livery stable owner.

56. Melvin Losier, 21, d. 3 February 1919, Yarmouth, sailor.

57. Mary Hurley, 26, d. 8 February 1919, Argyle Head, housewife.

58. Norman Wilson, 33, d. 1 January 1919, Hebron, station agent.

59. Beulah Doane, 33, d. 5 January 1919, Cape Forchu.

60. Sarah Cann, 41, d. 7 January 1919, Ohio, NS.

61. Harvey Stoddart, 14, d. 10 January 1919, Sandford.

62. Barbara Whitman, 1 year 7 months, d. 15 January 1919, Arcadia.

63. Lyndon Porter, 35, d. 4 January 1919, Port Maitland, merchant.

64. Evangeline Thibault, 36, d. 3 January 1919, Belleville, housework.

65. Margaret Van Amburg [*Emburg?*], 23, d. 20 February 1919, Pubnico, householder.

66. Alice Muise, 8, d. 29 January 1919, East Quinan.

67. Kingsley Tibbets, 42, d. 5 March 1920, Plympton, farmer.

68. George R. McCormack, 34, d. 6 March 1920, Wellington, farmer.

69. Elias Paterson, 62, d. 8 March 1920, died in Yarmouth Hospital, but from Digby, fisherman.

70. Mrs. Reta Smith, 27, d. 21 March 1920, Rockville, housewife.

71. Leola Hamilton, 22, d. 4 March 1920, Lower Argyle, housewife.

72. Willie Robichaud, 8, d. 16 May 1920, Wedgeport. *[He can only be found in the death register if one searches for his correct name, "Robichaud, Gervais Willie." He was nearly nine when he died, the son of Benjamin and Delphine LeBlanc Robichaud. HVS, Book 110, Page 224.]*

Chapter XX

SUMMATION

The Necessity of Accurate Statistics in Fighting Epidemics

IN 1918, DR. J. T. MACAULAY, city and district medical officer from Cape Breton County, was at a meeting of the Sydney Board of Health, held on October 26. He spoke against lifting the quarantine in Sydney. He was particularly insistent that schools remain closed. The Board of Health, he said, lacked the data to be effective, and until they got it, strategies could not be created to contain it.

Sydney Daily Post, 28 September 1918, p. 6. For the full report on this meeting, see the chapter on Cape Breton County.

He knew that without data, one cannot plan a campaign against an enemy—in this case, influenza.

I include Dr. MacAulay's statement of frustration, because our sourcebook still has the same problem, namely, lack of data on this most virulent epidemic. Even today, we still have no idea how to arrive at a figure for *cases* of influenza in Nova Scotia during the disease's 1918 to 1920 run, because no continuous coverage of patients exists, and no totally accurate counts from that time are available. We can only guess that the number of those infected with the virus at any one time or place was overwhelmingly greater than the number of deaths, a huge percentage greater. And while this is better than a disease that kills everybody, it does mean that for weeks and months, Nova Scotia society must have had to do without those who were ill, do without their skills, their labour, their contribution. Small towns, villages, and rural areas must have at times been so stricken that life—business and social life—was at a standstill. It's almost a surprise that any data at all was being sent in. So you will find less on that than I could wish. This project still needs your help!

Dr. Marble's lists have given this sourcebook a head start of at least twenty years of research. Keep in mind, however, that these sources are incomplete. The county lists of names featured here do not, in most cases, include his findings in newspaper obituaries or other reportage. Such names appear in his unedited alphabetical list of surnames, in the Appendix. They include names of some Nova Scotians who died outside the province, so the death total for this list will therefore be higher, and this should be taken into account. Please consider these sources not as final, but rather, as launching pads for further study. I encourage you to keep looking, keep collecting local memories. There is still much that could be studied, much that could be learned.

As mentioned earlier, Dr. Marble was directly copying the original registries, mistakes and all. Some of those ledger entries are duplicates. One woman even has three separate and slightly differing entries. There are death records for one person in two different counties. When a person died in Nova Scotia but far from home, the undertaker at the death scene, in preparing the body for shipping, would send in a report to his county registrar—the correct procedure, as the county of death determines who keeps the returns of death. But sometimes a second undertaker, in another county, the one who actually *buried* the body, also sent in a return of death to his registrar.

These lists, even though edited and amplified as they have recently been, are safer viewed as historical artifacts. They are not all-inclusive, in terms of deaths. They are not carved in stone.

Why? We went looking, via family memory, memoirs, or local information, for names of people whose deaths were never reported. We found some, and though they were not added to Dr. Marble's lists, you can read their stories in the relevant county chapters. Yet we can never be sure, no matter how long and hard we continue to look, that we have found them all. There weren't many. More research of this nature needs to be done, before such stories pass out of memory. As you can imagine, not every Nova Scotian has been interviewed about this.

Searching on the ground—browsing in local cemeteries, looking for dates of 1918 to 1920—proved less productive than we'd hoped. Remember that many people were hastily buried during this time, sometimes in mass graves, and they may have had no headstones. A hundred years have passed, so their descendants may be the only ones who still remember who they were and how they died. We were doing this work more out of curiosity than with any intelligent research plan.

We encourage individuals or historical societies across the province to listen to family knowledge, and to visit local cemeteries, looking for dates of 1918–20. They can then check for cause of death on the Nova Scotia Archives website described in the prologue. (Or stay home and do it online, looking at findagrave.com for Nova Scotia, for example.) When it comes to history, local memory is our biggest untapped provincial goldmine. Certainly, local memory has produced the most illuminating of our sourcebook information, the most riveting of our stories.

Another way the numbers don't tell the complete story is this: the Great Influenza, when it killed a pregnant woman, naturally killed her unborn child as well. Deaths in utero, stillbirths, and miscarriages are still deaths, and where the mother dies of flu, these deaths are also influenza-caused. Such deaths don't appear much in registries. We know about some through newspaper obituaries for the mother; usually when the child may have lived a few days.

Information on stillbirths and miscarriages, or deaths during pregnancy usually come to us via family memories. Miscarriages were never mentioned in death registers. Perhaps it was not the custom to record stillbirths, either: I have only seen a few. One such, in the Shelburne registry for 1918, showed a stillbirth entered and then slashed out. Finally, we know from Garry Shutlak, Nova Scotia Archives, of at least one newborn in *his* family, viable but living less than a day, who was not given either a birth *or* a death registration. This child's mother died of influenza almost immediately after he was born. I hope future studies will consider these sorts of omissions from the lists of the dead.

Another large group that could be studied for possible inclusion in the death totals are people in the registers whose cause of death is reported as pneumonia, many of whom almost certainly died of an influenza-caused pneumonia. See Chapter One for further information.

Dr. Marble had to err on the side of provability of data, and he rightly chose not to include names from the death registry which did not specifically mention influenza as a primary or secondary cause of death. Where these deaths were clusters of young adults (this influenza's preferred victims), all from one small village or attending the same church, or living on one particular island—and some of whom *are* labelled as influenza deaths, so we know it was in the village—I suggest that these "pneumonia" deaths are possible flu victims. Some Shelburne County people's deaths, especially, seem to be good candidates for a re-evaluation of the influenza death toll. It's not the kind of information we can prove or disprove, unless we go back in time and autopsy them all. But someone could examine the data and posit potential additions to the Nova Scotia death totals.

The thing that I noticed all the way through this collection of oral histories, the thing that impressed me the most was how people here consistently helped family, neighbours, and total strangers. It is this quality of Nova Scotians, to rise to the occasion with compassion, I think, that contributed most to our low death levels here, as compared with many other places.

Philadelphia, Pennsylvania, for example, had 759 deaths in *one day*—October 10, 1918—whereas the city of Halifax, in the entire three years of the Great Influenza had only 336. Halifax County, including the city deaths—the county with the highest total—had only 497 deaths in three years. Comparisons are odious, and there are too many factors to draw conclusions from this, I know, but compared to many cities, countries, even continents, Nova Scotia got off lightly.

John Barry. *The Great Influenza*. New York, Penguin Books, 2009: 329.

We had in Halifax, for the most part, some strong individuals in local governance: the Provincial Health Officer, Dr. W. H. Hattie; the Mayor of Halifax, Dr. Arthur C. Hawkins; Dr. Norman E. McKay, the chairman of the Board of Health and Quarantine Officer for the Port of Halifax. These three doctors in key positions knew exactly what to do and had the power to enforce it. Since Halifax had the largest population, and the largest port traffic, this counted for a lot. The city fielded a cast of medical personnel, both civilian and military—doctors, nurses, hospital staff—who worked themselves ragged, and who sometimes gave their lives taking care of the sick. Sydney had a good medical health officer in Dr. J. F. MacAulay, but he struggled with city aldermen who were better at arguing than at taking action. Rural communities, on the other hand, often made do with only one, or even no medical personnel at all. In a number of places, when influenza took out the local doctors, the people were petitioning for others to be sent—for help of any sort. Sometimes this was possible, sometimes they were left to cope alone.

The Great Influenza was a nightmare beyond our wildest imaginings, but Nova Scotia somehow survived. It survived because people helped each other—with common sense, with kindness, sometimes even by sheer bullheaded doggedness.

The Great Influenza Survivors, Nova Scotia, 1918–20

I wanted to end this sourcebook with a story about one family whose members were stricken by the influenza of 1918 to 1920 and who survived. Many Nova Scotians, though they had been seriously ill, did live through it.

Philip Hartling, Nova Scotia Archives, told me about the time in 1920 when his grandmother "had a really bad day." Her name was Margaret Gallagher Hartling. She and her husband, Ansel Hartling, lived in Port Dufferin in what is now Philip's own house. Their three children, Ethel, Florence, and Lloyd, were all down with Spanish flu, and Philip thinks the parents were as well. Everyone who came to help out during this crisis caught it too, and went home sick, leaving the older Hartlings to deal with the household as best they could.

It was February 25. A big windstorm was raging outside. Ansel told Margaret he had to go out to the barn for a while because the cow had gone into labour. When he finally returned, he announced that he had a terrible pain in his side. (Philip has been told that Ansel might have had pneumonia, brought on by Spanish Flu, which would account for that sort of pain.) His wife must have said something like, well, she'd gone into labour and was having pain too.

They were out in the kitchen, both in a fevered state, with three sick children upstairs, and to cap it all off, just then the windstorm blew out the kitchen window next to door to the dining room—frame, glass, and all. Margaret gave birth on the dining room table, to a third daughter, Mildred. Ansel boarded up the window as best he could. The cow was safely delivered of her calf. The children all recovered from the Spanish flu. Their parents almost certainly had the disease as well, but they too survived. Five years later, Philip's father, Gerald Hartling, was born on that same dining room table.

Philip Hartling to Ruth Whitehead, personal communication (at his retirement party), 28 March 2018. An email, 16 July 2018, provided specific details.

Ruth Holmes Whitehead
Halifax 2018-2020

CODA

The Centers for Disease Control and Prevention in Atlanta, Georgia, says it is not a question of whether this sort of influenza epidemic will occur again, but when. *"Influenza viruses are unpredictable—we can never be certain of when or from where the next pandemic will arise. However, another influenza pandemic is inevitable."*

www.cdc.gov/flu/pandemic-resource, March 11, 2019.

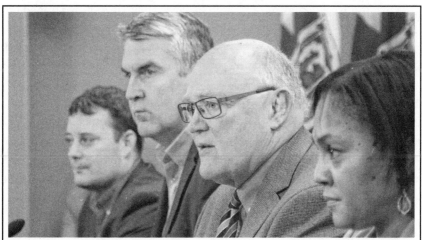

Nova Scotia has three presumptive cases of novel coronavirus (COVID-19) all related to travel. The individuals have been notified and are in self-isolation. Health and Wellness Minister Randy Delorey, left, Premier Stephen McNeil, Dr. Robert Strang, Nova Scotia's chief medical officer of health and deputy chief medical officer of health Dr. Gaynor Watson-Creed provided an update to the media Sunday afternoon. **ERIC WYNNE • THE CHRONICLE HERALD**

Province announces first presumptive cases

Cases are unconnected and all have been asked to self-isolate, Strang says

COVID-19 DEVELOPMENTS

• University classes suspended / **A3**

• Halifax airport to update pandemic plan / **A3**

• VIBERT: Listen to public health officials / **A4**

• U.S. told to hunker down by top health expert / **A8**

STUART PEDDLE
THE CHRONICLE HERALD
✉ speddle@herald.ca

the younger man returned from Europe on Tuesday, and the older man returned from

announced the cases at a news conference in Halifax on Sunday afternoon.

number — and all those indi-

A headline from the Halifax *Chronicle Herald*, on March 16, 2020, warns of the impending arrival of the COVID-19 pandemic in Nova Scotia. (*Courtesy the* Chronicle Herald)

A MERE THREE months after I sent this manuscript in to the publisher, I found myself living through a global pandemic—the COVID-19 virus had spread worldwide in just that time. Nova Scotia went into lockdown, and I into strict isolation. Once again the world seemed taken by surprise, even though we were continuously warned by the US Centers for Disease Control and Prevention, by numerous TED talks, by books such as John Barry's *The Great Influenza*, first published in 2005. While writing this story about the same pandemic's effect on Nova Scotia, I came across multiple anniversary documentaries on the so-called Spanish Flu, from multiple countries. All of them warned us that such a viral pandemic would (not "could") happen again. It's coming, they said, get ready!

My editor thinks an afterword appropriate. For days I've tried to write one, but I am left speechless. It's the nightmare of a history in which I had been immersed for two years which has suddenly become reality TV, playing out before my eyes. I have to write this cliffhanger now, however, because if I wait until the pandemic is over to add it, one or two more years may have passed. I may even be dead. I had hoped this book would come out by October 2020, one hundred years after the last Nova Scotian died in the 1918–20 outbreak. I wanted it to be a useful guide for what to do and what not to do. Now, we are fighting a pandemic after the fact, and we all have bigger things to worry about than a book launch.

The world is under siege. The number of people sick or dying is increasing exponentially. Schools and non-essential businesses close, then open, then close again; events are cancelled, crowds forbidden. I think our province is doing all it can, but there all still people acting as if this were a party with which they are now bored. If the second wave breaks over us, we *have* to quarantine ourselves. Our medical facilities will not be able to handle the numbers of sick and dying the province will experience if we do not follow instructions. Crowded situations are the perfect incubators and transmitters of the virus.

John Barry's opinion, as well as my own, is that the most important thing any government at any level can do in a situation like the Great Influenza or the COVID-19 epidemic is to tell people the absolute truth about what's going on, what the dangers are, and what measures they will have to take.

"We do not know what will happen. But we do know that of all the lessons from 1918, the clearest is that truth matters. A specialty among public relations consultants has evolved in recent decades called 'risk communication.' I don't care much for the term—it implies managing the truth. You don't manage truth; you tell the truth."

Barry, 2009: 480.

We need all levels of government to tell us the truth and insist on measures. Only then will we be frightened enough, finally, to pay attention to the strict quarantines necessary to stop this thing in its tracks. And then the rest is up to us. All of us.

Ruth Holmes Whitehead
September 4, 2020

ACKNOWLEDGEMENTS

In Nova Scotia: These people contributed in a major way to every chapter in this book: Dr. Allan Everett Marble, Chair of the Medical History Society of Nova Scotia, lent his unpublished research (Martin Hubley photocopy-digitized the entire fond). Sam Everett Howard, independent researcher, Halifax. Gordon Hammond, Special Projects Volunteer, Lake Charlotte Area Heritage Society, and Chris Hencklemann, computer genius. The staff of the Nova Scotia Archives, for help in the use of the website: Historical Vital Statistics (HVS) database; and for Newspaper Microfilms 1918-1920. Other individuals contributed magnificently to one or more chapters. My grateful thanks.

Annapolis County: Deborah Trask, Curator Emeritus, Nova Scotia Museum.
Antigonish County: Jocelyn Gillis, Curator; Liam Cogger, Intern; Antigonish Heritage Museum. The Cenotaph Project, Antigonish Heritage.
Cape Breton County: Dr. Jim St. Clair, university professor (retired); Rannie Gillis, writer and photographer.
Colchester County: Ashley Sutherland, archivist, Colchester Historeum, Truro. Dale Swann, Tatamagouche Museum. Janet Baker, Elizabeth Peirce, family histories.
Cumberland County: Harriet McCready; Linda Littlejohn; Edward Crane Gilbert; Parrsborough Shore Historical Society, Parrsboro. Frank Allan, book donor, Amherst. Dale and Eric Mills. Charles Thompson, memorialist, Truro.
Digby County: Angela (*famille LeBlanc*) Buckles, French translation.
Guysborough County: Ruth Legge, historical researcher, author; Jack Legge, facilitator, Liscombe Mills. Lewis MacIntosh and Lloyd Sinclair, local informants. Lois Ann Dort, Board Member, Guysborough Historical Society.
Halifax County: Elizabeth Peirce, author, Halifax. Bernie Francis, Mi'kmaw linguist, Halifax. Rosemary Barbour, Garry D. Shutlak, Barry Smith, Darlene Brine, Nova Scotia Archives. Philip Hartling, Nova Scotia Archives (retired) and Scott Robson, History Curator, Nova Scotia Museum (retired), Halifax. Janet Baker, author and oral history informant for six counties, Halifax. Martin Hubley, History Curator; Leslie Pezzack, Natural History Registrar (retired); Roger Lewis, Ethnology Curator; Katie Cottreau-Robins, Provincial Archaeologist; Joleen Gordon, Research Associate; Nova Scotia Museum of Natural History.

Roger Marsters, Maritime Museum of the Atlantic, Halifax. Karen Smith, Special Collections, Killam Library; Mark Lewis, Sir James Dunn Law Library; Eli Diamond, Department of Classics; Dalhousie University. Doug Pezzack (retired); Don Gordon (retired); Bedford Institute of Oceanography, Dartmouth. Chara Kingston, Army Museum, Halifax. Heather Ludlow, Legislative Library, Province House, Halifax. Sharon McDonald, independent researcher, Dartmouth. Susan McClure, Municipal Archives, Halifax. Angela Buckles, French translation. Brigitte Neumann, German translation. Fort Massey United Church and Rev'd Trevor Cleveland-Thompson, Halifax. Sarah Whitehead.

Hants County: Janet Baker, Ashley Sutherland, Elizabeth Peirce.

Inverness County: Dr. Jim St. Clair; Rannie Gillis.

Kings County: Kate MacInnes Adams, Kings County Museum, Kentville. Janet Baker; Ruth Legge. Borden Family descendants, Elizabeth Ann Cunningham, Bruce Jamieson.

Lunenburg County: Deborah Trask, Curator Emeritus, Nova Scotia Museum; Sharon McDonald, independent researcher; Sarah Whitehead.

Pictou County: Janet Baker. Jocelyn Gillis.

Queens County: Linda Rafuse, Director, Queens County Museum, Liverpool.

Richmond County: Gabriel LeBlanc, historian, author (2017) of *Mon Isle Madame*, D'Escousse; Caitlin McCready-Carswell; Lori Poirier Forgeron, West Arichat; Viola Samson, Samsons Cove; Lena Samson, Little Anse; Nicholas Boudreau, Petit-de-Grat. Harriet McCready, facilitator. Roger Marsters, schooner identification. Edward Crane Gilbert for salt trade history.

Shelburne County: Deborah Trask.

Victoria County: Pauline MacLean, researcher, Nova Scotia Highland Village, Iona.

Yarmouth County: Gwen Trask, Certified Genealogist—Canada, Yarmouth. Lisette Gaudet, archivist, Yarmouth County Museum and Archives. Deborah Trask. Roger Marsters.

In Ontario: Jim Burant, Library and Archives Canada, Ottawa (retired); Bennett McCardle, Library and Archives Canada, Ottawa.

And finally, my grateful thanks to Ali Moghadam, Staples, Halifax, for endless technical support when old computers failed and new computers did strange things.

Appendix

A LIST OF NOVA SCOTIANS WHO DIED IN THE INFLUENZA PANDEMIC OF 1918–1919

Allan E. Marble CG (C), Halifax, Nova Scotia, Canada, 2009
[These are Dr. Marble's unedited, unpublished notes, used by permission. See the county lists for an amended version, not by surname, but by county, to find specific people. His category, 'length of time ill,' is omitted here.]

"Notes: The total number of Nova Scotians who died from influenza was 2,051. [We both think it will be shown to have been much higher.] The influenza deaths identified from death certificates totaled 1,768. Sources: Nova Scotia Death Certificates and Nova Scotia Newspapers.

1. The names of people and places presented below are spelled as they appear in their death record (novascotiagenealogy.com) or in their death notice or obituary which appeared in a newspaper.

2. The reader will notice that some individuals listed below died of influenza according to a newspaper entry, but their death certificate does not indicate that influenza was the cause of their death. A check of their death certificate will most likely show that they died of pneumonia which usually followed an initial infection by the influenza virus.

3. It may be necessary to consult Place Names of Nova Scotia or a Gazetteer of Nova Scotia to determine the location of some of the places listed below.

4. Chronicle refers to the Morning Chronicle, *a Halifax newspaper.*

5. Abbreviations include: h (hours), d (days), w (weeks), m (months), y (years)

6. In the entries taken from newspapers, the place name following the name of the deceased is the place where that person died.

7. The question mark (?) in the age column indicates the age was given but could not be ascertained by the author, whereas the --- in the age column indicates that age was not given for that person.

Nova Scotian	Age	Place of Death	Date of Death
_____ , _____ , *Yarmouth, Chronicle, 8 September 1918, page 2 (a Gloucester fisherman).*			
_____ , _____ , *North Sydney, Sydney Daily Post, 2 October 1918, page 2 (two American seamen).*			
_____ , _____ , *Truro, Truro Daily News, 17 October 1918, page 4 (three deaths at Indian Reservation).*			
Unnamed Infant	13d	Martins River	14 FEB 1919
Abbott, Robert	63	Yarmouth	18 OCT 1918
Acker, Anthony	01	Shelburne	28 OCT 1918
Acker, Lucinda	02	Birchtown	05 NOV 1918
Adams, George	08	Halifax	02 NOV 1918
Adams, Orland	8d	Westchester	04 DEC 1918
Adams, Ralph	14m	Westchester	24 NOV 1918
Adams, Thomas	16	Halifax	23 OCT 1918
Adams, William	02	Halifax	16 NOV 1918
Albury, Edwin	18	Windsor	27 OCT 1918
Allander, Margaret	47	Halifax	01 NOV 1918
Allen, Mrs. Hallett, Springfield, Middleton Outlook, 15 November 1918, page 2 (née Demone).			
Allison, Fred	15	Five Mile River	03 FEB 1919
Allison, Pte Henry G., Vancouver, 38, Truro Daily News, 21 December 1918, page 2 (formerly of Upper Kennetcook).			
Almon, Jane C.	30	Georges River	15 NOV 1918

Amero, Mary	40	Doucetteville	13 DEC 1918

Amey, child, North Sydney, Sydney Daily Post, 4 December 1918, page 1 (child of Phillip Amey).

Amey, Eliza	04	North Sydney	02 NOV 1918

Amey, Mrs. Phillip, North Sydney, Sydney Daily Post, 4 December 1918, page 1.

Anderson, Belle	22	Springhill	07 NOV 1918
Anderson, Clarence	20	Harbour Bouchee	23 NOV 1918
Anderson, Joseph	4m	Mulgrave	18 DEC 1918
Anderson, Lucy	54	Hammonds Plains	08 NOV 1918
Andrews, Oscar	30	North Range	03 JUL 1919
Andrews, George	22	Halifax	08 NOV 1918
Andrews, Michael	6m	Trenton	17 MAR 1919
Andrews, Oscar	29	North Range	17 APR 1919
Anthony, Emma	27	Glace Bay	27 NOV 1918
Antle, Mary	42	Halifax	18 OCT 1918

Antony, Mrs. Tom., New York, 45, Westville Free Lance, 1 November 7. (She was a Cameron of Loch Broom, Pictou County).

Anvonell, Joseph	45	Sydney	14 OCT 1918
Arab, Helen	2m	Halifax	16 JAN 1919
Arbuckles, Charles	28	Ponds	08 JAN 1919
Arey, Alice	01	East Sable River	27 FEB 1919
Armsworthy, Clarence	21	Philip's Harbour	24 NOV 1918
Armsworthy, Margaret	26	Halifax	12 MAR 1919
Arnold, Eliza	58	Halifax	01 NOV 1918
Arsenault, Diminan	09	East Margaree	18 DEC 1918
Arsenault, Fred	---	Trenton	16 OCT 1918
Arsenault, Leo	04	Belle Cote	28 DEC 1918
Arsenault, Mary	3h	Little Bras D'or	NOV 1918
Arsenault, Mrs. Simon	72	East Margaree	30 DEC 1918
Arseneau, Albert	26	Pictou	28 NOV 1918
Arseneau, Joseph	3m	East Margaree	20 DEC 1918
Arthur, Margaret	23	Halifax	24 NOV 1918

Atkins [Atkinson], Selda, Darling's Lake, aged 7, Yarmouth Telegram, 29 November 1918, page 1.

Atkinson, Seldon [Selda]	06	Darling's Lake	29 NOV 1918
Attwood, Kathleen	03	Glace Bay	12 OCT 1918
Atwell, Albert	16	Malenson	23 FEB 1919
Atwell, Dennison	20	Morine Mountain	02 MAR 1919
Atwood, Doane	66	Newellton	08 NOV 1918
Aucoin, Marguerite	42	Cape Rouge	06 OCT 1918
Auntivine, Robert	21	Sydney	24 OCT 1918
Aylward, Annie	27	Falmouth	31 MAY 1919
Bacon, Almira	76	Hillgrove	11 APR 1919
Baglole, Alva	22	Halifax	20 FEB 1919
Bailey, George	04	Round Hill	30 JAN 1919
Bain, George	36	Yarmouth	19 JAN 1919
Baker, Ada	26	Halifax	31 DEC 1918
Baker, Arthur	21	East Jeddore	30 OCT 1918
Baker, Catherine	41	Glace Bay	14 DEC 1918
Baker, Harry	*31*	*Bridgewater*	*29 OCT 1918*

Halifax Evening Mail, 01 November 1918, page 6.

Bambrick, David	43	Melanson	10 NOV 1918

Bangay, Henry, Lockeport, aged 39, Liverpool Advance, 23 October 1918, page 2.

Banks, Victoria	18	Pictou	20 OCT 1918
Barber, George	49	City Home, Halifax	26 OCT 1918
Barkhouse, Grace	37	Canning	02 JAN 1919
Barrett, Charles	05	Halifax	15 OCT 1918

Barrett, Frank	30	Halifax	08 NOV 1918

Halifax Evening Mail, 9 November, page 1, (died at Willow Park Hospital).

Barrie, Melissa	54	Halifax	24 OCT 1918
Barrington, Edna	30	Sydney Mines	29 NOV 1918

Sydney Daily Post, 30 November 1918, page 1, (Mrs. John E. Barrington).

Barron, Anthony	43	Rawdon Gold Mines	26 MAY 1919
Batherson, Mary	63	North Sydney	05 DEC 1918
Batty, Harold	21	Halifax	25 OCT 1918
Bealer, Charles	35	Bridgewater	18 OCT 1918
Beals, Gladys	15	Preston	23 OCT 1918

Halifax Evening Mail, 26 October 1918, page 4.

Beazley, Minnie	10	Dartmouth	21 NOV 1918

Beck, Mrs. Lavinia, Lunenburg, Lunenburg Progress Enterprise, 30 October 1918, page 1.

Beckford, Margaret	35	Halifax	15 NOV 1918
Beddan, Eliza [see Beddow]	19	New Waterford	18 DEC 1918
Beddow, Eliza	19	Sydney Mines	16 DEC 1918
Beeler, Agnes	67	Scarsdale	18 OCT 1918

Beeler, Frederick, Annapolis Royal, 53. Halifax Evening Mail, 22 October 1918.

Beeler, James	53	Lequille	20 OCT 1918
Bell, Nancy	22	Riverdale	15 OCT 1918

Digby Courier, 25 October 1918, page 2 (Mrs. Percy Bell).

Belliveau, Evelyn	24	Joggins Mines	08 DEC 1918
Bennett, Almadine	3w	Parrsboro	27 FEB 1919
Bennett, Clarence	16	Sydney Mines	14 OCT 1918
Bennett, Margaret	23	Halifax	29 OCT 1918
Bennett, Samuel	42	Springhill	06 NOV 1918
Bennett, William	02	Canning	13 JAN 1919
Benoit, Bernadette	30	Charlos Cove	05 DEC 1918
Benoit, James	37	Petit de Grat	17 OCT 1918
Bent, David	25	Victoria	24 OCT 1918

Bent, Dorothy, Belleisle, aged 8, Bridgetown Monitor, 19 March 1919, page 4.

Bent, William E.	41	Belleisle	27 FEB 1919

Bridgetown Monitor, 5 March 1919, page 1.

Bentley, Charles, Westchester, aged 17, Amherst Daily News, 18 October 1918, page 2.

Bernard, Frederick	19	Trenton	17 OCT 1918

Berry, Frank, Sackville, N.B., Amherst Daily News, 26 October 1918, page 8 (of Amherst).

Best, FitzHerbert [Fitzhenry]	36	Sydney	08 OCT 1918
Bezanson, Nelson	31	Frauxville	26 OCT 1918
Biggs, S. A. B.	29	Sydney	10 OCT 1918
Billaed, Sarah	27	Halifax	23 OCT 1918
Bishop, Carl	16	Amherst	25 NOV 1918

Amherst Daily News, 26 November 1918, page 3.

Bishop, Etta	22	Greenwich	04 JAN 1919
Bjerrum, Soren	24	Yarmouth	27 SEPT 1918

Black, Frederick M., Amherst, Amherst Daily News, 10 March 1918, page 3.

Black, Lizzie May, Amherst, Amherst Daily News, 4 March 1919, page 5 (Mrs. Fred Black).

Black, Lillian	36	Liverpool	01 NOV 1918

Liverpool Advance, 6 November 1918, page 2 (Mrs. Lillian Black, aged 37)

Blakely, Acil	19	Goldboro	30 DEC 1918
Blanchford, Frank	27	Louisbourg	17 OCT 1918
Blinis, Muriel	22	Halifax	28 OCT 1918
Blinn, John	64	Corberrie	29 JUN 1919
Bonafant, Arsene	79	Grosses Coques	30 JUN 1919

Bonang, Joseph B., Dartmouth, 21, Halifax Evening Mail, 29 October 1918, page 2.

Bond, Ada	66	East Chester	06 MAR 1919

Bond, Mrs. Joseph	48	*Hazel Hill*	*19 NOV 1918*

Canso News, 30 November 1918, page 1 (died at Port Felix).

Bond, Rebecca	64	Little Bras d'Or	02 OCT 1918
Bonin, Peter	3m	Jordins Harbour	02 DEC 1918
Bonini, Nicholas	28	North Sydney	30 NOV 1918
Bonnar, Robert	40	North Sydney	08 DEC 1918

Boomer, Charlie, Brookfield, 10, Truro Daily News, 24 December 1918, page 2 (son of Wm).

Boomer, Willard	?	Halifax	19 DEC 1918

Boomer, William, Halifax, Truro Daily News, 24 December 1918, page 2 (of Brookfield).

Borden, Ellen	53	Sheffield Mills	11 JAN 1919

Bosse, Mrs. Frank, Mass., Amherst Daily News, 12 October 1918, page 3 (of Pugwash).

Oxford Journal, 10 October 1918, page 6 (her maiden name was MacLeod).

Bouchie, Jentie	3w	Petit de Grat	21 OCT 1918
Bouchie, Jervos	15m	Petit de Grat	17 OCT 1918
Bouchie, Marah	02	Petit de Grat	21 OCT 1918
Boudreau, Anita	02	Cape Auget	07 DEC 1918
Boudreau, Cathrine	16	Cabbage Cove	26 OCT 1918
Boudreau, Charles	10m	Cape Auget	19 NOV 1918
Boudreau, Clarence	17	Petit de Grat	03 NOV 1918
Boudreau, Francis	22	Boudreauville	27 OCT 1918
Boudreau, Godfrey	21	Boudreauville	21 OCT 1918
Boudreau, James	19	Halifax	05 NOV 1918
Boudreau, James	21	Halifax	05 NOV 1918
Boudreau, Joseph	25	Petit de Grat	19 OCT 1918
Boudreau, Joseph	6m	Poulamond	25 APR 1919
Boudreau, Leo	18m	Martinique	11 DEC 1918
Boudreau, Marie	76	Church Point	12 FEB 1919
Boudreau, Marie	09	Eastern Harbour	17 APR 1919
Boudreau, Mary	17	Little Ance	06 NOV 1918
Boudreau, Mary	27	Wedgeport	07 NOV 1918
Boudreau, Mary	18d	Cabbage Cove	22 FEB 1919
Boudreau, Romeo	11m	Arichat	04 FEB 1919
Boudreau, Sabine	26	Petit de Grat	26 OCT 1918
Boudreau, Sophie	12	Poulomond	27 OCT 1918
Boudreau, Veronica	01	Dominion	12 DEC 1918

Boudrot, Mrs. Barbara, North Sydney, aged 31, Sydney Daily Post, 25 November 1918, page 1.

Boudrout, Josephine	32	Sydney	11 OCT 1918
Boudville, Jean	22	Reserve Mines	06 OCT 1918
Boulter, Allen	47	Westchester Station	12 JAN 1919

Bourke, Louis, Halifax, Halifax Evening Mail, 30 October 1918, page 16 (an infant).

Bourque, Clodia	01	Amherst	06 NOV 1918
Bourque, Emerie	9m	Halifax	29 OCT 1918
Bourque, Marie	21	Eel Brook	20 DEC 1918
Boutilier, Doria	02	Tantallon	06 NOV 1918
Boutilier, Eliza	22	Halifax	06 JAN 1919
Boutilier, Ella	26	Mill Cove	25 FEB 1919
Boutilier, George	22	Sydney	04 NOV 1918
Boutilier, George	21	Halifax	19 DEC 1918
Boutilier, Gordon	27	Bedford	10 DEC 1918

Boutilier, Pte. Harold, France, aged 24, Halifax Evening Mail, 24 January 1919, page 9 (Black Pt).

Boutilier, Irene	35	Halifax	27 OCT 1918
Boutilier, Warren	8m	Boutilier's Point	29 JAN 1919
Boutilier, William	18	Milton	17 NOV 1918
Boyde, Catherine M.	20	Sydney Mines	26 NOV 1918
Boyer, Emma	23	West Arichat	06 MAR 1919

Boyer, Joseph   35   West Arichat   07 MAR 1919

Boylan, Nicholas, 37, Nova Scotia Hospital, 27 October 1918; Halifax Evening Mail, 28 October 1918, page 2.

Bradley, Mrs. Hugh   83   Whiteburn   04 AUG 1918

Bradley, John W.   27   Halifax   26 OCT 1918

Bradbury, Jacob   9m   Glace Bay   18 DEC 1918

Bradshaw, Mary, Windsor Forks, aged 13, Hants Journal, 18 December 1918, page 8.

Brawer, Annie   19   Sydney   04 OCT 1918

Breach, Margaret   ?   Halifax   30 NOV 1918

Breen, Calvin G.   17   Halifax   04 JAN 1919
   Halifax Evening Mail, 23 January 1919, page 1 (died at Marie Joseph).

Breen, Edward   54   Cape Jack   31 OCT 1918

Brennan, Thomas   31   North Sydney   15 OCT 1918

Brewer, Carmen   20   North Sydney   20 OCT 1918

Brewer, Sarah   05   Sydney Mines   03 NOV 1918

Briand, Charles   27   Halifax   10 JAN 1919

Bridge, John   40   Maccan   04 MAR 1919

Brightman, Alfred   45   Halifax   22 OCT 1918

Brigley, Wallace   14   Black Point   08 DEC 1918

Brisson, Arthur   18   Halifax   22 DEC 1918

Broadfoot, Harriet   24   Halifax   27 NOV 1918

Brock, George   21   Halifax   12 OCT 1918

Brooks, Beatrice   19   Glace Bay   27 OCT 1918

Brooks, Harry   28   Glace Bay   19 OCT 1918

Brown, Anastatia   28   Halifax   04 DEC 1918

Brown, Edna   20   Halifax   23 DEC 1918
   Halifax Evening Mail, 27 December 1918, page 1, (age given as 19).

Brown, Eliza   38   East Mapleton   19 NOV 1918

Brown, Elizabeth   31   Dartmouth   28 OCT 1918
   Halifax Evening Mail, 29 October 1918, page 2.

Brown, Ethel   02   Florence   11 NOV 1918

Brown, Gladys   01   Springhill   19 NOV 1918

Brown, Gordon   14   Halifax   10 MAR 1919

Brown, Grace   03   Italy Cross   25 OCT 1918

Brown, Harry   26   New Waterford   29 OCT 1918

Brown, Mrs. Hillary   28   New Victoria   23 OCT 1918

Brown, Howard   05   East Mapleton   15 NOV 1918

Brown, James   32   Florence   18 NOV 1918

Brown, Leonard   28   South Maitland   25 NOV 1918

Brown, Madge   03   Bramber   20 NOV 1918

Brown, Perry   16   Cheverie   06 NOV 1918

Brown, Thomas   84   Little River   06 MAR 1919

Brown, Tressa   41   Parrsboro   14 FEB 1919

Brown, Violet, Dartmouth, aged 2, Halifax Evening Mail, 04 November 1918, page 2.

Bruce, James R.   30   West Brooklyn   25 OCT 1918

Bruce, Mrs. James, Hilden, aged 47, Truro Daily News, 11 December 1918, page 1.

Bryan, Frederick   30   Halifax   08 NOV 1918

Buchanan, Eva   30   Ketch Harbour   19 MAR 1919

Buchanan, Margaret   62   Enslows Point   14 OCT 1918

Buckley, Joseph   30   St. Bernard   03 NOV 1918
   Digby Courier, 08 November 1918, page 2 (of Belliveau's Cove).

Budd, Bernice   33   Springhill   15 FEB 1919

Buideksson, August   40   Halifax   29 OCT 1918

Bull, Colin   36   Pictou   02 JAN 1919

Bullers, Charles,   47   Londonderry   24 JAN 1919

Bumpstead, Frederick   10   Amherst   11 JAN 1919

Burchell, Margaret   24   Halifax   24 OCT 1918

Burgess, Mary	04	Upper Musquodoboit	31 OCT 1918
Burgess, Mary	43	Upper Musquodoboit	08 NOV 1918
Burgoyne, Loraine	17	Halifax	21 OCT 1918
Burke, Annie	27	River Hebert	21 OCT 1918
Burke, Ida	*19*	*Halifax*	*19 OCT 1918*

Halifax Evening Mail, 21 October 1918, page 9.

Burke, Jerome	26	Portuguese Cove	06 NOV 1918
Burke, Mrs. John	21	Arichat	03 MAY 1919
Burke, Mary	8m	Arichat	31 APR 1919
Burke, Peter J.	*18*	*Halifax*	*07 OCT 1918*

Chronicle, 10 October 1918, page 3 (described as first to die in Halifax).

| Burke, Stanley | 01 | Lingan | 13 JAN 1919 |

Burns, Mrs. John, Berwick, aged 54, Berwick Register, 30 October 1918, page 2.

| Butcher, Richard | 28 | Sydney | 25 OCT 1918 |
| *Butler, Margaret Jane* | *34* | *Amherst* | *11 NOV 1918* |

Amherst Daily News, 12 November, 1918, page 3.

| *Byrne, Mrs. Mary* | *70* | *Halifax* | *NOV 1918* |

Halifax Evening Mail, 02 November 1918, page 7 (of Upper Water Street).

Cable, Sidney, Truro, aged 53, Halifax Evening Mail, 20 February 1919, page 13.

| Caccebetto, Rosa | 31 | Dominion | 05 MAR 1919 |

Cadogan, Mrs. Dr., ____, Marble Mtn, Sydney Daily Post, 25 December 1918, page 3 (nurse).

Cadman, Clarence	25	Halifax	20 DEC 1918
Cahill, Richard	24	Halifax	13 OCT 1918
Calder, Thomas	5m	Springhill	06 NOV 1918
Caldwell, William	72	City Home, Halifax	25 OCT 1918
Callow, Wentworth	14m	Oxford	04 NOV 1918
Cameron, Ann	60	North Sydney	02 NOV 1918
Cameron, David	11m	Trenton	26 MAR 1919

Cameron, Frank P., Amherst, aged 25, Amherst Daily News, 18 October 1918, page 2.

Cameron, Mary	36	Dominion	12 DEC 1918
Campbell, Annie	08	New Waterford	05 NOV 1918
Cameron, Annie	17	Mulgrave	26 FEB 1919
Campbell, Dan	20	Sydney	23 NOV 1918
Campbell, Mrs. Donald	70	Mabou Mines	13 DEC 1918
Campbell, Elizabeth	75	Little Bras d'Or	02 MAR 1919
Campbell, Leslie	18	Sydney	21 OCT 1918
Campbell, Margaret	60	Sydney	22 OCT 1918
Campbell, Mary	22	Glace Bay	07 DEC 1918
Campbell. Peter	27	New Waterford	10 DEC 1918
Campbell, William J.	14	North Sydney	30 SEPT 1918
Cann, Elizabeth	38	Yarmouth	23 SEPT 1918
Cann, Raymond	03	Comeau's Hill	05 NOV 1918
Cann, Sarah	*41*	*Ohio*	*07 JAN 1919*

Yarmouth Herald, 7 January 1919, page 1 (wife of William H. Cann).

| Cann, William | 31 | Sydney Mines | 03 DEC 1918 |

Cann, William T., Sydney, Amherst Daily News, 27 January 1919, page 3.

Canning, Mrs. Herbert	20	Thorburn	04 DEC 1918
Card, Annie	3m	Springhill	28 OCT 1918
Carlin, George	26	Sydney	29 NOV 1918

Carmichael, Agnes, Halifax, aged 3, Halifax Evening Mail, 30 October 1918, page 16.

Carmichael, James	29	Stellarton	11 DEC 1918
Carmichael, Sarah	04	Halifax	29 OCT 1918
Carnell, George	62	Glace Bay	01 DEC 1918
Carney, Harry	38	Halifax	28 DEC 1918
Carroll, David J.	21	Stellarton	22 NOV 1918
Carroll, Howard	20	Lantz Siding	07 JAN 1919

Carter, _____ , Lockhartville, *Halifax Evening Mail*, 23 January 1919, page 1 (a father).
Carter, _____ , Lockhartville, *Halifax Evening Mail*, 23 January 1919, page 1 (a mother).
Carter, _____ , Lockhartville, *Halifax Evening Mail*, 23 January 1919, page 1 (son of above).
Carter, _____ , Lockhartville, *Halifax Evening Mail*, 23 January 1919, page 1 (a daughter) [see Carty].
Carter, Charles, Massachusetts, *Canso News*, 26 October 1919, page 1 (of Canso).

Carter, Charles	21	Glace Bay	29 NOV 1918

Carter, Douglas G., Alberta, 24, *Amherst Daily News*, 3 March 1919, page 3 (of W. Leicester).

Carter, James	31	Halifax	24 OCT 1918
Carter, Truman J.	*2*	*Pugwash*	*03 DEC 1918*

Amherst Daily News, 27 December 1918, page 3 (name spelled Trueman).

Carty, Emmeline	84	Lockhartville	09 JAN 1919
Carty, John M.	75	Lockhartville	10 JAN 1919
Carty, Minnie	43	Lockhartville	10 JAN 1919
Carty, Theodore	16	Lockhartville	11 JAN 1919
Carver, Simeon	25	Waldon	26 FEB 1919
Casey, John	15	Springhill	13 NOV 1918
Cavanagh, Mrs. Lillian	*23*	*Halifax*	*21 OCT 1918*

Halifax Evening Mail, 22 October 1918 (described as Mrs. and 32 years old).
Westville Free Lance, 25 October 1918, page 8 (Mrs. J. L. Cavanagh, née McLean).

Cawes, Lucy	23	Halifax	10 OCT 1918
Chaisson, Alexander	30	Margaree Harbour	26 DEC 1918
Chaisson, Annie	02	Belle Cote	14 DEC 1918
Chaisson, Beatrice	07	Belle Cote	31 DEC 1918
Chaisson, Elizabeth	31	Reserve Mines	14 DEC 1918
Chaisson, Florence	8m	Belle Cote	11 DEC 1918
Chaisson, John	03	Belle Cote	13 DEC 1918
Chaisson, Lillie	06	Belle Cote	13 DEC 1918
Chaisson, Lucy	6m	Belle Cote	14 DEC 1918
Chaisson, Lucy Ann	04	Belle Cote	16 DEC 1918
Chaisson, Mary	18m	Belle Cote	14 DEC 1918
Chambers, Francis	68	Newport	26 DEC 1918
Chandler, Ida	28	Springhill	28 DEC 1918

Chanpoux, Rev., New Brunswick, Yarmouth Telegram, 13 Decemver 1918, page 1 (of Church Pt).

Chapman, Benjamin	63	Fort Lawrence	28 JAN 1919
Chase, Eliza	63	Halifax	21 OCT 1918
Chason, Thomas	34	Halifax	07 NOV 1918
Chetwynd, Robert	3m	Charlesville	08 APR 1919
Chiasson, Dennis	13	Grand Etang	08 DEC 1918
Chiasson, Elsie	31	Reserve Mines	13 DEC 1918
Chiasson, Francis	02	Glace Bay	05 DEC 1918
Chiasson, Mathilde	33	Eastern Harbour	23 OCT 1918
Chiasson, Mary	31	Little River	12 SEPT 1918
Chiasson, Mary	01	Glace Bay	21 DEC 1918

Chipman, Major Leverett deV., Halifax, Middleton Outlook, 27 December 1918, page 1.

Chisholm, Daniel	25	Nova Scotia Hospital	26 OCT 1918

Chisholm. Fred., Folly Mtn, Truro Daily News, 24 December 1918, page 2 (of Highland Village).

Chisholm, George	24	Great Village	14 DEC 1918
Chisholm, Hugh	45	New Glasgow	31 DEC 1918
Chisholm, Valentine	36	St. Andrews	04 NOV 1918
Chittick, John	3m	Sheet Harbour	07 MAR 1919
Chivers, Tilly	15	Shelburne	15 OCT 1918
Chorme, Marjorie	03	Sydney Mines	23 JAN 1919
Christie, Henry	15	Cape North	06 NOV 1918
Christie, Lowrie	*51*	*North Sydney*	*29 MAR 1919*

Halifax Evening Mail, 31 March 1919, page 9.

Christopher, John	29	Ketch Harbour	13 MAR 1919

Chung, Soo	38	Halifax	09 NOV 1918

Churchill, Miss Eva, Victoria, Yarmouth Herald, 21 January 1919, page 5 (of Yarmouth).

Churchill, Reginald	27	Port Maitland	16 OCT 1918

Chute, Mrs. A.B., South Berwick, Berwick Register, 13 November, 1918, page 2.

Chymist, Gertrude	*23*	*Lockeport*	*22 OCT 1918*

Liverpool Advance, 30 October 1918, page 2 (Mrs. Walter Chemist)

Clancey, Edgar	*31*	*Sydney*	*07 OCT 1918*

Halifax Evening Mail, 09 October 1918, page 1 (Edward Joseph Clancey).

Clancy, Cyril	05	Halifax	30 OCT 1918
Clark, Gordon	27	Stellarton	08 JAN 1919
Clark, Myrtle	25	Halifax	08 DEC 1918
Clarke, James	26	Sydney	03 OCT 1918
Clattenburg, Frank	47	Port Medway	23 MAR 1919

Clayton, Samuel, Preston, Halifax Evening Mail, 26 October 1918, page 4.

Clayton, Vernon, Western Canada, Bridgetown Monitor, 05 February 1918, page 4 (Young's Cove).

Cleary, James	32	Halifax	27 OCT 1918
Cleary, John	75	Enfield	05 JAN 1919
Clemens, Eric	27	Halifax	15 NOV 1918
Clements, Brenton	22	Mapleton	11 NOV 1918
Cleveland, Ernest	9m	Halifax	23 FEB 1919
Cleveland, Frank	19	Berwick	29 OCT 1918
Cleveland, Frank	26	Halifax	04 DEC 1918
Clow, Leith B.	---	Shelburne	11 NOV 1918
Coady, Mary	60	Margaree Harbour	22 DEC 1918
Coburn, Alonzo	41	Summerville	29 SEPT 1918
Cockell, Laura	28	Sydney	11 DEC 1918
Cohoon, Catherine	23	Halifax	26 NOV 1918
Cohoon, Maud	24	Dartmouth	28 NOV 1918
Colburne, Annie	33	Springhill	11 NOV 1918
Cole, Margaret	79	Maitland	31 AUG 1918
Collins, Kathlyn	26	Kentville	25 DEC 1918

Collins, Hatheway, Annapolis, Halifax Evening Mail, 25 October 1918, page 8.

Colp, Cora	*46*	*Eagle Head*	*01 DEC 1918*

Liverpool Advance, 4 December 1918, page 4 (Cora May Colp).

Colp, Willard	*19*	*Eagle Head*	*NOV 1918*

Advance, 4 December 1918, page 4 (age given as 18).

Colquhoun, Catherine, New York, Halifax Evening Mail, 28 November 1918, page 2 (of Halifax).

Colwell, Effie	01	Springhill	31 OCT 1918
Comeau, Ambroise	30	Grosses Coques	03 JAN 1918
Comeau, Blanche	3m	Meteghan River	29 APR 1919

Comeau, Fred, Little Brook, Digby Courier, 14 March 1919, page 5.

Comeau, Joseph B.	25	Meteghan River	27 OCT 1918
Comeau, Marie	3m	Meteghan	27 APR 1919
Como, Amos	38	Joggins Mines	16 MAR 1919
Condon, Eleanor	06	Sydney	17 DEC 1918
Connolly, Thomas	38	Halifax	15 NOV 1918
Connors, Thomas G.	*24*	*Dartmouth*	*22 OCT 1918*

Halifax Evening Mail, 23 October 1918, page 2 (Thomas George Connors).

Conrad, Crawford	21	Cherry Hill	17 OCT 1918
Conrad, Alice	17	Liverpool	20 OCT 1918
Conrad, Ray	23	New Dublin	24 OCT 1918
Conrod, Malcolm	22	Upper LaHave	02 NOV 1918
Conrod, Gertrude	19	East Chezzetcook	08 NOV 1918
Conrod, Rhoda	22	Chester	24 OCT 1918

Conway, John B., Amherst, Amherst Daily News, 23 December 1918, page 3.

Cook, Emily	60	Five Mile River	12 FEB 1919

Cooke, Mrs. Isabella, Centreville, 50, Sydney Daily Post, 20 November 1918, page 1.

Cooper, B. F.	31	Halifax	04 NOV 1918
Copan, Mary	8d	Halifax	03 NOV 1918
Cope, Annie	01	Windsor Junction	08 OCT 1918
Cope, Peter	6w	Indian Reserve	11 OCT 1918
Cope, Sarah	38	Windsor Junction	13 OCT 1918

Copeland, Mr., Halifax Evening Mail, 24 October 1918, page 6 (engineer on railway).

Copeland, Henry	18	Indian Reserve	29 JAN 1919

Copeland, Laurence P., Lunenburg, Lunenburg Progress Enterprise, 30 October 1918, page 5.

Copp, Viola	21	Great Village	22 OCT 1918
Corbett, James	49	Dominion	09 DEC 1918
Cordo, Ellen	21	Halifax	29 NOV 1918
Corkum, Earl	26	Louisbourg	22 OCT 1918
Corkum, Edwin	26	Jordan River	24 NOV 1918

Corkum, Maizie, Windsor, Lunenburg Progress Enterprise, 06 November 1918, page 5.

Cormier, Abraham	*76*	*Amherst*	*17 OCT 1918*

Amherst Daily News, 17 October 1918, page 8

Cormier, Mrs. Blair	35	Amherst	04 NOV 1918
Cormier, Bernice	7m	Amherst	24 OCT 1918
Cormier, Blair	35	Amherst	30 OCT 1918
Cormier, Catherine	12	Belle Cote	21 DEC 1918
Cotreau, Emilie	30	Wedgeport	27 NOV 1918
Cotter, Alexander	19	Halifax	22 NOV 1918
Coulter, Charles	52	Halifax	21 DEC 1918
Coulter, Lloyd	18d	Berwick	17 OCT 1918

Cowan, Mrs. Barbara, Saskatchewan, Yarmouth Telegram, 15 November 1918, page 1 (of Yarmouth).

Cox, Mary	*37*	*North Sydney*	*27 NOV 1918*

Sydney Daily Post, 30 November 1918, page 1 (Mrs. Arthur Cox, aged 32, died at Harbour View Hospital, Sydney).

Cox, Mildred	38	Medford	04 May 1919

Craig, James Henry, Dartmouth, aged 22, Halifax Evening Mail, 28 October 1918, page 2.

Craig, Susan,	*32*	*Dartmouth*	*21 OCT 1918*

Halifax Evening Mail, 22 October 1918, page 2 (name given as Ethel Craig).

Crawley, Joseph	09	Halifax	26 OCT 1918
Cress, Fred	40	Round Hill	02 FEB 1919
Crilly, John	21	North Sydney	28 SEPT 1918
Croat, Michael	06	Deepdale	08 FEB 1919
Croft, Cecil	20	Chester Basin	09 OCT 1918
Croft, Clarence	28	Chester Basin	07 OCT 1918
Cropley, Adelia	62	Nictaux	09 NOV 1918

Crosby, Miss Florence, Mass., Yarmouth Telegram, 18 October 1918, page 1 (of Yarmouth).

Crossley, Mary	32	Cheverie	02 NOV 1918
Crouse, Evelyn	08	West Clifford	25 DEC 1918
Crouse, Garland	04	LaHave	24 DEC 1918

Crouse, Mrs. Edmund, Lunenburg County, Halifax Evening Mail, 22 October 1918, page 6.
Crouse, Florrie, Lunenburg Progress Enterprise, 23 October 1918, page 1.

Crowe, Alexander	08	Springhill	02 NOV 1918
Crowe, George	23	Sandy Point	31 JAN 1919
Crowell, Bernard	19	Argyle	03 OCT 1918
Crowell, James	77	Yarmouth	07 Jan/. 1919
Crowell, Rayford	24	Clark's Harbour	09 NOV 1918
Cruise, George	65	Halifax	07 NOV 1918
Cudhea, Charles	02	Springhill	22 DEC 1918
Cummings, Donald	*30*	*Halifax*	*12 DEC 1918*

Halifax Evening Mail, 13 December 1918, page 2 (Donald A. Cummings).

Cummings, George	02	Stellarton	04 MAR 1919
Cummings, Jean W.	1m	New Waterford	29 SEPT 1918
Cummings, Mrs. Leah	30	Stellarton	05 MAR 1919
Cunningham, Alfred	02	Torbrook	06 MAY 1919
Currie, Laura	02	New Glasgow	31 MAR 1919
Curry, Josephine	24	Halifax	10 DEC 1918
Curry, Kenneth	*28*	*Hortonville*	*16 DEC 1918*

Halifax Evening Mail, 3 January 1919, page 11 (age given as 27).

Curry, Walter	42	Stellarton	12 NOV 1918
Curtis, Barbara	19	Sydney	16 OCT 1918
Curry, Gertrude	28	Port Morien	30 AUG 1918
Daley, Terence	41	Halifax	14 NOV 1918

Dakin, Percy B., Boston, aged 42, Digby Courier, 17 January 1919, page 1 (of Digby).

D'Arcy, John	*30*	*Sydney*	*20 OCT 1918*

Halifax Evening Mail, 22 October 1918, page 16 (died at Glace Bay).

Dauphinee, Lillian	21	Halifax	10 OCT 1918
Davidson, Blanche	18m	Stellarton	26 NOV 1918

Davidson, May, Montreal, 30, Amherst Daily News, 13 November 1918, page 3 (of Tidnish).

Davidson, William	28	Halifax	05 NOV 1918

Davies, Rev. Thomas, South Carolina, 41, Amherst Daily News, 4 January 1919, page 3.

Davis, Bernard	2d	Five Islands	05 NOV 1918
Davis, Cecil	02	Five Islands	05 NOV 1918
Davis, Mrs. David	32	Five Islands	05 NOV 1918
Davis, Frank	*36*	*Hantsport*	*20 DEC 1918*

Hants Journal, 25 December 1918 (died at Windsor).

Davis, Lemuel	*26*	*Sydney*	*04 OCT 1918*

Sydney Daily Post, 7 October 1918, page 4 (seaman Davis died at the Marine Hospital).

Davison, Eva	01	Gaspereaux	10 FEB 1919
Day, Alice	29	Halifax	31 DEC 1918
DeAdder, Annie	18	Middleton	22 DEC 1918
Deal, Henry	*61*	*Sentry*	*12 OCT 1918*

Halifax Evening Mail, 22 October 1918, page 6.

Dean, Thelma	11	Stellarton	15 DEC 1918
DeBattista, J.	27	Halifax	26 JAN 1919
DeBay, Ray	6m	DeBay's Cove	26 NOV 1918
DeCoste, Laurence	02	Stellarton	04 DEC 1918
DeGrish, Alonzo	30	North Sydney	20 DEC 1918
DeGuist, Alonzo	30	Halifax	20 DEC 1918
Deigan, Maria	*33*	*Halifax*	*06 JAN 1919*

Halifax Evening Mail, 6 January 1919, page 1 (Marie Irene Deigan).

Demings, Frank	21	Pugwash	06 OCT 1918
Demone, Annie	30	Lunenburg	19 JAN 1919
Demone, Archibald	*38*	*Lunenburg*	*17 OCT 1918*

Halifax Evening Mail, 22 October 1918, page 6.

Denteno, Albertina	29	Sydney	17 OCT 1918
D'Eon, Dorothy	04	Middle West Pubnico	30 OCT 1918

DeRabbie, John, Halifax, Canso News, 25 January 1919, page 1 (of Canso).
DesBrisay, William, Winnipeg, Halifax Evening Mail, 18 NOV 1918, page 3 (of Lunenburg).

Desmond, Beatrice	13	Parrsboro	23 OCT 1918
DesVeaux, Celeste	12	Little River	18 NOV 1918
DesVeaux, Elise	28	Belle Marche	16 NOV 1918
DeVany, Joseph	35	Centerlea	28 FEB 1919
Deveau, Benoit	01	Meteghan	09 JUN 1919
Deveau, Emile	16	Mavilette	26 MAY 1919
Deveau, Jéremé	30	Lake Doucette	28 OCT 1918
Deveau, Marguerite	17	Meteghan Station	06 NOV 1918

Deveau, Marie	96	Meteghan	23 MAR 1919
Devor, Charles	24	Little Bras D'or	19 NOV 1918
Devor, William	63	Little Bras D'or	20 NOV 1918
DeWolfe, Howard	7m	Lower Ship Harbour	25 NOV 1918
DeWolfe, Olive	21	Stellarton	25 NOV 1 18
DeYoung, Edward	*50*	*Halifax*	*28 OCT 1918*

Halifax Evening Mail, 29 October 1918, page 16 (died at the VGH).

DeYoung, Margaret	*44*	*Halifax*	*18 NOV 1918*

Halifax Evening Mail, 19 November 1918, page 1 (died in Willow Park Hospital).

DeYoung, Matilda	18	Eastern Passage	01 JAN 1919
Dickie, James	38	New Glasgow	06 NOV 1918
Dickson, Bryon	38	North Sydney	14 OCT 1918
Dickson, Thomas	10	New Waterford	01 NOV 1918

Dillman, Guy, England, Halifax Evening Mail, 6 December 1918, page 8 (of Dartmouth).

Dillman, Thomas	35	Halifax	28 OCT 1918
Dimenk, George	07	Halifax	05 JAN 1919
Dimock, Elsie	14	Scotch Village	10 APR 1919
Doane, Beulah	33	Cape Forchu	05 JAN 1919

Dodge, J. A., Kingston, aged 71, Middleton Outlook, 10 January 1919, page 3.

Dolan, Mary	27	Antigonish County	16 OCT 1918
Dolliver, Alfred	19	Bridgewater	05 NOV 1918
Doncaster, Cyril	02	Amherst	11 DEC 1918
Dooley, John	53	Westville	20 NOV 1918
Dooley, Marie	03	Halifax	28 NOV 1918
Dorion, Silvester	19	Charlos Cove	16 DEC 1918
Dorman, John	51	Billtown	06 MAY 1919
Dorrington, Joseph	27	Trenton	15 DEC 1918
Dorrington, Lewis	01	Beechville	14 SEPT 1918
Dorrington, Murray	13m	Beechville	11 SEPT 1918
Dotton, Frank	28	Oxford Junction	16 OCT 1918
Doucet, Joseph	07	Little Brook Station	24 MAY 1919
Doucet, Louise	87	Friar's Head	05 MAR 1919
Doucet, Philippa	26	Meteghan	07 NOV 1918
Doucet, Mrs. Simon	46	Belle Cote	22 DEC 1918
Doucet, Volucien	36	Tusket	16 SEPT 1918
Doucette, Abroise	25	Mavillette	25 NOV 1918
Doucette, Joshua	28	Wedgeport	09 NOV 1918
Douchwright, Lewis	30	Brookfield	20 DEC 1918
Douglas, David	*26*	*New Glasgow*	*03 NOV 1918*

Halifax Evening Mail, 05 November 1918, page 8 (of Stellarton, aged 25).

Douglas, Lillian S.	*06*	*Halifax*	*17 NOV 1918*

Halifax Evening Mail, 18 November 1918, page 3 (Lillian Sarah Douglas).

Downey, Alfred	02	Preston	25 OCT 1918
Downey, Lillie	01	Preston	25 OCT 1918

Downey, Paul, Preston, aged 1, Halifax Evening Mail, 26 October 1918, page 4.

Doyle, Florence	35	Arichat	15 FEB 1919
Doyle, John H.	54	Sydney	28 OCT 1918
Doyle, Mary	13m	Arichat	18 FEB 1919
Droesbeck, Alex	*25*	*Chignecto Mines*	*22 OCT 1918*

Amherst Daily News, 29 October 1918, page 4.

Drury, John A., Dartmouth, aged 30, Halifax Evening Mail, 6 November 1918, page 2.

Ducut, Fred [*Doucet*]	32	Halifax	17 OCT 1918
Dugas, Geneve	59	Belliveau's Cove	14 MAR 1919
Dugas, Edmund	24	Meteghan	19 OCT 1918
Duggan, Mary	47	Dingwall	30 DEC 1918
Dunn, Earl	05	Trenton	01 JAN 1919

Dunn, Rita	3w	Upper Clements	18 FEB 1919
Dunning, George	52	Sydney	24 DEC 1918
Dunphy, Vera	28	Amherst	31 OCT 1918
Durant, L.	23	Halifax	30 OCT 1918
Durling, Alonzo	19	Nictaux South	10 JAN 1919
Dwyer, Audrie	7m	Thorburn	26 DEC 1918
Dyer, Julia	10m	Stellarton	24 FEB 1919
Eager, Nellie	27	Wolfville	14 DEC 1918
Eagles, Miss Nellie	*27*	*Kentville*	*14 DEC 1918*

Berwick Register, 18 December 1918, page 3

Eastman, Eliza	34	North Sydney	27 OCT 1918

Eaton, George, Seattle, 30, Annapolis Spectator, 2 January 1919, page 1 (of Granville Ferry).
Eddy, Joseph, Sydney, Sydney Daily Post, 17 October 1918, page 1 (died at the Marine Hosp.).
Edgerly, Leda May, Mass., aged 21, Liverpool Advance, 26 February 1919, page 3 (of Liverpool).
Edwards, Alexander, Halifax, Truro Daily News, 23 December 1918, page 6.

Edwards, John	46	Sydney	28 DEC 1918
Ehman, Annie	*16*	*Halifax*	*31 DEC 1918*

Halifax Evening Mail, 10 January 1919, page 1 (Annie Ehmann, aged 17).

Timothe, Evangeline	53	Saulnierville	14 NOV 1918
Eisnor, Freeman	34	Lakeville	12 APR 1919

Elliott, Letitia, Dartmouth, aged 60, Halifax Evening Mail, 17 February 1919, page 2.
Elliott, Percy, Meadowville, aged 17, Pictou Advocate, 20 December 1918, page 8.

Ellis, Alonzo	31	Shubenacadie	07 JAN 1919
Ellis, George	09	PortMaitland	02 DEC 1918

Ells, Harley Edward, Port Greville, aged 3, Amherst Daily News, 21 November 1918, page 3.

Ellis, Jennie	58	Halifax	08 NOV 1918
Ells, Alfred	50	Canning	10 NOV 1918
Ells, Norman	*30*	*Amherst*	*24 NOV 1918*

Amherst Daily News, 25 November 1918, page 3.

Elms, Norman	18	New Glasgow	03 DEC 1918
Embree, Ida	34	Port Hawkesbury	05 OCT 1918
Embrie, Alberta	11	Oxford	29 NOV 1918
Emery, Charlotte	92	Bridgetown	14 NOV 1918
Emery, John	64	Westville	29 DEC 1918
Enslow, Mitchell	19	West Green Harbour	12 JAN 1919
Esau, Hilda	14	Londonderry	01 DEC 1918
Etter, Eleanor	33	Halifax	29 NOV 1918

Etter, Mrs. William G., River Philip, Amherst Daily News, 1 November 1918, page 3; Oxford Journal, 14 November 1918, page 1 (her maiden name was Baxter).
Evans, Florence, Halifax, Halifax Evening Mail, 30 October 1918, page 16.
Everett, Rev. H. Percy, Springhill, aged 30, Amherst Daily News, 28 October 1918, page 8.

Everill, Ada	16m	Chignecto	28 OCT 1918

Eville, Vivien Ariel, Boston, aged 19, Amherst Daily News, 4 October 1918, page 3 (of Halifax).

Fairn, Bessie	*39*	*Aylesford*	*17 DEC 1918*

Annapolis Spectator, 26 December 1918, page 1 (Mrs. Leslie R. Fairn).

Falt, Charles	20	Petite Riviere	09 NOV 1918
Fanning, Harold	01	Port Howe	16 JAN 1919
Fanning, Mrs. S.	*22*	*Canso*	*03 DEC 1918*

Canso News, 28 December 1918, page 2 (Mrs. Sylvester Fanning).

Farish, Capt. George	*37*	*Halifax*	*28 OCT 1918*

Liverpool Advance, 30 October 1918, page 2 (Captain George Cox Farish).

Farmer, Herbert	08	Liverpool	09 NOV 1918
Farmer, Winnie	06	Liverpool	07 NOV 1918
Farnam, D.	21	Halifax	29 JAN 1919
Farnell, Daniel	13	Sheet Harbour Road	16 NOV 1918

Farrell, Edward 09 North Sydney 01 JAN 1919
Farrington, Annie L., Lockeport, aged 16, Liverpool Advance, 23 October 1918, page 2.
Faulds, Sarah 42 Stellarton 16 NOV 1918
Feener, Carl 24 Italy Cross 05 NOV 1918
Feener, Matilda 65 Liverpool 31 OCT 1918
  Liverpool Advance, 6 November 1918, page 2 (Mrs. Matilda Feener).
Feetham, Ella 42 Halifax 14 NOV 1918
Fell, James 24 Lawlor's Island 06 OCT 1918
Feltmate, *Infant* 01 Eight Island Lake 21 DEC 1918
Ferguson, Malcolm 50 Sydney Mines 10 OCT 1918
Fewer, Francis 7m Halifax 09 NOV 1918
Finlayson, John 29 New Waterford 29 SEPT 1918
Finn, David 19 Sydney 23 OCT 1918
Fitch, Garfield 1m Conquerell Mills 11 MAR 1919
Fitzgerald, William T. 3 Halifax 11 OCT 1918
  Halifax Evening Mail, 12 October 1918, page 10.
Flannigan, Lizzie 35 Halifax 07 JAN 1919
  Halifax Evening Mail, 8 January 1919, page 1 (died at Influenza Hospital).
Flemming, Catherine 01 Hantsport 24 DEC 1918
Flemming, Georgina, Boston, Evening Mail; 12 October 1918, page 16 (nurse from Folly Mtn).
Flemming, Winnifred, Boston, Evening Mail; 12 October 1918, page 16 (nurse from Folly Mtn).
Fletcher, Ronald 7m Sydney 14 OCT 1918
Flick, Lottie J. 27 Halifax 28 OCT 1918
  Halifax Evening Mail, 28 October 1918, page 1.
Flinn, Luke G. 37 Halifax 15 NOV 1918
  Halifax Evening Mail, 19 November 1918, page 1.
Fogarty, Martin 17 Halifax 25 DEC 1918
  Canso News, 25 January 1919, page 1 (of Canso).
Fong, Sam 33 Halifax 17 NOV 1918
Foote, Edgar 19 Barney's River 27 NOV 1918
  Eastern Chronicle, 06 December 1918, page 1, (described as Robert Foote).
Forbes, Jean 02 Halifax 16 DEC 1918
Forbes, Lena 20 Louisbourg 02 DEC 1918
Ford, John 33 Meteghan 20 OCT 1918
Forsyth, Gordon 14m Halifax 10 NOV 1918
Fortier, Jules --- Lawlor's Island 27 SEPT 1918
Fougere, Francis 6m Poulamond 06 APR 1919
Fowler, Edith 06 Weymouth 08 DEC 1918
Fox, Harry 32 Yarmouth 09 JAN 1919
Fox, Leslie, Regina, 34, Yarmouth Herald, 21 January 1919, page 5 (of Yarmouth Co.).
Fox, Marjorie 13 Halifax 06 NOV 1918
Foyle, Dora 25 Halifax 05 DEC 1918
  Halifax Evening Mail, 7 December 1918, page 15.
Francis, Joseph 01 Milton 06 NOV 1918
Francis, Joseph 01 Halifax 24 DEC 1918
Frankland, John 42 Sydney 20 OCT 1918
Franklyn, Irene 6m Dayspring 24 OCT 1918
Fraser, Beatrice, Shawinigan Falls, Amherst Daily News, 24 October 1918, page 4 (of Truro).
Fraser, Bulah 10 Glen Margaret 08 DEC 1918
Fraser, Catherine, Saskatchewan, 22, Eastern Chronicle, 8 November 1918, page 4
Fraser, Mrs. David 35 New Glasgow 19 DEC 1918
Fraser, Edward H., Vancouver, 29, Eastern Chronicle, 17 December 1918, page 1 (of Eureka).
Fraser, George 20 Halifax 17 OCT 1918
Fraser, Hugh I., Toronto, aged 21, Pictou Advocate, 10 January 1919, page 8 (of Mabou).
Fraser, J. Austin, Seattle, 32, Hants Journal, 15 January 1919, page 1 (of Elmsdale). Truro Daily News,
  January 1919, page 3 (former member of the Yukon Legislature).

Fraser, Janet	42	Glen Margaret	01 DEC 1918
Fraser, John	8m	Halifax	21 OCT 1918
Fraser, Louis	43	Glen Margaret	30 NOV 1918
Fraser, Mrs. Marcella	38	Stellarton	23 JAN 1919
Fraser, Mary	*21*	*New Waterford*	*23 SEPT 1918*

Sydney Daily Post, 27 September 1918, page 5 (described as Miss Mary Fraser).

| *Fraser, Noel* | *27* | *Amherst* | *31 OCT 1918* |

Amherst Daily News, 30 October 1918, page 8.

| Frausel, James | 26 | Dayspring Poor Farm | 04 MAR 1919 |

Frauten, Rosie, Yarmouth, aged 17, Yarmouth Telegram, 20 December 1918, page 1.

| Frederick, Francis | 29 | French Village | 25 NOV 1918 |

Freeman, Mrs. Eliza, East Berlin, aged 25, Liverpool Advance, 2 October 1918, page 2.

Frellick, William	24	Western Head	01 NOV 1918
Frost, Raymond	20	Sydney	15 OCT 1918
Frotten, Mary	17	Argyle	19 DEC 1918
Fudge, Mary	88	Windsor	01 MAR 1919
Fulton, Elsie Ray	*14*	*Lakelands*	*01 NOV 1918*

Amherst Daily News, 15 November 1918, page 4.

Gaddon, Martin	12	Georges River	14 NOV 1918
Gaetz, Alvin	24	Head Chezzetcook	03 NOV 1918
Gaetz, Irvine	03	Grafton	05 DEC 1918
Gaetz, Rita	16	Seaforth	28 OCT 1918
Gallant, Margaret	7m	Belle Cote	13 FEB 1919
Garber, Martha	*34*	*Bridgewater*	*26 OCT 1918*

Lunenburg Progress Enterprise, 30 October 1918, page 5 (Mrs. Frank Garber).

Garcia, Jose	05	Glace Bay	17 DEC 1918
Gardiner, Elizabeth	22	Amherst	21 DEC 1918
Gardiner, Priscilla	38	North Sydney	24 OCT 1918
Gardner, Elizabeth	22	Amherst	21 DEC 1918
Gardner, Evelyn	09	Brooklyn	23 APR 1919
Gardner, Olethia [?]	02	Brooklyn	27 APR 1919
Garlock, Arthur H.	18	Sydney	28 SEPT 1918

Garrison, William, Indian Harbour, Halifax Evening Mail, 23 NOV 1918, page 6.

Gates, Evelyn	02	Upper Blandford	12 NOV 1918
Gates, Henry	59	Upper Blandford	28 NOV 1918
Gates, John	31	Glace Bay	01 DEC 1918

Gates, Rita E., Dartmouth, 16, Halifax Evening Mail, 29 October 1918, page 2.
Gaudet, Elisé, 23, St. Bernard, 31 OCT 1918; Digby Courier, 8 November 1918, page 2 (of Belliveau's Cove).
Gaudet, Fred, 21, St. Bernard, 03 NOV 1918; Digby Courier, 8 November 1918, page 2 (of Belliveau's Cove).

Gaudet, Rose	08	Saulnierville Station	01 NOV 1918
Gaudet, Rosie	43	Concession	31 OCT 1918
Gaum, Vincent	78	Blomidon	07 APR 1919
Gavel, Nina	6w	Saulnierville	29 OCT 1918
Gibson, Annie	24	Halifax	23 NOV 1918

Gideon, James, Calgary, aged 45, Liverpool Advance, 25 DEC 1918, p. 2 (of Liverpool).

Gidney, Myrtle	27	Mink Cove	23 NOV 1918
Gidney, Seymour	02	Sandy Cove	03 MAY 1919
Gielist, J.	40	Sydney	18 OCT 1918

Giffin, John V., Vancouver, aged 47, Liverpool Advance, 12 FEB 1919, p.4 (of Osborne).

Gilbert, Elizabeth	25	Sydney Mines	27 NOV 1918
Gilday, Clement	03	Glace Bay	22 DEC 1918
Gilday, Elizabeth	04	Glace Bay	20 DEC 1918
Gillingham, Bessie	19	New Waterford	03 DEC 1918
Gillis, Alex.	02	Glace Bay	04 DEC 1918
Gillis, Angus	47	New Waterford	06 DEC 1918
Gillis, Dougald	17	Upper Margaree	30 OCT 1918

Gillis, John	15	Upper Margaree	19 JAN 1919
Gillis, Michael	31	Florence	12 DEC 1918
Gillis, Minnie	19	Upper Margaree	17 JAN 1919
Gillis, Sarah	01	Reserve Mines	24 DEC 1918
Gilmet, Jessie	26	Glace Bay	10 DEC 1918

Glendenning, Amos J., Alberta, Amherst Daily News, 15 January 1919, page 4 (of Amherst).

Glode, Catherine	17m	Indian Reserve	16 OCT 1918
Glode, Sarah	05	Indian Reserve	16 OCT 1918
Gong, Ang	50	Halifax	02 NOV 1918
Good, Lillian	35	Sydney	22 DEC 1918

Goodick, Pearl, Lockeport, aged 17, Liverpool Advance, 23 October 1918, page 2.

Gooding, Albert	26	Sydney Mines	21 OCT 1918
Googoo, Annie	35	Georges River	27 OCT 1918
Googoo, Charles	30	Upper North Sydney	09 NOV 1918
Gordon, Harry	18	North Sydney	05 OCT 1918
Gordon, Henry	23	Halifax	24 JAN 1919
Gordon, Sarah	28	Oxford Junction	15 DEC 1918

Gorman, Mrs., Halifax, Halifax Evening Mail, 15 November 1918, page 1.

Gould, W. Bradley	*33*	*Nappan*	*11 JAN 1919*

    Amherst Daily News, 11 January 1919, page 5.

Goulden, Francis	01	Sandy Point	17 OCT 1918

Gouldworthy, Mary, Halifax, 30, Halifax Evening Mail, 11 December 1918, page 3 (Mrs. John).

Gouthro, Charles	39	Tracadie	05 DEC 1918
Gower, Victor	10w	Upper Ohio	10 JAN 1919
Goyetch, Irene	30	Arichat	03 JAN 1919
Grady, Victor	*21*	*Halifax*	*14 OCT 1918*

    Halifax Evening Mail, 15 October 1918, page 14.

Graham, Isabella	76	Halifax	23 FEB 1919
Graham, Joseph	*36*	*Dartmouth*	*24 OCT 1918*

    Halifax Evening Mail, 24 October 1918, page 2 (of Maynard Street in Halifax)

Graham, Louisa	31	Halifax	08 NOV 1918

Graham, Walter K., Vancouver, Truro Daily News, December 1918, page 3 (of Brookfield).

Grannon, Nora	33	Yarmouth	27 NOV 1918
Grant, Ernest	*22*	*Sunny Brae*	*22 OCT 1918*

    Eastern Chronicle, 25 October 1918, page 1 (died at Bridgeville of [sic] Abercrombie Road).

Grant, James	05	Preston	10 MAR 1919

Grant, Mrs. Leonard, Fox River, Amherst Daily News, 27 December 1918, page 3.

Graves, Abner	20	Nicholsville	22 JAN 1919
Gray, Arthur	01	Halifax	02 JAN 1919
Gray, Bessie	24	Westville	29 MAR 1919
Gray, Mrs. Florence	36	Newport Station	OCT 1918
Gray, Mary	29	Halifax	16 OCT 1918
Gray, Mary	67	Sambro	13 DEC 1918
Gray, Nellie A.	*28*	*Kentville*	*28 OCT 1918*

    Amherst Daily News, 29 October 1918, page 1 (died at Brockton, Mass.).

Greaves, Margaret	52	Sydney	18 OCT 1918
Green, Emma	19	North Sydney	19 OCT 1918
Greening, Annie	42	Melville Island	28 OCT 1918
Greenwood, William	39	Halifax	12 NOV 1918
Gregorie, Archibald	*26*	*Dartmouth*	*14 OCT 1918*

    Halifax Evening Mail, 15 October 1918, page 2.

Gregory, Catherine	27	Halifax	11 MAR 1919
Grono, Harold	21	Glen Haven	16 APR 1919

Grudbert, Joseph, North Sydney, Sydney Daily Post, 30 November 1918, page 1.

Guptell, Martha	14	Wallbrook	23 OCT1918

Gurts, John	36	Sydney	15 OCT 1918

Hagell, Miss Eleanor, Halifax, Sydney Daily Post, 16 December 1918, page 5 (of Sydney).

Haggart, Margaret	10m	Marshy Hope	25 NOV 1918
Hainey, Annie	33	Weymouth	17 NOV 1918
Hall, James	*55*	*River Hebert*	*10 OCT 1918*

Halifax Evening Mail, 21 October 1918, page 12.

Hall, Mrs. Ruth, Massachusetts, 25, Digby Courier, 24 JAN 1919, p. 5 (daughter of John Kee).

Hall, William	38	Sydney	24 DEC 1918
Ham, Eldred	30	Dartmouth	15 FEB 1919
Hamilton, Jessie	31	Wilmot	30 APR 1919
Hamm, Charles	17	Lequille	18 OCT 1918
Handspiker, Alice	*52*	*Mount Pleasant*	*02 JAN 1919*

Digby Courier, 3 January 1919, page 5.

Handspiker, Villa	7m	Digby	22 DEC 1918
Hanlon, Augustine	*39*	*Canso*	*28 NOV 1918*

Canso News, 28 December 1918, page 2 (Augustus in newspaper).

Hann, Helen G. 9m, Halifax, Halifax Evening Mail, 25 October 1918, page 1 (Helen Gertrude Hann).

Hanna, Victor	21	Halifax	17 JAN 1919
Hannam, Etta	24	Middleton	19 OCT 1918
Hannan, Elizabeth	04	New Waterford	06 DEC 1918
Hannigan, Ellen	32	New Waterford	19 DEC 1918
Hannon, Michael	31	Halifax	22 OCT 1918
Hanrahan, Kathleen	7m	Halifax	29 OCT 1918
Harding, Alexander	14	Descousse	09 FEB 1919
Harding, William	26	Halifax	21 OCT 1918
Hardstaff, Lillian	01	Halifax	27 OCT 1918

Harkins, Liliah, Philadelphia, 25, Truro Daily News, 3 February 1919, page 1 (of Nova Scotia).

Harloff, Hannah	04	North Sydney	06 SEPT 1918
Harlow, Ida	*47*	*Sable River*	*01 NOV 1918*

Liverpool Advance, 06 November 1918, page 2 (Mrs. Lewis Harlow, aged 49).

Harms, Heinrich	45	Amherst	14 JAN 1919
Harnish, Albert	*31*	*Hubbards*	*10 FEB 1919*

Halifax Evening Mail, 11 February 1919, page 3 (Albert L. Harnish, aged 32).

Harnish, Harold Clifford, France, Annapolis Spectator, 2 January 1919, page 1 (of Lequille).

Harnish, Margaret	35	East Dover	07 JAN 1919

Harper, Miss Hazel K., New Hampshire, Oxford Journal, 14 November 1918, page 1 (of Oxford).

Harrison, Freeda	35	Fenwick Mines	27 NOV 1918
Hart, Alice	10	Sambro	13 DEC 1918
Hart, Gladys	18	Sambro	09 DEC 1918

Hart, Ivan, Sydney, Sydney Daily Post, 30 September 1918, page 1.

Hartley, John	89	Middleton	13 JAN 1919
Hartling, Edward	21	Quoddy	28 NOV 1918
Hartling, Gladys	29	Jeddore	02 NOV 1918
Hauser, Daniel	54	Halifax	28 NOV 1918
Havelock, Mary	49	Springhill	13 NOV 1918

Hawes, Lucy, Halifax, aged 23, Evening Mail, 10 October 1918, page 1.

Hawley, Charles	86	Ingonish	23 OCT 1918
Hayes, Mary	19	Glace Bay	31 OCT 1918
Hays, Daisy	31	Halifax	05 DEC 1918
Hayward, Mary	40	Woodside	10 NOV 1918
Healey, Thomas	14m	Halifax	17 NOV 1918
Hebb, Maurice	29	Bridgewater	23 FEB 1919
Heckman, Annie	14	Central Woods Hbr	14 JULY 1918
Heighton, Francis	04	Pictou	09 DEC 1918
Hemeon, Bernard	*39*	*West Berlin*	*19 SEPT 1918*

Liverpool Advance, 2 October 1918, page 2 (died at Gloucester, Massachusetts).

Hemeon, Lois	48	West Berlin	15 NOV 1918
Hemming, Mary	25	Halifax	02 NOV 1918
Henderson, Ethel	20	Avonport	07 MAY 1919
Henderson, Harry	*28*	*Chignecto Mines*	*18 OCT 1918*

Amherst Daily News, 19 October 1918, page 4.

Henderson, James	48	Avonport	18 MAY 1919
Henderson, John	33	Sydney Mines	30 MAR 1919

Henderson, Mrs. John W., Mass., 28, Westville Free Lance, 8 November 1918, page 6 (she was Josie Gammon of West Branch, Pictou County).

Henderson, Nellie	27	Sydney Mines	13 MAR 1919
Hennessey, Ambrose	26	Halifax	19 OCT 1918
Henry, Emma	34	Beechville	02 NOV 1918
Henry, Zechariah	39	Beechville	28 OCT 1918
Henwood, Blanch	15	Black Rock	26 OCT 1918
Henwood, Lilla	13	Black Rock	20 OCT 1918
Heptidge, Bella	18	Halifax	31 DEC 1918
Herald, Willis	48	Sydney Mines	25 MAR 1919
Herget, Frances	07	Forties Settlement	30 OCT 1918
Hersey, Fred	18	Culloden	14 DEC 1918
Hervey, Fred	27	Victory	19 NOV 1918

Hewitt, Mrs. Sheldon, 31, Mass., Truro Daily News, 18 January 1919, page 7 (of New Annan).

Hicks, Harry	56	Bridgetown	23 MAR 1919
Higby, Mabel	28	Yarmouth	04 JAN 1919

Higgins, Estella Mabel, Belmont, aged 26, Truro Daily News, 7 January 1919, page 6.

Hilchey, Elsie	19	Halifax	22 OCT 1918
Hill, Dora	14	Bear River	20 FEB 1919
Hill, Gladys	8m	Beechville	25 OCT 1918
Hill. Mrs. John	25	Upper Economy	30 DEC 1918
Hill, Rose	13m	Louisdale	08 OCT 1918
Hill, Wanda	7m	Cove Road	31 DEC 1918
Hillborn, Pte.William	*19*	*Halifax*	*14 OCT 1918*

Halifax Evening Mail, 15 October 1918, page 14.

Hiller, Frank	50	North Sydney	02 NOV 1918
Hiltz, Ellica	36	Fraxville	02 MAR 1919
Hiltz, Frances	34	Forties Settlement	30 OCT 1918
Hiltz, James	49	Forties Settlement	24 OCT 1918
Hiltz, Maggie	14	Forties Settlement	29 OCT 1918
Himmelman, Georgina	32	LaHave Islands	05 JAN 1919
Himmelman, Pearl	18	Bridgewater	02 NOV 1918

Himmelman, Mrs. Pearl, Halifax, aged 18, Halifax Evening Mail, 21 NOV 1918, p. 1.

Himmelman, Rosa	*45*	*Lunenburg*	*27 OCT 1918*

Halifax Evening Mail, 01 November 1918, page 6, (described as Rosabelle).

Hirtle, Carrie	32	Dayspring	27 OCT 1918
Hodges, Maria	26	Georges River	20 NOV 1918
Hodgson, Lester	22	Goldboro	23 DEC 1918
Hoeg, Florence	49	River Hebert	10 NOV 1918

Hoffman, Maurice, Regina, Amherst Daily News, 18 January 1919, page 3 (of Amherst).

Hogan, Edmund	57	Weymouth	07 NOV 1918

Holder, Miss Harriet, Lunenburg, Halifax Evening Mail, 01 November 1918, page 9.

Holder, Harry	*32*	*Halifax*	*20 MAR 1919*

Halifax Evening Mail, 21 March 1919, page 16 (Henry L. Holder, aged 33).

Holland, Etta	26	Greenfield	02 JAN 1919
Holm, Charles	55	Sydney Mines	30 OCT 1918
Holmdees, Frank	29	Sydney Mines	20 JAN 1919
Holmes, Thomas	27	Halifax	23 JAN 1919
Hood, George	28	Stellarton	15 NOV 1918

Hooper, Florence	27	Sandy Cove	05 MAY 1919
Horobin, Edith	20	Dartmouth	12 JAN 1919
Hotchkiss, Ethel	19	Halifax	02 DEC 1918
Howard, George	31	Sydney	23 OCT 1918
Hubley, Daisy	09	French Village	16 FEB 1919
Hubley, Thomas	39	Halifax	07 DEC 1918
Hudson, *Infant*	5m	Hansford	27 NOV 1918
Hughes, Graham	17	Fox River	18 NOV 1918
Hughes, Mabel	*44*	*Fox River*	*16 NOV 1918*

Amherst Daily News, 21 November 1918, page 3 (Mrs. Robert Hughes).

Hughes, William	13	Westville	26 OCT 1918
Hume, Irene	*34*	*East Chester*	*20 FEB 1919*

Hants Journal, 12 March 1919, page 6 (Mrs.Edgar Hume, Irene Henrietta Dauphinee).

Humphrey, James	27	Halifax	04 OCT 1918
Hunter, Miss Edna	*23*	*Parrsboro*	*27 NOV 1918*

Amherst Daily News, 29 November 1918, page 3.

Hunter, Janet	29	Sydney Mines	08 FEB 1919
Huntley, Owen	38	Medford	31 DEC 1918
Hureau, John	19	[*resided*] Arichat	26 DEC 1918
Hurley, Mary	*26*	*Argyle Head*	*08 FEB 1919*

Yarmouth Herald, 11 February 1919, page 2, (wife of George A. F. Hurley).

Hurley, Michael	35	New Glasgow	19 NOV 1918
Hurst, Miss Emma	*28*	*Canso*	*18 NOV 1918*

Canso News, 30 November 1918, page 1.

Huskins, Victor	*18*	*West Green Harbour*	*28 OCT 1918*

Liverpool Advance, 30 October 1918, page 2, (age given as 17).

Hutchins, Vivian	03	North Sydney	02 DEC 1918

Hyson, Walter, Nfld, Evening Mail, 11 October 1918, page 14 (of Indian Point).

Illsley, Amelia	66	Halls Harbour	02 APR 1919

Irving, Lillian, Salt Lake City, 19, Eastern Chronicle, 4 February 1919, page 1 (of New Glasgow).

Isenor, Elias	2m	Lantz Siding	14 JAN 1919
Isenor, William	20	Lantz Siding	12 JAN 1919
Jacklin, George	16	Shelburne	31 OCT 1918
Jackson, Charles	17m	Dartmouth	27 FEB 1919
Jackson, Lena	23	Halifax	12 DEC 1918
Jackson, Mable	28	Lunenburg	07 NOV 1918
Jackson, Robert	28	Halifax	21 MAR 1919
Jacquard, Olive	72	Wedgeport	07 NOV 1918

Jaeger, Mrs. Emil, Minneapolis, 66, Hants Journal, 29 January 1918, page 8 (of Canaan).

Jarvis, Blanche	05	Weymouth Falls	25 OCT 1918
Jefferson, Jane	52	New Germany	01 NOV 1918
Jefferson, Mary M.	*28*	*Lawrencetown*	*30 OCT 1918*

Halifax Evening Mail, 08 November 1918, page 7 (Mrs. J. B. Jefferson).

Jenkins, Adelbert	38	Hebron	28 DEC 1918
Jennings, Douglas	3m	French Village	21 NOV 1918
Jewkes, May	40	Springhill	04 NOV 1918

Jobb, Weldon, Westchester, aged 16, Amherst Daily News, 28 October 1918, page 3; Oxford Journal, 7 November 1918, page 3 (age given as 17).

Jobe, Robert	18	Westchester Station	04 OCT 1918
Johnson, Annie	24	Stellarton	13 NOV 1918
Johnson, Annie	52	Pictou	22 DEC 1918

Johnson, Mrs. Avery, Springhill, Amherst Daily News, 14 February 1919, page 5.

Johnson, Ester	18	Ingramport	23 NOV 1918

Johnson, Gladys, Kemptown, aged 18, Truro Daily News, 13 January 1919, page 4.

Johnson, Hazel	18	Kemptown	11 JAN 1919
Johnson, Pauline	17	Halifax	31 DEC 1918

Johnson, Sophia	34	Springhill	02 FEB 1919

Johnson, William J., England, Truro Daily News, 26 February 1919, page 5 (of Glenholme).

Johnston, Alice	50	Barra Head	10 OCT 1918

Johnston, Evelyn, Alberta, 26, Westville Free Lance, 22 November 1918, page 3 (Barney's River).

Johnston, Jonathan L., England, Liverpool Advance, 13 November 1918, page 2 (Lockeport).

Johnston, Mary	15	Glen Margaret	05 DEC 1918
Johnston, Ronald	35	Sydney	08 NOV 1918
Johnstone, Mary	33	Sydney	16 OCT 1918
Johnstone, Mary	7m	Sydney	17 OCT 1918

Johnstone, Mrs. Wm, Mass., 48, Pictou Advocate, 14 February 1918, page 8 (of River John).

Jollymore, Ruth	12	Mill Cove	22 FEB 1919
Jones, Mrs. Gussie	27	West Cook's Cove	15 DEC 1918
Jordan, William	25	Eight Island Lake	04 DEC 1918
Julien, Mary	21	Middle Porter's Lake	31 OCT 1918
Julien, Theila	16	Halifax	06 DEC 1918

Kane, Susan, Preston, aged 23, Halifax Evening Mail, 4 November 1918, page 2.

Katcher, Eva	27	East River	29 OCT 1918
Keddie, Leveret	37	Middleton	28 JAN 1919
Keepens, Mary	38	Little Bras d'Or	16 OCT 1918
Kelly, Edith	19	Hortonville	16 DEC 1918
Kelly, Ethel	*23*	*Bridgetown*	*15 OCT 1918*

Bridgetown Monitor, 16 October 1918, page 4.

Kelly, Ignatius	01	Lingan	26 OCT 1918
Kelly, Lillie	03	Wentworth	29 OCT 1918
Kelly, Ralph	02	Wentworth	30 OCT 1918
Kelly, Sadie	8m	Wentworth	28 OCT 1918
Kennedy, Firman	16	Halifax	09 DEC 1918
Kennedy, John	30	Inverness	13 SEPT 1918

Kennedy, Lily May, Halifax, 9 months, Halifax Evening Mail, 19 November 1918, page 1.

Kennedy, Murdo	37	Inverness	03 SEPT 1918
Kent, Dora	14m	Amherst	22 OCT 1918
Kerninerzott, Zaccho	34	Glace Bay	21 DEC 1918
Kilcup, Eugene	8m	Aldershot	10 MAY 1919
King, William	18	Pugwash	29 OCT 1918
Kinney, Florence	28	Yarmouth	15 DEC 1918
Kippin, Emma	32	Sydney	25 NOV 1918

Kirby, Miss. Hazel, Chapman Settlement, 17, Amherst Daily News, 20 November 1918, page 3.

Knickle, Elizabeth	3w	Lunenburg	17 FEB 1919
Knickle, Mrs. Mary	96	Blue Rocks	13 NOV 1918

Knickle, Mrs. Pearl, Lunenburg, Lunenburg Progress Enterprise, 30 October 1918, page 1.

Knowlton, Elizabeth	*37*	*Halifax*	*13 DEC 1918*

Halifax Evening Mail, 14 December 1918, page 23 (Mrs. Lorway Knowlton).

Koritern, Mary	45	Yarmouth	27 OCT 1918
Kraft, Ida	52	Halifax	20 DEC 1918
Kraft, Ida	52	Louis Head	28 DEC 1918
Laba, Charles	01	Halifax	14 FEB 1919
LaBelle, Hercules	27	Halifax	03 NOV 1918

LaFleur [?], Alex., Sydney, 21, Sydney Daily Post, 01 November 1918, page 7 (Emergency Hosp.).

Lahey, Charles	22	Main-a-Dieu	16 MAR 1919
Lahey, George	8m	Main-a-Dieu	29 OCT 1918
Laidlaw, Edith	17	Halifax	06 DEC 1918
Lairsey, John	02	Sydney	19 OCT 1918
Lake, Beulah	24	Kempt Shore	07 NOV 1918
Lake, Eva	*34*	*Walton*	*26 MAR 1919*

Halifax Evening Mail, 31 March, page 3 (Mrs. Howard Lake).

Lake, Lt. G.	38	Sydney	25 OCT 1918

Lake, Gerald	4m	Walton	08 APR 1919
Lake, Howard	*34*	*Walton*	*27 MAR 1919*
Halifax Evening Mail, 31 March 1919, page 3.			
Lake, Juaneta	1m	Cheverie	15 NOV 1918
Lake, Stella	08	Summerville	21 May 1919
Lake, Viola	06	Summerville	22 May 1919
Lamb, Cecil F., Mass., aged 19, Amherst Daily News, 04 October 1918, page 3 (of Parrsboro).			
Landry, Alfred	27	Tracadie	17 FEB 1919
Landry, Allen J.	*29*	*Halifax*	*20 NOV 1918*
Amherst Daily News, 22 November 1918, page 3 (age given as 27).			
Landry, Joseph	2m	Petit de Grat	03 JAN 1919
Landry, Minnie	30	Petit de Grat	25 OCT 1918
Landry, Philomène	*20*	*Amherst*	*20 NOV 1918*
Amherst Daily News, 21 November 1918, page 3 (described as "Miss").			
Landry, Theresa	05	Poulomond	07 NOV 1918
Lane, Gertrude	35	Truro	17 DEC 1918
Langford, Donald	17	Danvers	16 OCT 1918
Langford, Donald	16	Danvers	17 OCT 1918
Langill, Mrs. Burton	21	Trenton	02 DEC 1918
Langill, Joshua	55	Tancook	13 MAR 1919
Langille, Anthony	58	Centreville	15 OCT 1918
Langille, Christine	24	Westville	25 NOV 1918
Langille, George	4m	Blue Rocks	11 NOV 1918
Langille, Mary	*45*	*Lunenburg*	*30 NOV 1918*
Lunenburg Progress Enterprise, 04 December 1918, page 1 (Mrs. Whidden Langille).			
Lanigan, Ellen	64	Halifax	20 JAN 1919
Lannigan, Elizabeth	*24*	*Halifax*	*27 OCT 1918*
Liverpool Advance, 06 November 1918, page 2 (died in Infectious Diseases Hosp.).			
Lansburg, Laurie	*30*	*Kemptown*	*16 JAN 1919*
Truro Daily News, 18 January 1919, page 7 (identified as Laurie Landsburg).			
Lapierre, Flora	16	Grand Desert	23 MAR 1919
Lapierre, Judith	45	Grand Desert	23 MAR 1919
Larson, Gustave	28	Halifax	04 DEC 1918
Lawrence, Amos J., Alberta, 32, Truro Daily News, 10 February 1919, page 1 (of Southampton).			
Lawlor, Bridget	69	Ogden	11 MAR 1919
Lawson, Edwin	54	St. Mary's [River]	29 OCT 1918
Lawson, William	38	Halifax	11 DEC 1918
Leach, Sidney C.	*37*	*Halifax*	*22 OCT 1918*
Halifax Evening Mail, 22 October 1918, page 1 (Sidney Charles Leach).			
Leahy, Mrs. Margaret	*38*	*Halifax*	*06 DEC 1918*
Halifax Evening Mail, 7 December 1918, page 15 (Mrs. William Leahy).			
Lean, Alfred	50	Florence	19 NOV 1918
LeBlanc, Alexander	06	Inverness	12 SEPT 1918
LeBlanc, Amelia	38	Belle Cote	17 DEC 1918
LeBlanc, Caroline	74	Belle Cote	25 DEC 1918
LeBlanc, Elise	40	Meteghan River	13 NOV 1918
LeBlanc, Eloise	31	Amherst	12 DEC 1918
LeBlanc, Germain	03	Belle Cote	19 DEC 1918
LeBlanc, Jeremie	39	Abrams River	11 NOV 1918
LeBlanc, Lloyd	12	Wedgeport	04 NOV 1918
LeBlanc, Louise	28	Eastern Harbou	28 JUL 1919
LeBlanc, Margaret	17	Belle Cote	16 DEC 1918
LeBlanc, Mrs. Patrick	31	East Margaree	26 DEC 1918
LeBlanc, Paul	45	Westville	16 NOV 1918
LeBlanc, Placide	80	Belle Cote	17 DEC 1918
LeBlanc, Simon	4m	Little Bras D'or	28 OCT 1918

Name	Age	Place	Date
LeBlanc, Mrs.Thomas	45	Margaree Harbour	13 DEC 1918
LeBlanc, Wilfred	03	Margaree Harbour	14 DEC 1918
LeBlanc, Zelda	34	River Hebert	14 OCT 1918
LeBlanch, Mertie	*34*	*Halifax*	*14 OCT 1918*

Halifax Evening Mail, 15 October 1918, page 14.

Name	Age	Place	Date
LeFlenn, Alexander	21	Sydney	29 OCT 1918
Leforte, Charles	3m	Inverness	14 SEPT 1918
Leforte, Hattie	23	Inverness	02 SEPT 1918
Legere, Malinda	36	Joggins Mines	30 MAR 1919
Legere, Peter	01	Springhill	03 NOV 1918
LeGoff, Mary	2m	Alder Point	21 NOV 1918
Lemieux, William	20	Halifax	01 NOV 1918
LeMoine, John C.	28	North Sydney	14 NOV 1918
Leprayley, Selina	8m	Shelburne	18 MAR 1919
Leslie, Helen	17	Upper Musquodoboit	26 OCT 1918
Levi, Carl	25	Halifax	29 OCT 1918
Levy, Bradis	12	Halifax	18 DEC 1918
Levy, Clifford	25	Little Tancook	20 MAR 1919
Levy, Gladys	11	Feltzen South	22 JAN 1919
Levy, Victor	12	Halifax	23 NOV 1918

Lewis, Avery, Lockeport, aged 19, Liverpool Advance, 23 October 1918, page 2.

Name	Age	Place	Date
Lewis, John	50	Glace Bay	14 NOV 1918

Lewis, Mary Lavinia, Lockeport, aged 18, Liverpool Advance, 23 October 1918, page 2.

Name	Age	Place	Date
Lightfoot, Helen	05	Prince Albert	28 OCT 1918
Lilley, Alma	10m	Halifax	29 SEPT 1918
Lingard, Cecil	*71*	*Truro*	*31 OCT 1918*

Halifax Evening Mail, 2 November 1918, page 1 (died Willow St. Hosp.).

Name	Age	Place	Date
Lively, Charles	20	Halifax	12 DEC 1918
Livingstone, Ellen	38	Glace Bay	21 OCT 1918
Livingstone, George	03	Westville	17 NOV 1918

Lockhart, Edwin, Idaho, Truro Daily News, 09 December 1918, page 4 (of Londonderry).
Lockwood, Terence C., England, Oxford Journal, 30 January 1919, page 3 (of Lockeport).
Logan, Lorne, B.C., 19m, Amherst Daily News, 22 November 1918, page 3 (of Amherst).

Name	Age	Place	Date
Lohez, Joseph	5m	Stellarton	17 FEB 1919
Lohnes, Aesop	25	Jordan River	24 NOV 1918
Lohnes, Donald	08	South Milford	02 NOV 1918
Lohnes, George	*32*	*Riverport*	*06 DEC 1918*

Halifax Evening Mail, 10 December 1918, page 13 (brother to Melbourne).

Name	Age	Place	Date
Lohnes, Jervois	*26*	*Back Sentry*	*26 OCT 1918*

Lunenburg Progress Enterprise, 06 November 1918, page 5 (Jervous Warren Lohnes).

Name	Age	Place	Date
Lohnes, Melbourne S.	*29*	*Bridgewater*	*08 DEC 1918*

Bridgewater Bulletin, 10 December 1918, page 4.
Lohnes, Warren, Lunenburg, Halifax Evening Mail, 01 November 1918, page 6.

Name	Age	Place	Date
Long, Elizabeth	20	Little Bras D'Or	19 NOV 1918
Long, Mary	26	Little Bras D'Or	28 OCT 1918
Long, Morris	45	Glace Bay	13 OCT 1918
Longard, John	37	Halifax	04 DEC 1918
Lopie, George	53	Beechville	26 OCT 1918

Lorette, Philcos, Amherst, aged 19, Amherst Daily News, 23 October 1918, page 8.

Name	Age	Place	Date
Losier, Melvin	*21*	*Yarmouth*	*03 FEB 1919*

Digby Courier, 7 February 1918, page 4 (of Chatham, NB).

Name	Age	Place	Date
Lovell, Harriet	28	North Sydney	09 OCT 1918
Lovett, Rita	*09*	*Tufts Cove*	*01 NOV 1918*

Halifax Evening Mail, 04 November 1918, page 2.

Name	Age	Place	Date
Lowe, Helen	23	Bridgetown	19 OCT 1918
Lowry, Emma	7m	Martinique	01 JAN 1919

Lucas, Osborne	35	Halifax	23 DEC 1918
Luffman, Edith	6m	North Sydney	27 MAR 1919
Lundy, Frank	19	Halifax	15 OCT 1918
Lurie, Herman	23	Halifax	26 NOV 1918
Lush, Mabel	*27*	*Halifax*	*18 DEC 1918*

Halifax Evening Mail, 19 December 1918, page 1.

Lutz, Bessie	---	Lake George	10 JAN 1919
Lyman, Bessie	65	Cambridge	01 JAN 1919

Lynn, Eva L., Truro, aged 24, Halifax Evening Mail, 7 November 1918, page 8 (Mrs. J. B.).
   Truro Daily News, 4 November 1918, page 4 (died at the Ainslie Hospital).

MacAulay, Frank	*32*	*East Noel*	*21 NOV 1918*

Hants Journal, 18 December 1918, page 8 (died in the Emergency Hospital in Halifax).

MacAulay, Mary	32	New Waterford	30 DEC 1918

MacDonald, North Sydney, two children of D. D. MacDonald; Sydney Daily Post, 30 September, 1918, page 1.

MacDonald, Alex. W.	16	St. Joseph's	01 FEB 1919

MacDonald, Albert, New York, Pictou Advocate, 7 February 1919, page 8 (of Durham).

Macdonald, Bessie	23	Halifax	02 JAN 1919

MacDonald, Daniel, New Brunswick, Sydney Daily Post, 27 November 1918, page 3 (Cape Breton).

MacDonald, Hugh	18	West Bay	23 FEB 1919
MacDonald, John	24	Halifax	08 NOV 1918

MacDonald, John, Halifax, aged 27, Halifax Evening Mail, 15 November 1918, page 1.

MacDonald, John	20	West Bay	28 FEB 1919
MacDonald, Louise	23	West Gore	02 JAN 1918
MacDonald, Lydia	02	New Waterford	17 DEC 1918
MacDonald, Margaret	*23*	*Halifax*	*08 NOV 1918*

Halifax Evening Mail, 15 November 1918, page 1 (died in the Influenza hosp.).
MacDonald, Rev. Ronald A., Glace Bay, 37, Sydney Daily Post, 4 November 1918, page 1.
MacDonnell, Dr. W. S., England, Truro Daily News, 7 December 1918, page 1 (of Whitney Pier); Yarmouth
   Telegram, 13 December 1918, page 1 (native of Sydney and Dalhousie grad of 1910).

MacDougall, Isabell	04	Thorburn	10 DEC 1918
MacEachern, Dan	07	New Waterford	02 OCT 1918
MacEwan, John	18	Liverpool	23 NOV 1918
MacGillivray, James	70	New Victoria	29 NOV 1918
MacGillivray, Orville	28	New Waterford	07 DEC 1918

MacIntosh, Mrs. Jessie, Lunenburg, Halifax Evening Mail, 1 November 1918, page 9.
Macintosh, Miss Jessie, Ontario, Liverpool Advance, 6 NOV 1918, p. 2 (of Lunenburg).

MacIsaac, Mary	27	New Waterford	04 DEC 1918
Mack, Maud	50	Lunenburg	11 OCT 1918

MacKay, Mrs. Alex., Mount Thom, 53, Pictou Advocate, 20 December, 1918, page 8.
MacKay, Gordon, PEI, aged 30, Pictou Advocate, 27 December 1918, page 8 (of Hardwood Hill).

MacKay, Mrs. M.H.	*37*	*West Bay*	*02 JAN 1919*

Halifax Evening Mail, 8 January 1919, page 1 (Euphemia MacKay, aged 38).

MacKie, Mrs. Katie	30	Glace Bay	03 JAN 1919
MacLean, William	47	Riversdale	15 JAN 1919

MacLeod, Cuthbert F., Pugwash Jct., aged 21, Amherst Daily News, 18 January 1919, page 3.
MacLeod, Eva Isabel, Halifax, Oxford Journal, 12 December 1918, page 6 (matron at Dr. Mader's Hospital).

MacLeod, Isabelle	31	Westville	29 NOV 1918
MacLeod, Jane	71	Burnside	04 NOV 1918
MacMillan, Anthony	*41*	*Pine Hill Hospital*	*29 OCT 1918*

Halifax Evening Mail, 01 November 1918, page 9 (Sgt. A. McMullan, aged 38).
Macneil, Rev. Joseph, Vancouver, 35, Sydney Daily Post, 06 November 1918, page 1 (Grand Narrows).

MacQueen, Annie	19	New Waterford	10 NOV 1918
Madden, Mertis	27	Baccaro	05 JAN 1919
Madigan, H.	---	Lawlor's Island	21 OCT 1918

Magee, Malcolm 30 Halifax 11 DEC 1918
Mahar, Frances, Wellington, Halifax Evening Mail, 26 October 1918, page 4.
Maher, Mrs. James, Mass., 30, Amherst Daily News, 19 October 1918, page 3 (of Amherst).
Mahin, John R. 24 Sydney 10 OCT 1918
Maillet, Mrs. Esther 37 Mavilette 14 JAN 1919
Mailman, Teresa 02 Halifax 09 OCT 1918
    Halifax Evening Mail, 10 October 1918, page 1.
Malanda, Eric --- Halifax 03 MAR 1919
Malanda, Mary 42 Halifax 05 MAR 1919
Malguen, Tesire 38 New Waterford 05 DEC 1918
Mallett, Mrs. Edith, Mavilette, aged 38, Digby Courier, 24 January 1919, page 5.
Malzard, Jean 5d Arichat 28 FEB 1919
Manette, Joseph 23 Halifax 27 OCT 1918
Maniah, Rosey 15 Stellarton 03 NOV 1918
Mannng, Ruth, Sussex, aged 4, Truro Daily News, 08 January 1919, page 4 (from Falmouth).
Manslip, Cassie 20 Amherst 13 NOV 1918
Manson, Annette 54 Centreville 25 JAN 1919
Manuel, Jacob 01 Canso 25 NOV 1918
Marchand, Barbara 29 Louisdale 27 JAN 1919
Marchand, Marie 62 Port Royal, C.B. 28 OCT 1918
Marriott, Ruby 27 North Williamston 20 DEC 1918
Marsden, Walter J., Halifax, aged 8 months, Halifax Evening Mail, 16 November 1918, page 12.
Marsh, Mrs. J.B., Boston, Berwick Register, 23 October 1918, page 2 (of Berwick).
Marshall, Catherine 47 Halifax 25 OCT 1918
Marshall, Edgar, Hampton, aged 16, Bridgetown Monitor, 15 January 1919, page 4.
Marshall, Ingram 29 Middleton 03 NOV 1918
Marshall, Isabell 39 South Range 20 APR 1919
Marshall, Joseph 16 Hampton 11 DEC 1918
Marshall, O., Dartmouth, Halifax Evening Mail, 24 October 1918, page 2.
Marshall, Stuart E., Connecticut, Halifax Evening Mail, 09 January 1919, page 9 (of Middleton).
Martell, Albert --- Cabbage Cove 24 OCT 1918
Martell, Deline 47 L'Ardoise 03 NOV 1918
Martell, Henry 19 Rockdale 08 OCT 1918
Martell, Louise 2m West L'Ardoise 27 MAR 1919
Martell, Margaret 25 New Waterford 04 DEC 1918
Martell, Mary 07 Cabbage Cove 21 OCT 1918
Martell, Philomen 2m West L'Ardoise 31 MAR 1919
Martell, Sabeth --- Cabbage Cove 03 NOV 1918
Martell, Virginia 20 Halifax 10 MAR 1919
Martell, Rev. William 32 Bridgewater 14 DEC 1918
    Bridgewater Bulletin, 17 December, page 4, (Rev. William R. Martell.)
Martell, Willie --- Cabbage Cove 21 OCT 1918
Martin, Daniel 04 Halifax 05 DEC 1918
Martin, Mrs. Mary 79 Stellarton 03 DEC 1918
Martin, Therese 03 New Waterford 15 DEC 1918
Mason, Florence 39 Lunenburg 19 OCT 1918
    Halifax Evening Mail, 22 October 1918, page 6 (Mrs. Angus Mason).
Mason, Francis, Lunenburg, Lunenburg Progress Enterprise, 30 October 1918, page 1.
Mason, Mrs. Harold, Falkland Ridge, Middleton Outlook, 15 November 1918, page 2.
Mason, Mrs. Henry 23 Eight Island Lake 30 NOV 1918
Mason, Jennie 23 Halifax 05 DEC 1918
Mason, John D., British Columbia, 34, Truro Daily News, 18 January 1919, page 7 (from Alton).
Mason, Morris 24 Eastern Points 18 OCT 1918
    Halifax Evening Mail, 22 October, page 6.
Mason, Philip 09 Eastern Points 25 OCT 1918
Matheson, Alexander 18 Sydney 31 OCT 1918

Matheson, Donald	01	Sydney	26 OCT 1918
Matheson, John	75	Westville	26 NOV 1918
Matheson, Sarah	70	Louisbourg	18 JAN 1919
Mathews, Percy	02	Debert	28 NOV 1918
Mathias, Percy	17	Halifax	22 NOV 1918
Matsusaki, Matsutaro	34	Halifax	21 DEC 1918
Matthews, Alice	54	East Ragged Island	17 MAR 1919
Matthews, Dudley	03	Shelburne	25 OCT 1918
Matthews, James	5m	Jordan River	09 OCT 1918
Matthews, James	33	Springhill	31 DEC 1918
Mattie, Charles	06	New Glasgow	18 DEC 1918
Maxner, Frederick	54	Windsor	23 OCT 1918
Maxwell, John	26	Glace Bay	20 DEC 1918

McAndrews, John, Mass., Middleton Outlook, 11 October 1918, page 2 (of Port George).

McArthur, Margaret	59	Sydney Mines	05 DEC 1918
McAskill, Kate Ann	36	Sydney	31 OCT 1918
McAskill, Neil	35	Englishtown	20 MAY 1919
McAulay, George	33	Halifax	12 FEB 1919
McCallum, Robert S.	41	New Glasgow	02 DEC 1918
McCarthy, Gordon	02	Conquerell	09 MAR 1919
McCarthy, Sarah	27	Shelburne	21 NOV 1918
McCaul, Eva L.	*32*	*Delap's Cove*	*28 NOV 1918*

Annapolis Spectator, 12 December 1918, page 3 (Evangeline died in Massachusetts).

McCaul, William	33	Lawlor's Island	18 DEC 1918

McCoy, L. F., Kentville, aged 34, Kentville Advertizer, 25 October 1918, page 4.

McCrae, Florence	33	Halifax	13 NOV 1918
McCreadie, R.	31	Sydney	16 OCT 1918
McCuish, Rose	16	Port Hood	24 DEC 1918
McCulloch, Maggie	16	Noel Road	25 OCT 1918
McDaniel, William	25	Margaree Forks	07 NOV 1918
McDaniels, William	27	Georges River	07 NOV 1918
McDonald, Agnes	31	Little Judique	24 DEC 1918
McDonald, Alice	10	Glace Bay	19 DEC 1918
McDonald, Angus	35	Stirling, C.B.	23 NOV 1918
McDonald, Angus	52	Plaster North Shore	11 MAY 1919
McDonald, Annie	39	Sydney Mines	11 DEC 1918
McDonald, Annie	04	Evansville	01 JAN 1919
McDonald, C.	45	Reserve Mines	14 DEC 1918
McDonald, Catherine	16	Catalone	17 NOV 1919
McDonald, Clarence	5m	Grantville	05 APR 1919
McDonald, Daniel	16	Trenton	29 NOV 1918
McDonald, Daniel	14	Little Judique	27 DEC 1918
McDonald, Daniel	35	Glace Bay	01 JAN 1919
McDonald, Daniel	20	Mira	05 APR 1919
McDonald, Donald	68	Inverness Asylum	13 JUL 1919
McDonald, Harriet	03	Glace Bay	21 OCT 1918
McDonald, Hugh	23	Loganville	21 OCT 1918
McDonald, J. Herbert	---	Antigonish County	--- OCT 1918
McDonald, Jean	30	Sydney	14 OCT 1918
McDonald, John	29	Sydney	12 OCT 1918
McDonald, John	8m	Dominion	10 DEC 1918
McDonald, John	24	Little Judique	26 DEC 1918
McDonald, John	8m	Stellarton	31 DEC 1918
McDonald, John L.	32	Shubenacadie	27 JAN 1919
McDonald, John W.	2d	Heatherton	23 DEC 1918
McDonald, Katie	30	Stirling, C.B.	23 NOV 1918

McDonald, Mrs. M.R.	30	Sydney Mines	15 NOV 1918
McDonald, Malcolm	---	Little Bras d'Or	08 DEC 1918
McDonald, Margaret	20	Halifax	08 NOV 1918
McDonald, Margaret	59	Glace Bay	29 NOV 1918

McDonald, Margaret, Mass., Eastern Chronicle, 7 February 1919, page 7 (of Port Hood).

McDonald, Margaret	09	Maryvale	05 MAR 1919
McDonald, Marjary	26	Inverness	01 SEPT 1918
McDonald, Mary	05	Sydney Mines	18 DEC 1918
McDonald, Mary	14	Glace Bay	24 DEC 1918
McDonald, Mary D.	26	Halifax	29 OCT 1918
McDonald, Mary	50	Black River	26 FEB 1919

McDonald, Richard, Canso, aged 62, Canso News, 29 March, 1919, page 1.

McDonald, Roderick	30	Point Tupper	19 OCT 1918
McDonald. Ronald	30	Glace Bay	03 NOV 1918
McDonald, Walter	*49*	*Halifax*	*06 DEC 1918*

Halifax Evening Mail, 10 December 1918, page 2 (spelled MacDonald).

| *McDonald, Wilbert* | *22* | *Truro* | *17 NOV 1918* |

Halifax Evening Mail, 18 November 1918, page 3 (Truro Emergency Hospital).

McDonald, William	29	Glace Bay	09 JAN 1919
McDonnell, Alex.	24	South West Ridge	15 MAY 1919
McDonough, Alfred	35	Halifax	01 NOV 1918
McDougall, Annie	62	Centennial	21 DEC 1918
McDougall, John J.	28	Sydney	22 OCT 1918
McDougall, Mary	18	Sydney	19 NOV 1918
McDougall, Mary J.	10	New Waterford	27 SEPT 1918
McDougall, Saidie	*21*	*North Sydney*	*29 NOV 1918*

Sydney Daily Post, 3 December 1918, page 1 (Miss Sadie MacDougall of Margaree).

McDougall, Sarah	23	Margaree Forks	29 NOV 1918
McEachern, Alex	27	Port Hood	27 NOV 1918
McEachern, Alex	26	Judique	14 DEC 1918
McEachern, Alex	08	Port Hood	26 APR 1919
McEachern, Gordon	48	New Glasgow	28 DEC 1918
McEachern, Howard	17	Stellarton	05 MAR 1919
McEachern, James	52	Inverness	04 SEPT 1918
McEachern, Joseph	23	Trenton	15 NOV 1918
McFarlane, James	06	Glace Bay	06 NOV 1918
McFhie [*McPhee*], Mary	54	Upper Big Tracadie	15 MAR 1919
McGovern, Chester	24	Joggins Mines	21 NOV 1918
McGovern, William	28	Joggins Mines	17 NOV 1918
McGowan, Martha	58	Hunt's Point	16 MAR 1919
McGrath, Albert	19	Boularderie	16 NOV 1918

McGrath, Alfie, Amherst, aged 17, Amherst Daily News, 23 October 1918, page 8.
McGrath, Charles, Amherst, aged 26, Amherst Daily News, 28 October 1918, page 8.

McGrath, George	27	Halifax	19 JAN 1919
McGrath, Josephine	35	Dartmouth	16 OCT 1918
McGrath, Mary	21	New Waterford	23 SEPT 1918

McInnes, James, Halifax, aged 20, Halifax Evening Mail, 26 October 1918, page 4.

McInnes, John	83	McInnes Mountain	29 DEC 1918
McInnes, Rachel	78	McInnes Mountain	08 DEC 1918
McInnis, Alexander	77	Musquodoboit Hbr	04 DEC 1918
McInnis, Elizabeth	72	Ball's Creek	26 MAR 1919
McInnis, John	33	Pictou	05 DEC 1918
McInnis, Margaret	18	Sydney	09 DEC 1918
McIntosh, George	*53*	*Lockeport*	*16 OCT 1918*

Liverpool Advance, 23 October 1918, page 2 (his age was given as 50).

McIntosh, Rev. John   32   Bridgewater   23 FEB 1919
    Bridgewater Bulletin, 25 February 1919, page 3.
McIntosh, Minnie, Lockeport, aged 19, Liverpool Advance, 23 October 1918, page 2.
McIntyre, Christina   32   Sydney   09 OCT 1918
McIntyre, Hector   30   Glace Bay   12 OCT 1918
McIntyre, Johanna   9m   Sydney   12 OCT 1918
McIntyre, John, Sydney, Sydney Daily Post, 10 October 1918, page 1.
McIsaac, Allan   06   Dunvegan   28 MAR 1919
McIsaac, Christina   37   Chocolate Lake   19 SEPT 1918
McIsaac, John   33   Inverness   07 SEPT 1918
McIver, Donald   26   Halifax   17 NOV 1918
McIvoy, Earl   22   Dartmouth   03 NOV 1918
McKay, Bertha   27   Riversdale   09 MAR 1919
McKay, Eldora   03   Springhill   31 OCT 1918
McKay, Harry   34   Onslow   09 DEC 1918
McKay, James   84   Abercrombie   24 MAR 1919
McKay, Miss Lilias, Maryland, Halifax Evening Mail, 09 December 1918, page 7; (New Glasgow) Eastern
    Chronicle, 06 December 1918, page 1 (Lillian McKay, nurse at a Military Hospital).
McKay, Mrs. Neil   45   Cape Dauphin   08 APR 1919
McKay, Thomas   18   St. Paul's   09 JAN 1919
McKeigan, James   08   Glace Bay   30 SEPT 1918
McKeigan, Dan   33   Sydney   13 DEC 1918
McKenna, Andrew   21   Halifax   26 FEB 1919
McKenzie, Angus   35   Stellarton   10 JAN 1919
McKenzie, Mrs. Angus, Truro, Halifax Evening Mail, 31 October 1918, page 2 (Willow St. Hospital).
McKenzie, Arabella   28   Sydney River   16 NOV 1918.
McKenzie, Clinton S., British Columbia, aged 18, Truro Daily News, 07 December 1918, page 1 (of Maitland,
    Hants County. Died in Connaught Hospital in Prince George).
McKenzie, Edith   9m   Stewiacke   09 DEC 1918
McKenzie, Elma   02   Stellarton   31 MAR 1919
McKenzie, Emma   ---   Brookside   30 OCT 1918
McKenzie, Harry   29   Halifax   30 OCT 1918
McKenzie, Jean   18m   Stellarton   25 MAR 1919
McKenzie, John   27   Piedmont   22 NOV 1918
McKenzie, Dr. John J. 45   Pictou   12 OCT 1918
    Halifax Evening Mail, 12 October 1918, page 1 (Health Officer for Pictou).
McKenzie, Julia   52   Jordan Ferry   15 FEB 1919
McKenzie, Mary   24   Sydney Mines   28 DEC 1918
McKinnon, Addie   26   South River Road   11 SEPT 1918
McKinnon, Bertha M.   38   *Truro*   *05 NOV 1918*
    Halifax Evening Mail, 7 November 1918, page 10 (age given as 40). Truro Daily News, 05 November 1918,
    page 8 (née Bertha Fisher. Died in Emergency Hospital).
McKinnon, Mary   30   Margaree Harbour   29 DEC 1918
McKinnon, William   78   Marshalltown   15 DEC 1918
McKnight, Miss Gladys, Kings Co., Amherst Daily News, 12 March 1919, page 4.
McLanders, John, British Columbia, aged 75, Truro Daily News, 27 December 1918, page 6 (Waldegrave,
    Colchester County).
McLaughlin, Amos   54   Pleasant Hills   08 FEB 1919
McLauchlin, Herbert   33   Lochaber   19 MAR 1919
McLaughlin, James   27   Bridgetown   15 JAN 1919
McLean, Alexander   71   Scotsville   22 AUG 1919
McLean, Beatrice   37   Sydney Mines   08 DEC 1918
McLean, Dan C. Jr., East Lake Ainslie, 18, Sydney Daily Post, 10 December 1918, page 1.
McLean, Hector   24   *North Sydney*   *13 OCT 1918*
    Sydney Daily Post, 16 October 1918, page 1 (son of Dr. McLean).
McLean, John   22   Georges River   05 DEC 1918

McLean, John J.	35	Sydney Mines	26 NOV 1918
McLean, Katie	35	Whycocomagh	03 JAN 1919

McLean, Kenneth Willie, Riverside, aged 47, Truro Daily News, 5 February 1919, page 4.

McLean, Mabel	04	Glace Bay	10 NOV 1918
McLean, Malcolm	20	Hubbards	13 NOV 1918

McLean, Willie Arthur, Central West River, 29, Eastern Chronicle, 29 November 1918, page 1.

McLellan, Jennie	*17*	*Cambridge*	*10 DEC 1918*

Truro Daily News, 24 December 1918, page 2 (Jennie McLennan, aged 17, died at Five Islands on 19 December).

McLellan, Lillian	35	Central Economy	14 JAN 1919
McLellan, James	15	Glace Bay	17 FEB 1919
McLellan, Mary Ann	25	S.W. Margaree	10 OCT 1918
McLennan, Emmaline	05	Alder Point	12 NOV 1918
McLeod, _____	21	Pugwash	29 DEC 1918
McLeod, Anthony	01	Glace Bay	27 DEC 1918
McLeod, Christina	23	Sydney	03 OCT 1918
McLeod, Flora	21	Upper South West	18 JAN 1919
McLeod, J.	40	Sydney	24 OCT 1918
McLeod, Walter	17	Glace Bay	24 DEC 1918

McManaman, W. Henry, East Mines Station, 30, Amherst Daily News, 29 October 1918, page 7.

McMillan, Mary	26	Sydney	26 NOV 1918
McNamera, Emanuel	13m	L. River Inhabitants	07 OCT 1918
McNeil, Angus	58	North Sydney	07 OCT 1918
McNeil, Annie	28	Sydney	16 OCT 1918
McNeil, Dan	17	Sydney	04 DEC 1918
McNeil, Irvin	18	Bass River	27 MAR 1919
McNeil, Lizzie	22	Ben Eoin	09 DEC 1918
McNeil. Margaret	14	New Waterford	12 DEC 1918
McNeil, Mary	11	Rockingham	19 NOV 1918
McNeil, Mary	03	Glace Bay	20 DEC 1918
McNeil, Michael	28	North Sydney	03 DEC 1918
McNeil, Michael	26	Halifax	13 DEC 1918
McNeil, Peter J.	05	Glace Bay	03 SEPT 1918
McNeil, Stephen	19	Shenacadie	25 DEC 1918
McPhail, Annie	36	Heatherton	01 JAN 1919
McPhail, Florence	31	Heatherton	24 DEC 1918
McPhee, Daniel	36	Sydney Mines	05 DEC 1918
McPhee, Helen	14	West Gore	19 NOV 1918
McPhee, Saran A.	42	Dominion	09 OCT 1918
McPherson, Emma	50	New Aberdeen	28 OCT 1918
McPherson, Murdoch	33	Glace Bay	01 NOV 1918
McPherson, Veronica	01	Williams Point	23 FEB 1919
McPherson, Murray	35	Springhill	08 NOV 1918

McQuarrie, Daniel, Truro, Halifax Evening Mail, 25 October 1918, page 2 (Willow St. Hospital).

McQuarrie, Florence	30	Port Hastings	16 JAN 1919
McQuarrie, John	38	Hopewell	08 DEC 1918
McQuarrie, John	42	Port Hastings	26 DEC 1918
McQueen, Annie	27	Sydney	25 NOV 1918
McRae, Catherine	87	Sydney Forks	20 OCT 1918
McRae, Fred	30	St. Joseph's	22 NOV 1918
McRae, James	3m	Louisdale	08 OCT 1918
McRae, Mabel	*32*	*Sydney*	*16 DEC 1918*

Sydney Daily Post, 17 December 1918, page 5 (Mrs. Dr. John McRae, née Mabel Fletcher).

McRae, Maria	76	Sydney Mines	28 MAR 1919
McRitchie, Catherine	18	St. Ann's	28 OCT 1918
McRory, _____	10d	Skye Mountain	15 JAN 1919

McRory, Effie   19   Skye Mountain   22 JAN 1919
McVarish, Christena   22   Dominion   22 DEC 1918
Meek, Mrs. Geddie, Red Deer, 47, Hants Journal, 15 January 1919, page 1 (of Windsor).
Meikle, Duncan   35   Sydney   05 DEC 1918
Melanson, Ada   08   Springhill Junction   28 OCT 1918
Melanson, Florence   32   Corberrie   30 JAN 1919
Melanson, Gladys   08   Marshalltown   15 DEC 1918
Melanson, Maggie   18   Amherst   26 NOV 1918
Melanson, Margaret   *77*   *Amherst*   *15 FEB 1919*
    Amherst Daily News, 18 February 1919, page 5.
Melanson, Viney   31   Plympton Station   24 DEC 1918
Melvin, Annie   25   East River   30 OCT 1918
Metcalf, Lillian   41   Sydney Mines   08 NOV 1918
Michael, Mrs. Stephen 50   Barra Head   01 OCT 1918
Michele, François   *29*   *Lawlor's Island*   *OCT 1918*
    Chronicle, 02 October 1918, page 2 (was on a French Cable Ship).
Miles, Dorothy   6w   Shelburne   29 JAN 1919
Millard, Margaret   15   Liverpool   13 FEB 1919
Miller, Mrs. _____   26   Hubbards   21 DEC 1918
Miller, Bedford   *39*   *Springhill*   *31 OCT 1918*
    Oxford Journal, 07 November 1918, page 3 (age given as 29).
Miller, Eral   03   Northfield   22 DEC 1918
Miller, Fannie   45   Sydney   12 DEC 1918
Miller, Harry   36   New Aberdeen   13 DEC 1918
Miller, Henry   87   Upper Kennetcook   09 MAY 1919
Miller, Miss Nellie *23*   *Dartmouth*   *02 NOV 1918*
    Halifax Evening Mail, 04 November 1918, page 2.
Mills, Charles   *30*   *Shulie*   *01 DEC 1918*
    Amherst Daily News, 7 January 1919, page 3 (died at River Hebert).
Mills, Elisha R.   *21*   *Pugwash*   *10 NOV 1918*
    21 Amherst Daily News, 15 November 1918, page 6 (of Truro).
Mills, Grace   07   Amherst   23 DEC 1918
Mills, Helen M., Amherst, aged 7, Amherst Daily News, 03 December 1918, page 4.
Mills, Cpl. Roy A., Toronto, 24, Amherst Daily News, 12 February 1919, page 3 (of Joggins).
Mills, Pte. William *32*   *Halifax*   *31 OCT 1918*
    Amherst Daily News, 7 January 1919, page 3 (death given as 30 November).
Mills, Wilson   02   Bramber   13 NOV 1918
Minn, William   28   Halifax   15 NOV 1918
Mitchell, Mabel   19   Dartmouth   24 FEB 1919
Mitchell, Pearl   46   Chester   19 OCT 1918
M'Neil, Captain Angus J., Sydney Daily Post, 08 October 1918, page 1 (died at Hamilton Hospital).
Mobley, Mrs. Nellie   29   Glace Bay   29 DEC 1918
Moffatt, Brian   25   Dominion   31 OCT 1918
Moffatt, Mrs. Isabel   34   Glace Bay   16 OCT 1918
Moir, Franklyn C., Boston, aged 13, Evening Mail, 1 October 1918, page 2 (of Halifax).
Moir, William   13   Halifax   29 SEPT 1918
Mombourquette, Alexina, Lower L'Ardoise, Halifax Evening Mail, 08 January 1919, page 1.
Monk, Florence   26   Halifax   21 NOV 1918
Montague, Ethel B.   *34*   *Dartmouth*   *11 DEC 1918*
    Halifax Evening Mail, 11 December 1918, page 14 (Mrs. William J. Montague).
Montgomery, Hilda   *30*   *Bridgewater*   *25 FEB 1919*
    Yarmouth Herald, 25 February 1919, page 2 (formerly of Yarmouth, aged 35).
Moody, Rodney   25   Wallace   04 FEB 1919
Moore, Mrs. _____   32   Economy   08 JAN 1919
Moore, Arietta, New York, 13, Bridgewater Bulletin, 24 December 1918, page 4 (of Bridgewater).

Moore, Charles	22	Oxford	03 NOV 1918

Amherst Daily News, 17 December 1918, page 5.

Moore, Eddie, Oxford Junction, aged 22, Oxford Journal, 6 February 1919, page 2.

Moore, Frank	30	Kentville	04 FEB 1919
Moore, John	56	Halifax	23 OCT 1918
Moore, John	19	Halifax	29 OCT 1918

Moore, Marion, New York, 16, Bridgewater Bulletin, 24 December 1918, page 4 (of Bridgewater).

Mooring, Bessie V., Halifax, 27, Halifax Evening Mail, 13 December 1918, page 2 (Mrs. Henry).

Moran, Leo	---	South Ingonish	20 DEC 1918
Moran, Myrtle	21	Trenton	18 DEC 1918

Morehouse, Harry, Middleton, aged 34, Middleton Outlook, 8 November 1918, page 2.

Morgan, Ada	02	Dartmouth	15 OCT 1918
Morgan, Augustus	32	Port Latour	22 OCT 1918
Morgan, Effie	35	Sydney	16 DEC 1918
Morgan, Harold	4m	Stellarton	21 NOV 1918
Morgan, Susanna	36	Glace Bay	21 OCT 1918
Moriarity, Hilda	6m	Halifax	13 SEPT 1918

Morine, Arthur, Cornwallis, Truro Daily News, 17 February 1919, page 2.

Morine, Mrs. Edith	*42*	*Kentville*	*02 DEC 1918*

Truro Daily News, 17 February 1919, page 2 (wife of Arthur Morine).

Morine, Robie	*20*	*Kentville*	*16 DEC 1918*

Truro Daily News, 17 February 1919, page 2 (son of Arthur Morine).

Morris, Charles	61	Chester	03 NOV 1918

Morris, Dimock, Advocate, Amherst Daily News, 30 October 1918, page 4.

Morris, Giles	49	Joggins Mines	14 NOV 1918
Morris, Lucinda	*32*	*Bridgewater*	*08 NOV 1918*

Lunenburg Progress Enterprise, 13 November 1918, page 1 (Miss Lucinda Morris).

Morris, Philip, Lunenburg, Halifax Evening Mail, 1 November 1918, page 6.

Morris, William	40	Joggins Mines	16 NOV 1918
Morrison, Angus	19	Leitches Creek	20 DEC 1918
Morrison, Catherine	28	Port Hastings	12 JAN 1919

Morrison, Clarence F., B.C., 26, Halifax Evening Mail, 19 November 1918, page 1 (of Glenholme).

Morrison, Lillian L.,	*25*	*Halifax*	*09 OCT 1918*

Amherst Daily News, 21 October 1918, page 3.

Morrison, Samuel	40	Sydney	22 OCT 1918

Morse, Beaumont, Vancouver, Amherst Daily News, 2 January 1919, page 5 (son of Dr. Morse).

Morse, Percy	37	Bloomington	25 MAR 1919
Morton, Annie	31	Yarmouth	21 DEC 1918
Morton, William	02	Yarmouth	11 JAN 1919
Moses, Edward	17	Lequille	17 OCT1918
Moses, Nathan	36	Ohio	27 DEC 1918

Mosher, Andrew, Giltown, Halifax Evening Mail, 12 December 1918, page 3 (Musqudoboit Hbr).

Mosher, Dolly	*35*	*Middleton*	*11 NOV 1918*

Middleton Outlook, 20 December 1918, page 2 (Mrs. Zenas Mosher).

Mosher, Sydney	21	Hantsport	29 OCT 1918
Mososka, Anthony	70	Sydney Mines	25 DEC 1918
Mossman, Hector	*29*	*Riverport*	*30 OCT 1918*

Halifax Evening Mail, 1 November 1918, page 6.

Mossman, J. Wilfred, Lunenburg Progress Enterprise, 23 October 1918, page 1.

Mossman, James	*35*	*Rose Bay*	*16 OCT 1918*

Halifax Evening Mail, 22 October 1918, page 6 (J. Wilfred Mossman).

Mott, Thomas	---	Dartmouth	15 OCT 1918
Moulaison, Augustin	3m	Surette Island	18 DEC 1918
Moulaison, George	09	Sluice Point	07 DEC 1918
Moulaison, Rose	09	Sluice Point	21 DEC 1918
Mountain, Mary	26	Halifax	31 OCT 1918

Mowbray, Thomas	80	Halifax	29 OCT 1918
Moxon, Alexander	29	Halifax	27 OCT 1918
Moxon, Charles	37	Halifax	06 NOV 1918
Muir, Jennie	26	Westville	20 DEC 1918
Muise, Alfred	24	Belleville	25 SEPT 1918
Muise, Alice	08	East Quinan	29 JAN 1919
Muise, Pte. Cyrial W.	*54*	*Digby*	*06 DEC 1918*

Bridgetown Monitor, 11 Dec. 1918, page 3 (returned soldier).

Muise, Harriet	16	Yarmouth	09 NOV 1918
Muise, Judith	36	Belleneck	09 NOV 1918
Muise, Laura	02	Belleneck	14 NOV 1918
Muise, Sarah	*55*	*Digby*	*09 DEC 1918*

Bridgetown Monitor, 11 December 1918, page 3 (wife of Pte. C. W. Muise).

Mullen, Elizabeth	06	Easton	14 OCT 1918
Mullen, Ellsworth	*25*	*Havelock*	*12 OCT 1918*

Digby Courier, 08 November 1918, page 4 (died at Hillsdale).

Mullen, Lennie	30	Havelock	18 OCT 1918
Mulloy, Alphonses	36	Halifax	14 OCT 1918
Mumford, Lloyd	29	Halifax	18 OCT 1918
Munro, Clara	03	Beechville	27 OCT 1918
Munro, Peter	26	Beechville	24 OCT 1918
Munro, Robert	02	Kentville	08 MAY 1919

Munro, Sinclair, Groveland, 23, Westville Free Lance, 29 November 1919, page 1.

Munro, Stella	3m	Beechville	25 SEPT 1918
Munroe, Arthur	02	Halifax	24 NOV 1918
Munroe, John	15	Beechville	03 NOV 1918
Munroe, Joseph	21m	Canso	25 NOV 1918
Munroe, Laurence	06	Trentonq	25 NOV 1918

Munroe, Peter, Nova Scotia Hospital, aged 1, Halifax Evening Mail, 26 October 1918, page 4.

Munroe, Mrs. Robert	34	Canso	29 DEC 1918

Murphy, Fred C., San Francisco, Hants Journal, 11 December 1918, page 1 (of Scotch Village).

Murphy, Henry	3m	Mineville	11 DEC 1918
Murphy, John	64	City Home, Halifax	25 OCT 1918
Murphy, Marion	02	Halifax	21 OCT 1918
Murphy, William	29	Sydney	22 OCT 1918
Murphy, William	26	South Bar	23 OCT 1918
Murphy, William	27	Halifax	24 NOV 1918
Mury, Louis	14	West Arichat	08 FEB 1919

Myatt, Simon, Tufts Cove, aged 29, Halifax Evening Mail, 6 November 1918, page 2.

Myette, Bridget	21	Halifax	29 DEC 1918
Myette, Herbert	19	Grand Desert	25 NOV 1918
Naas, Olive	*21*	*Sentry*	*28 OCT 1918*

Halifax Evening Mail, 1 November 1918, page 6 (Mrs. Harris Naas).

Naugle, Alice	35	Eastern Passage	11 NOV 1918
Naugle, George	*41*	*Devil's Island*	*13 DEC 1918*

Halifax Evening Mail, 17 December 1918, page 2 (died on 16 December).

Naugler, Henry	19	Whynot Settlement	18 OCT 1918
Naylor, Frank	22	Halifax	30 OCT 1918
Nearing, Stella	22	Halifax	29 DEC 1918

Nelligan, John D., Ontario, 28, Halifax Evening Mail, 30 November 1918, page 2 (of Halifax).

Nelson, Adeliade	16	Londonderry	02 FEB 1919
Nelson, Mary	02	Yarmouth	12 NOV 1918
Neville, Myrtle	16m	Sydney	10 OCT 1918
Newberry, Weston	29	Halifax	15 FEB 1919
Newell, William M.	50	Halifax	16 DEC 1918
Newman, Robert	21	Springhill	01 JAN 1919

Neys, Ward	20	Lawlor's Island	19 DEC 1918
Nicholas, Joe	08	Barra Head	11 OCT 1918
Nicholas, Michael	01	Barra Head	15 OCT 1918
Nicholas, Mrs. Paul	35	Barra Head	08 OCT 1918
Nichols, David	25	Halifax	10 DEC 1918

Nicholson, Miss Jean, New York, Amherst Daily News, 04 February 1919, page 5 (of Gulf Shore).

Nicholson, Margaret	34	North Sydney	11 OCT 1918
Nickerson, Adelbert	37	East Pubnico	11 OCT 1918
Nickerson, Albert	01	Baccaro	28 OCT 1918
Nickerson, Alford	16	Malden	01 JAN 1919
Nickerson, Douglas	9m	Cape Sable Island	02 NOV 1918
Nickerson, Fred	44	Weymouth	22 FEB 1919
Nickerson, Minard	19	Clark's Harbour	12 NOV 1918
Nickerson, Percy	35	Cape Sable Island	28 OCT 1918
Nickerson, Russell	30	Clark's Harbour	17 OCT 1918
Nickerson, Winnifred	30	Upper Woods Hbr	07 OCT 1918
Niles, W.H.	22	New Glasgow	13 DEC 1918
Noble, Lucy	34	Halifax	17 OCT 1918

Noiles, Mrs. Arthur, aged 29, Amherst, Amherst Daily News, 1 November 1918, page 3.

Norka, Desire	38	New Waterford	05 DEC 1918
Norman, Roberta	27	Glace Bay	13 NOV 1918
Norwood, Edmund B.,	*42*	*Hubbards*	*30 DEC 1918*

Bridgewater Bulletin, 7 January 1919, page 2 (was physician).

Nyjoke, Ala	01	Sydney	11 DEC 1918
O'Brien, Harold	22	Murphy's Cove	09 DEC 1918
O'Brien, Mary L.	*25*	*Dartmouth*	*21 OCT 1918*

Halifax Evening Mail, 22 October 1918, page 2 (Mary Louisa O'Brien).

O'Brien, Sophine	05	Chignecto Mines	30 OCT 1918
O'Brien, Stephen	39	Halifax	05 NOV 1918
O'Brien, Wreatha	3m	Gardiner Mines	07 DEC 1918
O'Connell, Joseph	02	Halifax	02 NOV 1918
O'Day, Dennis	15	Port Morien	14 DEC 1918
O'Handley, Margaret	73	Sydney	30 OCT 1918
O'Hanley, Frank	*37*	*Dartmouth*	*25 OCT 1918*

Halifax Evening Mail, 25 October 1918, page 2.

O'Hara, Genevieve	04	New Waterford	17 DEC 1918
O'Hearn, John	30	Dartmouth	03 NOV 1918

O'Hearn, Philip, Dartmouth, aged 30, Halifax Evening Mail, 4 November 1918, page 2.

Oickle, Harvey	25	Greenland	11 FEB 1919
Oickle, Ruth	4m	Greenland	26 FEB 1919
Oickle, Winnie	25	Victory	14 NOV 1918
Oikle, Nellie	10m	Shelburne	04 MAR 1919
O'Leary, Theresa	*45*	*Windsor Forks*	*04 DEC 1918*

Hants Journal, 18 December 1918, page 8 (Mrs. George O'Leary).

Olive, John	01	Reserve Mines	12 JAN 1919
Olsen, Carl	28	Sydney	01 NOV 1918
Olsen, Richard	*---*	*Lawlor's Island*	*30 SEPT 1918*

Chronicle, 2 October, 1918, page 2, (an American sailor).

On, Jeu	28	Halifax	04 NOV 1918
O'Neil, Veronica	36	Glace Bay	27 OCT 1918
O'Neill, Ernest	19	Plympton	28 DEC 1918
O'Toole, Mrs. Mary	30	Glace Bay	08 NOV 1918

Oulton, Thomas, Amherst, aged 27, Halifax Evening Mail, 21 October 1918, page 12.

Oxner, Harry	17	Lunenburg	03 NOV 1918
Oxner, William	34	Lunenburg	01 JAN 1919
Paddock, Lydia	37	Glace Bay	07 JAN 1919

Palmer, Nora	*30*	*Morristown*	*02 OCT 1918*

Berwick Register, 16 October 1918, page 2 (Mrs. Carol Palmer).

Papineau, Alphonse	*23*	*Amherst*	*03 NOV 1918*

Amherst Daily News, 04 November 1918, page 3 (a soldier).

Parks, James	82	Port George	22 DEC 1918
Parks, Nora	*28*	*Halifax*	*20 OCT 1918*

Halifax Evening Mail, 21 October 1918, page 9.

Patriquin, Elizabeth	35	Greenville Station	22 OCT 1918
Patriquin, Barbara	32	Londonderry	01 DEC 1918

Patriquin, Mrs. Noble, West Wentworth, aged 35, Amherst Daily News, 30 October 1918, page 3.

Patterson, David	8m	Economy	18 JAN 1919
Patterson, Mary	04	Benacadie	23 JAN 1919
Paul, Anthony	09	Springhill Junction	14 OCT 1918
Paul, Catherine	11	Indian Reserve	05 NOV 1918
Paul, Jonas	64	Herring Cove	11 OCT 1918
Paul, Joseph	39	Springhill Junction	10 OCT 1918
Paul, Joseph	27	Springhill Junction	23 NOV 1918
Paul, Joseph	78	Windsor Junction 1	3 OCT 1918
Paul, Katie	28	Windsor Junction	20 OCT 1918
Paul, Sarah	73	Windsor Junction	19 OCT 1918
Pearl, Jessie	16	Arlington	19 JAN 1919
Pearson, John	33	Stellarton	18 MAR 1919
Peck, Augustus	32	Glace Bay	20 NOV 1918
Peddle, Francis	34	Glace Bay	14 OCT 1918
Peeler, Robert	29	North Sydney	09 DEC 1918
Peers, Wesley	62	Wallace	26 FEB 1919
Pembroke, George	18	Chester	12 OCT 1918
Penny, Andrew	23	New Waterford	09 DEC 1918

Penny, Mrs. Fred, Mahone Bay, Halifax Evening Mail, 16 October 1918, page 12.

Penny, Hector	69	New Glasgow	22 DEC 1918
Penny, Josephine	22	Halifax	30 NOV 1918
Penny, Rhoda	58	New Glasgow	12 DEC 1918
Perkins, Clifford	38	Sydney	11 OCT 1918

Perkins, William, Sydney, Sydney Daily Post, 15 October 1918, page 5.

Pero, Hubert	14	Alder Point	25 NOV 1918
Pero, Lillian	12	Alder Point	12 NOV 1918
Perry, David	38	Roseway	21 JAN 1919

Perry, Delbert G., Mass., Yarmouth Telegram, 29 November 1918, page 1 (of Port Maitland).

Peters, Andrew	22	Halifax	28 FEB 1919

Peters, Annie, Halifax, 22, Halifax Evening Mail, 04 March 1919, page 10 (from PEI).

Peters, Clarence	04	Glace Bay	09 JAN 1919
Petipas, Joseph	24	Tracadie	30 NOV 1918
Petipas, Mrs. Joseph	24	Tracadie	10 DEC 1918
Petipas, Lena	27	Halifax	08 NOV 1918
Petitpas, Rebecca	48	Poirierville	09 MAY 1919
Petrie, Catherine	14	Sydney	28 OCT 1918
Petrie, Margaret	72	New Victoria	18 DEC 1918
Petropolis, Chris	16	Halifax	06 OCT 1918
Pettigrew, John	17	Springhill	06 FEB 1919
Phalen, Diana E.	85	East Port Medway	12 JAN 1919
Phelan, James	81	Arichat	16 MAR 1919
Phillips, Wilbert	32	Halifax	24 NOV 1918
Pictou, Mary	17m	Bear River	08 FEB 1919
Pictou, Oliver	15	Bear River	08 FEB 1919
Pike, Mrs. Wesley	50	North Sydney	13 MAR 1919
Pinch, David	43	Wallbrook	07 DEC 1918

Pinch, Gertrude   14   Wallbrook   31 OCT 1918
Pinch, Gladys   06   Wallbrook   11 NOV 1918
Pipes, Carl   *28*   *Amherst*   *21 OCT 1918*
    Amherst Daily News, 21 October 1918, page 4.
Pirie, Allan   18m   Halifax   06 NOV 1918
Podowaka, Ignac   27   Sydney   29 DEC 1918
Poirier, Casimer   28   Descousse   23 JAN 1919
Poole, Frank, Petit de Grat, 24, Chronicle, 02 October 1918, page 1 (fisherman from Nfld).
Porter, Frances   87   Upper Selma   01 MAY 1919
Porter, James, Saskatchewan, 35, Yarmouth Telegram, 22 November 1918, page 1 (of Hebron).
Porter, Lyndon   35   Port Maitland   04 JAN 1919
Porter, Thomas   27   Sydney Mines   25 MAR 1919
Pothier, Alfred   *22*   *Yarmouth*   *07 NOV 1918*
    Halifax Evening Mail, 10 November 1918, (died at Yarmouth Hospital).
Pothier, Lawrence   17   Yarmouth   29 DEC 1918
Pothier, Peter Camille, Wedgeport, aged 25, Yarmouth Herald, 25 February 1919, page 2.
Potter, Miss Rose A., Los Angeles, Pictou Advocate, 24 January 1919, page 1 (of Scotsburn).
Pottie, David   32   Sydney   14 OCT 1918
Powell, Mable   24   Dartmouth   31 OCT 1918
Power, Hilda   03   Halifax   08 DEC 1918
Power, William, Portuguese Cove, 28, Halifax Evening Mail, 21 November 1918, page 1.
Power, William J., Halifax, Halifax Evening Mail, 14 December 1918, page 23 (Influenza Hospital).
Power, William   45   Halifax   15 DEC 1918
Powers, James A.   26   Alder Point   14 NOV 1918
Powill, Mrs. J. J., Halifax, 31, Halifax Evening Mail, 28 October, 1918, page 4.
Pratt, Viola Myrtle   09   Belmont   30 DEC 1918
Prince, Elida   59   Lunenburg   09 NOV 1918
Prudence, Ronald L., Halifax, Halifax Evening Mail, 20 March 1919, page 4.
Pulsiver, Annie   13   Beaver Bank   21 JAN 1919
Purdy, Frank   03   Halifax   02 NOV 1918
Purdy, Harry   *27*   *Sydney*   *18 NOV 1918*
    Oxford Journal, 21 November 1918, page 1 (of Little River, Cumberland County).
Purdy, Pte. Jacob W., Calgary, Oxford Journal, 28 November 1918, page 11 (of Belmont).
Purdy, Marion Elizabeth, Amherst, 26, Amherst Daily News, 4 January 1919, page 3; Oxford Journal, 2
    January 1919, page 1 (described as Miss and that she died at Millvale).
Pyche, Leander, Canso, Canso News, 28 February 1919, page 1.
Pyke, Stella   *19*   *Halifax*   *14 JAN 1919*
    Halifax Evening Mail, 16 January 1919, page 1 (Miss Stella Pyke).
Pyne, Agnes M.   32   Digby   16 DEC 1918
Pyne, Percy   35   Digby   22 DEC 1918
Quinan, Patrick   25   Lawlor's Island   15 OCT 1918
Quinn, Francis   17   Sydney Mines   10 DEC 1918
Quinton, Edward   18   Cape Sable Island   15 OCT 1918
Ramey, Lucy   5m   South Berwick   05 NOV 1918
Rand, William   83   Sheffield Mills   27 MAY 1919
Rankin, Albert   23   Scotch Hill   18 DEC 1918
Rankin, Hughena   36   New Glasgow   10 NOV 1918
Rankine, Hughena G., 26, Westville, Westville Free Lance, 15 November 1918, page 4.
Raugell, Margaret   26   Halifax   25 OCT 1918
Ray, Ethel, Halifax, 18, Halifax Evening Mail, 3 December 1918, page 16 (in Isolation Hospital).
Ray, Harold   25   Yarmouth   08 NOV 1918
Rector, Christy   10   Maccan   27 NOV 1918
Rector, Clarence M.   *27*   *Westville*   *07 DEC 1918*
    Amherst Daily News, 17 December 1918, page 5.
Rector, Harry   08   Maccan   26 NOV 1918

Rector, Wesley   09   Maccan   01 DEC 1918
Reid, Dr. John G., Ontario, aged 29, Pictou Advocate, 19 January 1919, page 8 (of Brule).
Rhynold, George   39   Canso   28 NOV 1918
        Canso News, 28 December 1918, page 2.
Rice, Alma   12   Lake LaRose   31 MAR 1919
Rice, Charles   45   Westchester   02 OCT 1918
Rice, Cyril   38   Glace Bay   01 DEC 1918
Rice, Mrs. Mary, Halifax, Halifax Evening Mail, 2 December 1919, page 4.
Richard, Angus   29   New Glasgow   02 DEC 1918
Richard, Annie   30   Charlos Cove   13 DEC 1918
Richard, David   28   Charlos Cove   15 DEC 1918
Richard, Joseph, Moncton, Amherst Daily News, 23 October 1918, page 8 (of Amherst).
Richard, Julia   34   Charlos Cove   14 DEC 1918
Richards, John   41   Woodside   16 NOV 1918
Richards, John   69   North Sydney   15 DEC 1918
Richardson, Elizabeth 57   Indian Harbour   04 NOV 1918
Rideout, William   05   North Sydney   19 MAR 1919
Riley, Lavenia   01   Mapleton   24 NOV 1918
Rines, Rossie, Vancouver, 32, Halifax Evening Mail, 23 December 1918, page 1 (of Maitland).
Ringer, _____   9d   Shelburne   21 JAN 1919
Ripley, Ezra Richard, Fenwick, aged 22, Amherst Daily News, 5 November 1918, page 3.
Ripley, Torlyer   03   Springhill   21 NOV 1918
Roach, Alice   19   Frauxville   31 OCT 1918
Roach, Ardella   37   Western Head   11 OCT 1918
Roach, Joseph   02   Dartmouth   31 OCT 1918
        Halifax Evening Mail, 2 November 1918, page 1 (age given as 2 years, 6 months).
Roach, Mrs. Leander, Western Head, aged 34, Liverpool Advance, 23 October 1918, page 2.
Roach, Margaret   59   Fraxville   02 MAR 1919
Roach, Mary   84   Western Head   16 OCT 1918
Roach, Maud   49   Yarmouth   25 MAR 1919
Roache, _____, Lockeport, aged 11, Liverpool Advance, 23 October 1918, page 2.
Roache, Louise   13   Western Head   18 OCT 1918
Robar, Mary   5m   East Clifford   31 DEC 1918
Robar, Ronald   03   North River   24 NOV 1918
Robard, George   68   Yarmouth   23 OCT 1918
Robbie, James   18   Halifax   15 DEC 1918
Robertson, Annie E.   04   Sydney   12 DEC 1918
Robertson, Bernard   34   Bridgewater   21 OCT 1918
        Amherst Daily News, 21 October 1918, page 4.
Robertson, Jessie   22   Westville   17 NOV 1918
Robertson, R.B.H., Lockeport, aged 34, Liverpool Advance, 23 October 1918, page 2.
Robichaud, Robert   15m   Meteghan   24 OCT 1918
Robinson, Charles   27   Bridgetown   23 JAN 1919
Robinson, Florence   20   Waterville   23 NOV 1918
        Berwick Register, 27 November 1918, page 2 (Mrs. Lester Robinson).
Robinson, George   64   Bridgetown   28 JAN 1919
Robinson, Glena   28   Halifax   05 DEC 1918
Robson, Sgt. Stewart, Halifax, Halifax Evening Mail, 7 November 1918, page 16.
Roche, Lucy   23   Rockdale   15 NOV 1918
Rodney, Ernest   03   Weymouth   27 NOV 1918
Rogers, Thomas   45   Halifax   29 OCT 1918
        Halifax Evening Mail, 30 October 1918, page 16.
Rogers, William   67   City Home, Halifax   25 OCT 1918
Roma, Evangeline   46   West Chezzetcook   09 NOV 1918
Roma, Joseph   21   West Chezzetcook   19 OCT 1918
Romans, Kate   39   Halifax   08 NOV 1918

Rombolt, Mary	40	Meteghan	30 OCT 1918
Ronayze, Alexander	17	Sydney Mines	05 DEC 1918
Ronayze, John	29	Sydney Mines	08 DEC 1918
Rood, Ethel	25	Halifax	09 DEC 1918
Rooker, Dora	26	Halifax	30 DEC 1918

Rose, Rev. Isaac A., Vermont, Truro Daily News, 26 February 1919, page 5 (of South Maitland).

Ross, William	53	Roxville	02 APR 1919

Rounsefel, Mrs. Frances G., Halifax, Halifax Evening Mail, 28 December 1918, page 12.

Roven, James	31	Halifax	24 NOV 1918
Rowlands, Lillian	1m	Brookfield	27 DEC 1918
Roy, Evelyn	45	Liverpool	17 NOV 1918
Roy, F.	17	Mill Cove	15 FEB 1919
Rudderham, Mary	68	North Sydney	07 DEC 1918
Rudolph, Mary	19m	Pictou	11 FEB 1919
Rumley, Florence	05	Stellarton	20 NOV 1918
Rumley, Margaret	16	Roman Valley	24 MAR 1919
Rushton, Mrs. Olive	57	Westchester Station	22 NOV 1918
Russell, Robert	31	Westville	30 NOV 1918
Russell, William	01	Halifax	22 OCT 1918
Ryan, Alice	*30*	*Sydney*	*26 NOV 1918*

Truro Daily News, 27 November 1918, page 4 (Miss Dolly Ryan, aged 30).

Ryan, Henry	7d	Halifax	14 NOV 1918
Ryan, J.T.	34	Halifax	16 OCT 1918
Saccary, Joseph	18	Glace Bay	05 DEC 1918

Sampson, _____, Halifax Evening Mail, 04 November 1918, page 14 (son of Mrs. Felix).
Sampson, Mrs. Felix, Halifax Evening Mail, 04 November 1918, page 14.

Samson, Albany	23	Petit de Grat	21 OCT 1918
Samson, Cecelia	22	Petit de Grat	05 NOV 1918
Samson, Georgina	25	Descousse	07 DEC 1918
Samson, Gorgie	01	Cabbage Cove	21 OCT 1918
Samson, Lena	24	Petit de Grat	25 OCT 1918
Samson, Leon	18	Petit de Grat	01 NOV 1918
Samson, Lucy	53	Cabbage Cove	21 OCT 1918
Samson, Martha	29	Petit de Grat	21 OCT 1918
Samson, Mary	33	Petit de Grat	31 OCT 1918
Samson, Wilfred	25	Cabbage Cove	23 OCT 1918
Sanford, Matilda	75	Walton	30 MAR 1919
Sargent, George	33	Halifax	23 JAN 1919
Saulnier, Louis	3m	Meteghan	31 MAR1919
Saulnier, Louise	03	Meteghan	19 OCT 1918
Saulnier, Marc	80	Meteghan Center	03 JUN 1919
Saulnier, Marie	05	Meteghan	08 NOV 1918
Saulnier, William	29	Halifax	21 DEC 1918
Saulnier, **		1918	
Sayyean, Howard	21	Sydney	20 OCT 1918

Scales, Fred, Canso, Canso News, 28 December 1918, page 2.
Scanlon, Edward   *02*   *Halifax*   *09 OCT 1918*
    Halifax Evening Mail, 10 October 1918, page 1 (child of Edward Scanlan).
Schaffner, Melville A., Saskatoon, 45, Halifax Evening Mail, 4 March 1919, page 2 (of Truro).

Schlosser, Rosie	17	Maccan	24 OCT 1918
Schultz, Elizabeth	75	City Home, Halifax	29 OCT 1918
Scott, Abbie	19	River Hebert	13 DEC 1918
Scott, Elphege	32	Halifax	05 OCT 1918
Scott, Harold	17	Westchester	14 OCT 1918
Seale, Charles	32	New Glasgow	02 DEC 1918
Seaman, Lida	22	Chignecto Mines	30 OCT 1918

Selby, Arnold   05   Avonport`   13 MAY 1919
Severy, Elizabeth Ann, Los Angeles, Yarmouth Herald, 11 March 1919, page 2 (She was a Flint and formerly from
    Plymouth, Yarmouth County).
Sevigne, Elmer   01   Halifax   22 NOV 1918
Shaffelburg, Helen   16   Halifax   17 FEB 1919
Shanahan, Mrs. Sarah 28   St. Peter's   27 FEB 1919
Shanks, Katherine   60   Halifax   29 OCT 1918
Shannon, Violet   *35*   *Halifax*   *14 OCT 1918*
    Halifax Evening Mail, 15 October 1918, page 14.
Shannon, William   38   Halifax   15 OCT 1918
Shatford, Beatrice   *18*   *Halifax*   *05 DEC 1918*
    Halifax Evening Mail, 11 December 1918, (died at Willow Park Hospital).
Shears, Mrs. Jane, Halifax, aged 27, Halifax Evening Mail, 17 December 1918, page 3 (Mrs. John).
Shephard, Margaret   29   Florence   18 OCT 1918
Shephard, Robert   *26*   *Dartmouth*   *13 NOV 1918*
    Halifax Evening Mail, 14 November 1918, page 2 (died in the Emergency Hospital).
Sherlock, R.   26   Halifax   15 OCT 1918
Shields, Frederick   51   Canso   01 DEC 1918
Shrader, Mrs. David *64*   *Canso*   *20 NOV 1918*
    Canso News, 30 November 1918, page 1 (Shrider in newspaper).
Sibley, Hilda   *23*   *Meaghers Grant*   *15 NOV 1918*
    Truro Daily News, 14 December 1918, page 2 (née Hilda Mannelle).
Sibley, James Kent   30   Meaghers Grant   29 NOV 1918
Simmonds, Mrs. James, Lockeport, aged 33, Liverpool Advance, 30 October 1918, page 2.
Simmons, Tressa   27d   Dominion   12 DEC 1918
Simpson, Mrs. J. F., Mass., Amherst Daily News, 18 February 1919, page 5 (of Little River).
Singer, Nicholas   75   Kennetcook   05 APR 1919
Skidmore, John K.   *32*   *Mulgrave*   *08 DEC 1918*
    Oxford Journal, 12 December 1918, page 6 (of Pirate Harbour, Guysboro Co.)
Skinner, Charles   34   New Glasgow   28 NOV 1918
Skinner, Kenneth   *24*   *Digby*   *07 DEC 1918*
    Bridgetown Monitor, 11 December 1918, page 3.
Skinner, Mrs. Laura   32   Guysboro   27 DEC 1918
Skinner, Sarah   30   North Sydney   26 OCT 1918
Slaunwhite, Annie   24   Terence Bay   21 DEC 1918
Slaunwhite, Catherine 20   Halifax   28 OCT 1918
Smith, Arthur   1 day   Truro   18 FEB 1919
Smith, Bessie   30   Barrington   15 OCT 1918
Smith, Blanche, Christie's Point, Yarmouth Telegram, 20 December 1918, page 1.
Smith, Blanche   21   Baccaro   12 DEC 1918
Smith, Christina   63   Joggins Mines   31 MAR 1919
Smith, Clarence   16   North Sydney   23 NOV 1918
Smith, Clinton   03   Baccaro   12 DEC 1918
Smith, Edward   07   Halifax   12 NOV 1918
Smith, Edward,   26   Yarmouth   23 DEC 1918
Smith, Elizabeth O. *19*   *East Apple River*   *22 NOV 1918*
    Amherst Daily News, 26 November 1918, page 3 (described as "Miss").
Smith, Fernwood, Christie's Point, Yarmouth Telegram, 20 December 1918, page 1, (son of Blanche).
Smith, Miss Flossie, Winnipeg, Hants Journal, 18 December 1918, page 8 (from Stanley).
Smith, Frank   29   Smithville   30 JAN 1919
Smith, Mrs. Frank L., Vancouver, Halifax Evening Mail, 28 November 1918, page 2 (of Halifax); Truro Daily
    News, 29 November 1918, page 2 (she was a nurse at Ladner Hosp. in B.C.).
Smith, George   19   Canso   30 NOV 1918
Smith, Goldie   04   Cape Sable   17 SEPT 1918
Smith, Hannah   86   Smithville   12 JAN 1919
Smith, Hilda   26   Port Latour   27 OCT 1918

APPENDIX   ᵛᵗ   393

Smith, Horace	43	Smithville	19 JAN 1919

Smith, Miss Irene, Cape Sable Island, 23, Yarmouth Telegram, 18 October 1918, page 1.

Smith, Pte James T., Sydney, Sydney Daily Post, 30 September, page 1 (died in Moxham Hospital).

Smith, Miss Jennie	20	*Fenwick*	*01 NOV 1918*

Amherst Daily News, 1 November 1918, page 3.

Smith, John	02	Canso	03 DEC 1918
Smith, John	18	Aldershot	09 MAY 1919
Smith, Laurie	28	Port Mouton	27 JAN 1919
Smith, Leah May	*15*	*Pugwash*	*04 JAN 1919*

Amherst Daily News, 9 January 1919, page 4.

Smith, Leonce	18	Saulnierville Station	21 OCT 1918
Smith, Leslie	24	Grand Pre	23 OCT 1918
Smith, Rella	29	Amherst	18 FEB 1919
Smith, Thomas	77	City Home, Halifax	29 OCT 1918

Smith, Vera, New Jersey, 16, Eastern Chronicle, 22 October 1918, page 1 (of New Glasgow).

Smith, William	8m	Bridgewater	04 NOV 1918
Smyth, Angus	29	Judique	11 DEC 1918
Smythe, Raymond	04	Judique	16 DEC 1918
Snair, Kitchener	03	Black Point	19 DEC 1918
Snair, Madge	01	Black Point	05 FEB 1919
Snow, Wilfred	21	Canard	26 OCT 1918
Somers, Moses	28	Briley Brook	18 FEB 1919
Sound, Oriah	18m	Halifax	19 NOV 1918
Speakman, Thomas	28	Halifax	26 JAN 1919
Spence, Alden	14	Springhill	28 DEC 1918
Spencer, D'Arcy	68	Halifax	11 MAY 1919

Spencer, Miss Valetta, Halifax, ca.30, Sydney Daily Post, 25 October 1918, page 1 (of Sydney).

Spurr, Elizabeth	71	Melvern Square	09 APR 1919
Squires, Norman	04	North Sydney	27 OCT 1918
Stacey, James	38	Gabarus	19 JAN 1919
Stanford, James	65	Chester	11 NOV 1918

Stanley, A., Lockeport, aged 3, Liverpool Advance, 23 October 1918, page 2.

Stanley, Stella	02	Lydgate	17 OCT 1918
Stark, Wallace	04	Digby	18 DEC 1918
Stark, Wallace	33	Digby	19 DEC 1918
Steadman, Edith	*42*	*Halifax*	*23 DEC 1918*

Halifax Evening Mail, 24 December 1918, page 1 (Willow Park Influenza Hospital).

Steele, Bridget	18	Halifax	12 DEC 1918
Stephens, Charles	50	Sydney	05 OCT 1918
Stephens, William	01	Lydgate	23 OCT 1918
Stevens, Arthur D.	*33*	*Halifax*	*21 OCT 1918*

Halifax Evening Mail, 22 October 1918 (Arthur D. Stevens, 32).

Stevenson, Wilfred, Saskatoon, 20, Westville Free Lance, 17 January 1919, page 6 (of Brule).

Stewart, Ella	52	Amherst	19 MAR 1919
Stewart, Katie	27	Gabarus	10 JAN 1919
Stewart, M.W.	35	Sydney Mines	09 DEC 1918
Stimers, Louise	35	Halifax	10 NOV 1918
Stialchuk, Metro	53	Sydney Mines	30 OCT 1918
Stockley, Gordon	24	Halifax	17 OCT 1918
Stoddart, Harvey	14	Sandford	10 JAN 1919
St.Peter, Olive June	*12*	*Maccan*	*04 NOV 1918*

Amherst Daily News, 05 November 1918, page 3.

Stubbart, Germain	70	Belle Cote	22 DEC 1918

Sulis, Fred Orville, New York, 25, Bridgetown Monitor, 08 January 1919, page 4 (of Deep Brook).

Sullivan, John	28	Kentville	26 MAR 1919
Surette, Celenie	27	Wedgeport	23 OCT 1918

Surette, Charles	23	Wedfeport	24 OCT 1918
Surette, Clemente	17	Middle West Pubnico	05 OCT 1918
Surette, Monde	36	Yarmouth	10 DEC 1918
Surette, Percy	5m	Yarmouth	11 DEC 1918
Surette, Stephen	52	Middle West Pubnico	18 OCT 1918

Sutherland, Frank, Massachusetts, Canso News, 26 October 1918, page 4 (of Canso).

Sutherland, Irene	17	River John Road	21 DEC 1918
Sutherland, John	*22*	*Lockeport*	*15 OCT 1918*

Halifax Evening Mail, 16 October 1918, page 14 (son of Fred Sutherland).

Sutherland, Max	*16*	*Lockeport*	*16 OCT 1918*

Halifax Evening Mail, 16 October 1918, page 14 (son of Fred Sutherland).

Sutherland, Murray, Sask., aged 32, Amherst Daily News, 29 October 1918, page 3 (of Aulac).

Sutherland, Murray	32	Westville	01 DEC 1918
Swanwick, Gertrude	35	Springhill	28 OCT 1918
Sweeny, Kenneth	28	Yarmouth	09 NOV 1918
Swindell, Margaret	66	Burlington	02 FEB 1919
Symonds, Mrs. Geo.	34	Lockeport	21 OCT 1918
Tanner, Leslie	*16*	*Lunenburg*	*10 OCT 1918*

Halifax Evening Mail, 11 October 1918, page 8.

Tanner, Mary	*20*	*Blue Rocks*	*21 OCT 1918*

Halifax Evening Mail, 22 October 1918, page 6 (daughter of Ernest Tanner)

Tanner, Mrs. Robert	66	Central Cariboo	02 NOV 1918

Tarr, J. Stanley, Mass., aged 33, Liverpool Advance, 9 October 1918, page 2 (of Western Head)

Taunt, Rose	33	West Dover	13 May 1919
Taylor, Agnes	23	Margaree Harbour	20 DEC 1918
Taylor, David	32	Bridgetown	11 JAN 1919
Taylor, George	37	Lawlor's Island	11 OCT 1918
Taylor, James	72	Cross Roads	29 APR 1919

Taylor, Lee, Massachusetts, 29, Amherst Daily News, 7 January 1919, page 3 (of Apple River).

Taylor, Sophie	61	Medford	06 JAN 1919
Taylor, William	47	Middleton	26 JAN 1919
Teed, Ernest	15	Pugwash	26 DEC 1918
Teed, Lewis	21	Pugwash	26 DEC 1918
Tefler, Leonard S.	*34*	*Bridgewater*	*25 OCT 1918*

Liverpool Advance, 30 October 1918, page 2 (age given as 33).

Theriault, Helen	02	Alder Point	27 OCT 1918
Thibault, Evangeline	36	Belleville	03 JAN 1919
Thibault, Grace	25	Saulnierville Station	27 OCT 1918
Thibault, Joseph	30	Accaciaville	10 APR 1919
Thibodieu, Charles	54	Meteghan Center	05 APR 1919
Thomas, Adelaide	02	Indian Reserve	17 OCT 1918

Thomas, Austin, Thomasville, 53, Yarmouth Herald, 14 January 1919, page 5.

Thomas, Charles	*24*	*New Glasgow*	*08 DEC 1918*

Westville Free Lance, 13 December 1918, page 4 (of St. Peter's, Cape Breton).

Thomas, Howard	20	Halifax	17 OCT 1918

Thomas, James, British Columbia, 30, Sydney Daily Post, 4 December 1918, page 1 (of N. Sydney).

Thomas, Mrs. Minnie	26	Thompson	19 NOV 1918
Thomas, Oliver	33	Cape Negro	20 JAN 1919
Thompson, _____	01	Dominion	25 DEC 1918
Thompson, Augustus	*49*	*Yarmouth*	*01 OCT 1918*

Halifax Evening Mail, 2 October, 1918, page 13 (from Gloucester, Mass.)

Thompson, Edward	40	City Home, Halifax	28 OCT 1918
Thompson, Irma	*17*	*West Middle Sable*	*20 OCT 1918*

Liverpool Advance, 30 October 1918, page 2 (described as Erma Thompson).

Thompson, Lola, Trenton, Truro Daily News, 3 January 1919, page 7.

Thompson, Melville	13m	Westville	25 NOV 1918

Thomson, Alexander	36	Westville	26 DEC 1918
Thomson, Leola	20	Trenton	05 DEC 1918

Thurber, Delta Maude, Freeport, aged 20, Digby Courier, 24 January 1919, page 5.

Tipping, Norman	32	Great Village	15 DEC 1918
Tipping, Stewart	30	Great Village	19 DEC 1918

Tobin, Jack, Europe, Pictou Advocate, 7 March 1919, page 1 (of Pictou).

Tobin, Peter Jr.	26	Halifax	24 OCT 1918
Todd, Florence	22	Halifax	21 OCT 1918
Toiley, James	*8m*	*Stellarton*	*01 NOV 1918*

Pictou Advocate, 8 November 1918, page 1 (described as a child of James Tolly).

Townsend, Mrs. Frank, Lockeport, aged 35, Liverpool Advance, 23 October 1918, page 2.

Townsend, Kathleen	17	*Lydgate*	*14 October 1918*

Liverpool Advance, 23 October 1918, page 2.

Townsend, Roy, Lockeport, aged 4, Liverpool Advance, 30 October 1918, page 2.

Trahan, Celestin	71	Meteghan	-- MAY 1919
Trahan, Harvey	20	Meteghan	30 OCT 1918
Trefery, Arnold	03	Stellarton	04 DEC 1918
Trefery, Vivian	8m	Stellarton	07 DEC 1918
Troop, Ralph	32	Granville Ferry	13 MAY 1919
Tugman, Ernest	21	New Waterford	14 DEC 1918
Tully, William B.	38	Kentville	23 OCT 1918
Tupper, Jessie	36	Stellarton	05 DEC 1918
Tupper, John D.	*18*	*Stellarton*	*04 DEC 1918*

Eastern Chronicle, 10 December 1918, page 1 (died in the Emergency Hospital).

Turbide, Mrs. Annie	31	Alder Point	16 NOV 1918
Turbide, Clement	24	Pictou	15 DEC 1918
Turner, Effie	37	Frauxville	19 NOV 1918
Turner, Elizabeth	42	Halifax	09 DEC 1918
Tyler, Augusta	38	Inglewood	31 DEC 1918
Underwood, Charles	37	Mapleton	20 OCT 1918
Vallie, Mary	21	New Waterford	24 NOV 1918
Van Amburg, Marg.	23	Pubnico	20 FEB 1919
Van Buskirk, Eliz.	28	Springhill	31 DEC 1918
Van Emburg, Edith	3m	Yarmouth	18 DEC 1918
Van Tassell, Mrs. A.	23	Mount Pleasant	14 DEC 1918
Van Tassell, Agustus	01	Mount Pleasant	16 DEC 1918
Van Tassell, Dustin	6m	Digby	23 DEC 1918
Van Tassell, Norman	*18*	*Digby*	*-- DEC 1918*

Bridgetown Monitor, 11 December 1918, page 3.

Van Tassell, William	03	Mount Pleasant	16 DEC 1918
Vaughan, David W.	38	Halifax	23 NOV 1918
Vaughan, Mary	14	Windsor Forks	02 DEC 1918
Veinotte, Ethel	17	Mahone Bay	07 JAN 1919
Velenori, Marie	01	New Waterford	30 SEPT 1918

Vernon, Mrs. E.D., Truro, Halifax Evening Mail, 02 January 1919, page 14 (née Annie Dobson).

Vidito, Howard	04	Torbrook	01 APR 1919

Vignault, Capt. Samuel, Mulgrave, 40, Halifax Evening Mail, 25 November 1918, page 1.

Vigneau, Elizabeth	66	Alder Point	25 NOV 1918
Vogler, Franklin	3m	Ingramport	02 DEC 1918
Vokey, Eileen	6m	Glace Bay	12 JAN 1919
Wadden, Clarence G.	03	Glace Bay	02 JAN 1919
Wade, Oliver	67	Springhill	01 JAN 1919
Waetaetas, Joseph	10m	Stellarton	10 NOV 1918
Wagner, _____	16m	Dominion	11 DEC 1918
Wagner, William	36	Dominion	18 DEC 1918

Wagstaff, Miss Lillian, Chicago, 41, Annapolis Spectator, 09 January 1919, page 7 (of Granville).

Waldron, James	57	Halifax	10 MAR 1919

Walker, Archibald, Vancouver, 35, Eastern Chronicle, 17 January 1919, page 1 (of New Glasgow).

Walker, Florence	42	Halifax	15 NOV 1918
Walker, Harriet	28	*Dartmouth*	*26 OCT 1918*

Halifax Evening Mail, 28 October 1918, page 2 (wife of Norman Walker).

Walker, Ruine	10m	Halifax	16 MAR 1919

Walker, Samuel L., Los Angeles, 29, Truro Daily News, 22 November 1918, page 2 (of Gay's River).

Walkins, Mrs. Peter	86	Hazel Hill	09 NOV 1918
Wall, Edward	24	Sydney	01 NOV 1918

Walsh, Daniel, Truro, 38, Truro Daily News, 05 December 1918, page 7 (died at Willow St. Hospital).

Walsh, Elizabeth	40	Point Tupper	21 OCT 1918
Walsh, James	50	New Waterford	18 SEPT 1918
Walsh, Wellington	42	Avonport	04 MAY 1919
Walton, Freeman	45	New Ross Road	04 FEB 1919
Wambolt, Beatrice	26	Halifax	18 NOV 1918
Ward, Thomas	28	*Halifax*	*28 NOV 1918*

Halifax Evening Mail, 29 November 1918, page 1.

Wareham, George	41	New Waterford	25 SEPT 1918
Wareham, Samile	31	Glace Bay	01 DEC 1918

Warner, Ruth, Dartmouth, Halifax Evening Mail, 17 February 1919, page 2.

Warren, Heather	20	Glace Bay	17 DEC 1918
Warren, William	38	Sydney	08 DEC 1918
Waterman, Walter	07	Middleton	13 JAN 1919

Waters, Pte Lowell E., Sydney, Sydney Daily Post, 1 October 1918 page 1 (died in hospital).

Watkins, Sarah	17m	Yarmouth	21 OCT 1918
Watton, Annie	74	Kings County	29 OCT 1918
Watton, Hannah	38	Victoria	15 OCT 1918
Weagle, Selina	30	Avonport	14 MAY 1919
Wear, Norman	17	Victoria Beach	03 DEC 1918
Weatherby, Freda	6m	Lower Truro	06 MAR 1919
Webb, Aloysus	27	Harbour Bouche	17 NOV 1918
Webb, Hazel	16m	Fenwick Mines	26 NOV 1918
Webber, Kathleen J.	35	Middle Sackville	01 MAR 1919

Halifax Evening Mail, 4 March 1919, page 11, (obituary, she was a teacher).

Weeks, William	25	Ship Harbour	01 NOV 1918

Weir, Norman, Victoria Beach, 18, Digby Courier, 13 December 1918, page 2.

Weir, Mrs. Walter, New Glasgow, Halifax Evening Mail, 1 November 1918, page 9.

Welsh, Daniel	38	Truro	04 DEC 1918
Welsh, Joseph	28	Thorburn	02 DEC 1918
Wentzell, Clayton F.	19	Riverport	01 JAN 1919
Wentzell, Maggie	27	*Sentry*	*16 OCT 1918*

Halifax Evening Mail, 22 October 1918, page 6 (Mrs. William Wentzell).

West, Charles, Mass., aged 28, Liverpool Advance, 9 October 1918, page 2 (of Liverpool).

Westburn, Ruth	01	Halifax	20 OCT 1918
Westhaver, Grace	20	Chester	26 SEPT 1918
Wheadon, Minnie	01	Walton	16 NOV 1918
White, Edith	27	North West Arm	22 JAN 1919

White, Mrs. John, Halifax, aged 40, Halifax Evening Mail, 4 December 1918, page 16.

White, Mary	41	Halifax	30 NOV 1918
White, Maud	27	*Halifax,*	*14 NOV 1918*

Halifax Evening Mail, 15 November 1918, page 1 (died at Willow Park Hospital).

White, Robert	4m	Joggins Mines	22 NOV 1918
White, Wallace	36	Whiteside	30 NOV 1918
White, Walter	02	Little Bras d'Or	12 OCT 1918
White, Walter	25	Halifax	23 OCT 1918
Whitman, Barbara	19m	Arcadia	15 JAN 1919

Whitten, Lottie	17	Yarmouth	13 DEC 1918
Whitzman, Mendel	34	Halifax	10 NOV 1918

Whynact, Mrs. Frank, Halifax Evening Mail, 22 October 1918, page 6 (née Hilda Mason).

Whynot, Hattie	*28*	*Liverpool*	*18 NOV 1918*

    Liverpool Advance, 20 November 1918, page 3 (Hattie May Whynot).

Whynott, Kenneth	22	Windsor	11 DEC 1918
Whyte, Mrs. Mary	45	Stellarton	23 MAR 1919
Wier, Rita	07	Halifax	27 NOV 1918
Wile, Bernard	*41*	*Wileville*	*30 OCT 1918*

    Halifax Evening Mail, 8 November 1918, page 1.

Wile, Edna	06	Wileville	21 FEB 1919
Wile, Ida	41	Wileville	22 NOV 1918
Wile, Myrtle	01	Bridgewater	28 OCT 1918
Wile, Nelson	72	Bridgewater	04 FEB 1919
Wile, Uriah	47	Wileville	06 JAN 1919

Wilkins, Linford, Port Lorne, aged 23, Bridgetown Monitor, 25 December 1918, page 4.
Williams, Edward, Truro, aged 45, Truro Daily News, 5 February 1919, page 2.

Williams, George	02	South Bay	14 MAY 1919

Williams, Mrs. Joseph F., Lockeport, aged 32, Liverpool Advance, 21 October 1918, page 2.

Williams, Mary	56	Kentville	05 APR 1919
Williams, Patrick	32	South Bay	16 MAY 1919
Williams, Robert	59	Fall River	19 FEB 1919

Williams, William Earl, Lockeport, aged 2, Liverpool Advance, 30 October 1918, page 2.
Wilson, Mrs. Charles, Bear River, 51, Bridgetown Monitor, 11 December 1918, page 3.

Wilson, Lt. Colin	*30*	*Halifax*	*20 OCT 1918*

    Halifax Evening Mail, 21 September 1918, page 9 (listed as Lt. Calvin Wilson).

Wilson, Henry	34	Sydney	04 OCT 1918
Wilson, Hugh	03	Springhill	29 NOV 1918

Wilson, Rev. Joseph E., Amherst, Amherst Daily News, 04 November 1918, page 3.

Wilson, Katherine	54	Springhill	02 NOV 1918
Wilson, Norman	33	Hebron	01 JAN 1919

Wilson, Trueman, Alberta, 38, Halifax Evening Mail, 19 November 1918, page 1 (of Belmont).

Wiltshire, Rev. James	28	Sydney	25 DEC 1918
Wimpers, Ellen	5m	Halifax	12 DEC 1918
Winchester, Georgie	*41*	*Digby*	*01 NOV 1918*

    Halifax Evening Mail, 4 November 1918, page 7 (Mrs. W. S. Winchester)

Winters, Mrs. Fred., Lunenburg, Lunenburg Progress Enterprise, 30 October 1918, page 4; Middleton Outlook, 15 November 1918, page 2 (formerly Miss Grimm of Springfield).

Winters, Ivan	*27*	*[The] Ovens*	*06 OCT 1918*

    Halifax Evening Mail, 08 October 1918, page 6, (ill for only two days)

Winters, Regina	45	Bridgewater	19 FEB 1919

Withers, Capt. Nelson, Saint John, 58, Yarmouth Herald, 11 February 1919, page 2 (of Yarmouth).

Wolfe, Harold	02	East Jordan	29 NOV 1918
Wood, Ruth	03	Westville	20 NOV 1918

Wood, Miss Stella, 26, River Hebert, 10 DEC 1918; Amherst Daily News, 14 December 1918, page 4

Wood, Mrs. W.W.	40	Maccan	04 MAR 1919
Woodward, Willard	26	Middleboro	09 NOV 1918
Woodworth, Kathleen	02	Lockhartville	08 JAN 1919
Works, Evelyn	38	Stellarton	11 DEC 1918
Works, Joseph	*23*	*Truro*	*26 OCT 1918*

    Halifax Evening Mail, 28 October 1918, page 1.

Wotton, Mrs. Hannah, Aylesford, aged 37, Berwick Register, 13 November 1918, page 2.
Wotton, Mrs. John N., Aylesford, aged 74, Berwick Register, 13 November 1918, page 2.
Wright, Harry, Dartmouth, aged 32, Halifax Evening Mail, 9 November 1918, page 2.
Wright, Mrs. J. A., Vancouver, aged 33, Truro Daily News, 20 November 1918, page 1, (nee Maggie Annand of Gay's River)

Wright, Kathleen	20	Beechville	25 OCT 1918
Wyatt, Hilda	29	Tufts Cove	05 NOV 1918
Wynacht, Hilda	21	Lunenburg	20 OCT 1918
Wynacht, Linda	26	Middle South	17 DEC 1918
Wynot, Medora	*32*	*Bridgewater*	*06 NOV 1918*

Liverpool Advance, 6 November 1918, page 2 (Madora May Wynacht, aged 38).

| Yetman, Joseph | 28 | Halifax | *01 DEC 1918* |

Halifax Evening Mail, 2 December 1918, page 2 (was a barber, aged 27).

York, Ethel	04	Digby	24 OCT 1918
York, Mrs. Stillman	21	Digby	02 OCT 1918
Yorke, Walter	10m	North Sydney	14 MAR 1919
Young, Anna	18	Bayers Settlement	02 NOV 1918
Young, Annie	34	North Sydney	13 DEC 1918
Young, John	20	Strathlorne	11 MAR 1919
Young, Kathleen	28	Middleton	04 NOV 1918
Young, Lorne	29	Lake Paul	14 JAN 1919
Young, Lulu	*17*	*Green Harbour*	*18 OCT 1918*

Liverpool Advance, 23 October 1918, page 2 (died at Lockeport).

Young, Morris	11	Burlington	05 JUN 1919
Young, N.A.	5m	Little Bras D'or	13 MAR 1919
Young, Rosavilla	26	Martin's Brook	08 NOV 1918
Young, Vaughan	*07*	*Weymouth*	*26 OCT 1918*

Middleton Outlook, 15 November 1918, page 2 (formerly Flossie Kathleen King)
Young, William, Marble Mountain, Halifax Evening Mail, 8 January 1919, page 1.
Zinck, Florence, Mahone Bay, Halifax Evening Mail, 14 February 1919, page 3.

Zwicker, Charles	18	Camperdown	05 MAR 1919
Zwicker, Everett	06	Camperdown	09 MAR 1919
Zwicker, John	03	Camperdown	09 MAR 1919
Zwicker, Rufus	*32*	*Dartmouth*	*31 OCT 1918*

Halifax Evening Mail, 1 November 1918, page 2.

SANDRA KIPIS

RUTH HOLMES WHITEHEAD has worked since 1972 for the Nova Scotia Museum, since 2003 as a Curator Emerita and Research Associate. She has authored or co-authored twenty books, including *Stories from the Six Worlds*, *The Old Man Told Us*, *Black Loyalists*, and *Ancestral Images*. In 1995, she was awarded a Doctorate of Laws, honoris causa, by St. Francis Xavier University. In 2014, Dr. Whitehead was inducted into the Order of Nova Scotia. She lives in Halifax.